National Symposium on Family Issues

Volume 10

Series editors
Susan M. McHale
Valarie King
Jennifer E. Glick

More information about this series at http://www.springer.com/series/8381

Jennifer E. Glick • Susan M. McHale
Valarie King
Editors

Rural Families and Communities in the United States

Facing Challenges and Leveraging Opportunities

Springer

Editors
Jennifer E. Glick
Population Research Institute
Penn State
University Park, PA, USA

Susan M. McHale
Social Science Research Institute
Penn State
University Park, PA, USA

Valarie King
Department of Sociology
Penn State
University Park, PA, USA

ISSN 2192-9157 ISSN 2192-9165 (electronic)
National Symposium on Family Issues
ISBN 978-3-030-37688-8 ISBN 978-3-030-37689-5 (eBook)
https://doi.org/10.1007/978-3-030-37689-5

This Springer imprint is published by the registered company Springer Nature Switzerland AG
The registered company address is: Gewerbestrasse 11, 6330 Cham, Switzerland

Preface

The landscape of family life is ever changing. The strategies needed to maintain family economic stability, health, and general well-being vary across space and place. Although the rural-urban divide is often portrayed as the most important geographic distinction, there is tremendous diversity across rural communities. As the demographic composition of the U.S. changes, our rural communities also change. So, in contrast to some depictions, families in rural areas are from diverse racial, ethnic, linguistic, and cultural origins. Furthermore, the challenges facing rural areas are not uniform—some rural areas are resource constrained, losing services and social supports. Other areas host opportunities that support healthy families and child well-being.

The 2018 National Symposium on Family Issues brought together an interdisciplinary slate of researchers to address how economic and demographic shifts across rural communities, and the diversity within these communities, shape family relationships and development. The focus on the challenges ahead gives us a look into the future of work, parenting, and health across the rural landscape in the U.S. Research also reveals resiliency and strategies that may help rural families thrive as their communities change.

The volume begins with a focus on the broad trends in rural economies and how conditions of work impact individual well-being and family functioning. There is no doubt that the labor market realities facing families in rural areas are changing rapidly. But there is no one portrait of a rural place in the U.S., and economic and demographic shifts change opportunities and constraints. Research also implicates the policies of the past and the legacy of long-term rural poverty that make the challenges of responding to broader economic shifts even more challenging. Fewer job opportunities encouraged out-migration and accelerated rural aging. At the same time, the growth of some rural areas as new migrant destinations diversified the population of some communities. The chapters in Part I demonstrate the long run implications of demographic, policy, and political shifts in the U.S. from the mid-twentieth century and point to the possibilities for rural development in the future.

These historical shifts across diverse rural areas set the stage for the current economic and health challenges facing families today. Thus, Part II of this volume presents research on these current pressing issues and the emerging needs of rural communities. The authors demonstrate the threat to work and prosperity brought about by increasing automation of the workplace and the need for education and training opportunities as rural economies are transformed. And, in keeping with the focus on diversity across rural areas, the authors demonstrate how shifts in mortality and mobility are creating distinct age structures across the rural continuum. Finally, this theme of the complexity and diversity of rural communities in the U.S. sheds light on the variation in opioid use disorders and opioid mortality across rural areas. It is clear that this is a multidimensional problem that is not limited to one simplistic cause or solution.

In Part III, the volume turns to work that demonstrates the resilience of diverse families in rural spaces with a focus on family roles, relationships, and development pathways. These in-depth and longitudinal analyses assess risks and resilience for children and adolescents of Latino, African American, and Anglo-American origins in several different regions of the country. For some, family life in rural areas means fewer economic opportunities but greater social support as extended family buffers one another. For others, being present in rural America reflects recent migration and adaptation to new environments. Thus, there is variability in the way the rural context shapes, challenges, and supports family processes and youth development. The research presented here illustrates how families navigate these challenges and proposes new frameworks for studying diverse communities settled across the rural-urban continuum today.

The 2018 National Symposium on Family Issues was a unique opportunity to hear from scholars from varied disciplinary backgrounds who are investigating different challenges facing rural families in the U.S. today. We hope that their work highlighted in this volume will set the stage for new scholarship and policy recommendations that recognize that there is no one-size-fits-all prescription for the diversity of challenges facing rural communities.

University Park, PA, USA

Jennifer E. Glick
Susan M. McHale
Valarie King

Acknowledgments

The editors are grateful to the organizations at Penn State that sponsored the 2018 Family Symposium and this resulting volume, including the Social Science Research Institute (SSRI); Population Research Institute (PRI); the departments of Sociology and Criminology; Human Development and Family Studies; Agricultural Economics, Sociology, and Education; Psychology; and the Clinical and Translational Science Institute, Child Study Center and Prevention Research Center. The editors also gratefully acknowledge essential core financial support in the form of a five-year grant from the Eunice Kennedy Shriver National Institute of Child Health and Human Development (NICHD; R13-HD048150), as well as ongoing advice from Regina Bures at NICHD. The support of our partners enabled us to attract outstanding scholars from a range of backgrounds and disciplines from the community of researchers, practitioners, and policy-makers on whom the quality of the series depends.

The efforts of many individuals went into planning the 2018 symposium and producing this volume. Our internal advisory board, consisting of Dawn Witherspoon, Nancy Luke, Doug Teti, Kevin Thomas, Mayra Bamaca, Greg Fosco, Patricia Miranda-Hartsuff, and Sarah Damaske, were helpful from the early stages of brainstorming for the 2018 symposium. In addition, we are very grateful to Stephen Matthews, Lori Francis, and Brian Thiede for moderating symposium sessions. We also thank the staff in the Population Research Institute and the Social Science Research Institute at Penn State including Sherry Yocum, Angela Jordan, Diane Diviney, Rebecca Shultz, and Rachel Charney. Finally, the Symposium and book would not have been possible without Carolyn Scott's organizational skills, commitment, and attention to the many details that go into developing an engaging conference and producing a scholarly volume.

Jennifer E. Glick
Susan M. McHale
Valarie King

Contents

Part I Family Life and Work in Rural Communities

Rural Poverty: Research and Policy for U.S. Families 3
Ann R. Tickamyer

Changes in Work and Family Across the Rural U.S. 27
Marybeth J. Mattingly

Employment and Wages in the Places Left Behind 47
Mark D. Partridge, Rodrigo Pérez-Silva, and Sydney Schreiner

Part II Economic and Health Challenges Facing Families in the Rural U.S.

Rural Job Loss to Offshoring and Automation 89
Srikant Devaraj, Emily J. Wornell, Dagney Faulk, and Michael Hicks

Opioid Crisis in the Rural U.S. 117
Shannon M. Monnat

Demographic Components of Aging in the Nonmetropolitan U.S., 1980–2017 145
John Cromartie

Part III Family Roles, Well-Being, and Development Pathways in Rural Areas

Rural African Americans' Family Relationships and Well-Being 169
Velma McBride Murry, Shauna M. Cooper, Marketa Burnett, and Misha N. Inniss-Thompson

Early Development and Family Life in Rural America 201
Lynne Vernon-Feagans and Margaret M. Swingler

Latino Prosocial Development in the Rural U.S. 237
Gustavo Carlo, Madison Memmott-Elison, and Lisa J. Crockett

Rural Families in the U.S.: Theory, Research, and Policy 253
Matthew M. Brooks and Sabrina T. Voltaire

Index 269

Contributors

Matthew M. Brooks Penn State, University Park, State College, PA, USA

Marketa Burnett University of North Carolina at Chapel Hill, Chapel Hill, NC, USA

Gustavo Carlo University of Missouri, Columbia, MO, USA

Shauna M. Cooper University of North Carolina at Chapel Hill, Chapel Hill, NC, USA

Lisa J. Crockett University of Nebraska-Lincoln, Lincoln, NE, USA

John Cromartie United States Department of Agriculture, Economic Research Service, Kansas City, MO, USA

Srikant Devaraj Ball State University, Muncie, IN, USA

Dagney Faulk Ball State University, Muncie, IN, USA

Michael Hicks Ball State University, Muncie, IN, USA

Misha N. Inniss-Thompson Vanderbilt University, Nashville, TN, USA

Marybeth J. Mattingly Federal Reserve Bank of Boston, Boston, MA, USA

Madison Memmott-Elison University of Missouri, Columbia, MO, USA

Shannon M. Monnat Syracuse University, Syracuse, NY, USA

Velma McBride Murry Vanderbilt University, Nashville, TN, USA

Mark D. Partridge The Ohio State University, Columbus, OH, USA

Rodrigo Pérez-Silva Centre for Economics and Social Policy, Universidad Mayor, Santiago, Chile

Sydney Schreiner The Ohio State University, Columbus, OH, USA

Margaret M. Swingler University of North Carolina at Chapel Hill, Chapel Hill, NC, USA

Ann R. Tickamyer Penn State, University Park, PA, USA

Lynne Vernon-Feagans University of North Carolina at Chapel Hill, Chapel Hill, NC, USA

Sabrina T. Voltaire Penn State, University Park, PA, USA

Emily J. Wornell Ball State University, Muncie, IN, USA

About the Editors

Jennifer E. Glick, Ph.D. is Arnold S. and Betty G. Hoffman Professor in Sociology and Director of the Population Research Institute at Penn State.

Susan M. McHale, Ph.D. is Director of the Social Science Research Institute and Distinguished Professor of Human Development and Family Studies and Professor of Demography at Penn State.

Valarie King, Ph.D. is Professor of Sociology, Demography, and Human Development and Family Studies and Associate Head of the Department of Sociology and Criminology at Penn State.

Part I
Family Life and Work in Rural Communities

Rural Poverty: Research and Policy for U.S. Families

Ann R. Tickamyer

Popular perceptions of *rural America*, its residents, families, and communities are deeply contradictory. It is the land and people left behind and the center of our current political storm. It is the "rural idyll" of green pastures, sweeping landscapes, and quiet prosperity, and the home of deep poverty, deaths of despair, and environmental ravage. It is both agricultural and industrial, but its problems are most especially de-industrial. It is viewed as the bastion of white people with strong ties to conservative values, politics, morality, and religion and the historical home for minority racial and ethnic enclaves, indigenous populations, and the destinations for both new and old immigration with diverse culture, language, and practices. It is continually "forgotten" but also overrepresented in both U.S. myth and politics—"flyover country" and the "heartland." In reality, there is no one *rural America* in the U.S. today, but rather diverse places and populations with equally diverse backgrounds, goals, and opportunities, all too often united by economic distress.

One condition of the rural U.S. that is often overlooked or misunderstood is the depth, extent, and forms of poverty found there. Historically, poverty was associated with the plight of the rural poor in such isolated places as Appalachia, the Mississippi Delta, Southwestern colonias, and native lands and reservations. More than 50 years ago, *The People Left Behind,* published by The President's National Advisory Commission on Rural Poverty (1967), focused on exposing the deprivations of rural poverty as an opening shot in what became the War on Poverty. However, as attention was drawn to the conditions of urban ghettos, struggles for civil rights and racial justice, and growing attention to urban crowding, crime, and substance use, rural issues became increasingly marginalized and urban poverty became the target of both benign and malign attention of research, the public, and policy makers. Yet,

A. R. Tickamyer (✉)
Penn State, University Park, PA, USA
e-mail: art14@psu.edu

J. E. Glick et al. (eds.), *Rural Families and Communities in the United States*,
National Symposium on Family Issues 10, https://doi.org/10.1007/978-3-030-37689-5_1

rural poverty persisted in the background at disturbing rates, sometimes brought out as a counter to urban problems, but too often forgotten, neglected, or dismissed.

In 1993, the Rural Sociological Society (RSS) undertook a heroic effort to update knowledge of rural poverty by documenting the existence, persistence, sources, and consequences of rural poverty after years of neglect. Publication of *The Task Force on Persistent Rural Poverty* remains a landmark event in demonstrating the plight of rural peoples and places (RSS Task Force, 1993). It took another quarter of a century and a recession that rivals only the Great Depression of the 1930s for damage to the economy and family and community well-being to once again update and assess conditions of poverty in the rural U.S. *Poverty in the United States*, published by Columbia University Press in 2017, brought together numerous distinguished scholars from multiple disciplines with expertise on rural issues (some of whom are authors of this volume) to provide a comprehensive view of the state of poverty in rural places and among rural families and communities (Tickamyer, Sherman, & Warlick, 2017). Coverage includes the history, geography, demography, economics, policy, and the causes and consequences of poverty for rural peoples and places in the U.S.

Drawing on contributions to this volume and a symposium of the Rural Policy Research Institute (Rural poverty, 50 years after *The People Left Behind*—A research conference. Looking backward and forward. March 21–22, 2018, Washington, DC), this chapter builds on the current state of knowledge to lay out the issues facing scholars of poverty and the impact of poverty on rural families and communities with a focus on the links between research and policy dimensions. Issues include:

- Spatial perspectives: What is rural and what is unique about rural? What are the ways to evaluate claims of rural versus urban versus suburban poverty? What are the links?
- Measurement perspectives: How do the ways we define and measure poverty influence understanding of who is poor and what to do about it?
- Theoretical perspectives: Why do the same tired themes and discredited explanations persist?
- Are we missing the boat by focusing on poverty or income? Should we be more concerned with poverty versus inequality or income versus wealth?
- Policy: Is there rural policy, and should there be rural policy? What are place-based approaches versus other approaches to policy? What do we know and what do we need to know to address rural poverty in all its diversity?
- What else do we need to do in order to address widespread rural poverty and deprivation?

Addressing these issues requires confronting the contradictory perceptions and misperceptions that make rural poverty an insidious and persistent problem that reaches beyond the borders of the rural U.S.

Geography and Demography of the Rural U.S.

The opening chapter of *Rural Poverty in the United States* (Tickamyer et al., 2017) begins with a chapter titled, "Where is Rural America and Who Lives There?" (Johnson, 2017). The challenges associated with studying rural America start with the definition of rural. Although everyone *knows* what rural and urban mean, in research the terms are technical concepts that do not always correspond to popular usage. One of the problems of research on the rural U.S. is that data collection and availability do not necessarily correspond to either popular usage or scientific measures. Thus, many studies of rural people and places use the nonmetropolitan county designation as a proxy for rural. To quote the USDA Economic Research Service (ERS), one of the most definitive sources on the rural U.S.:

> …nonmetropolitan (nonmetro) areas, (are) defined by the Office of Management and Budget (OMB) on the basis of counties or county-equivalent units (e.g., parishes, boroughs). Counties are the standard building block for publishing economic data and for conducting research to track and explain regional population and economic trends. Estimates of population, employment, and income are available for them annually. They also are frequently used as basic building blocks for areas of economic and social integration, such as labor-market areas. (USDA, ERS, n.d.-d, "Nonmetro Counties," para. 1)

The obverse, a metropolitan area designation, works well for urban areas with distinctions made between central cities and outlying urban regions tied to the core city. Rural or nonmetro, however, ends up something of a leftover category that includes huge variation in population density, economic base, and size of communities. Nonmetro counties are divided into micropolitan areas if commuting patterns link them to an urban cluster with 10-49,999 persons and noncore, i.e., all the rest. Sometimes metro and nonmetro classifications produce contradictory results. For example, large swathes of agricultural land may exist within close enough proximity to urban areas to be labeled a metro county. Remote exurban outposts that were formerly solidly rural may become the newest additions to the metropolitan embrace. Both ERS and the U.S. Census Bureau create rural–urban continuum codes that recognize degrees or variations in urbanization (cf. USDA, ERS, n.d.-c). Rural and urban boundaries are permeable, subject to processes of shifting, blurring, and crossing making rural–urban distinctions less and less meaningful other than at polar opposites (Lichter & Ziliak, 2017).

There are other official definitions of rural, most notably the Census Bureau designation based on population size and density. Rural is defined as open country with fewer than 500 people per square mile and places with a population of less than 2500. This definition is less useful to researchers interested in the socioeconomic characteristics of rural people and places because of the absence of other data available for that scale. The fact that substantial amounts of social, economic, and political data are collected and available over time at the county level make this the "go to" measure for research on the rural U.S. For this chapter, unless otherwise noted, rural is defined as nonmetropolitan, and the two terms will be used interchangeably.

In aggregate, rural population characteristics differ from those of metropolitan residents. The rural population is older, whiter, less educated, and poorer. These averages mask the great and growing diversity of rural populations, especially among low income and poor residents, with large and increasing numbers of Hispanics as well as substantial numbers of African Americans, Native Americans, and new immigrants of various backgrounds. Overall, the rural population of the U.S. exceeds 50 million people, lives in places that cover 75% of its territory, and displays the diversity found in the rest of the nation (Johnson, 2017).

Rural Poverty Measures and Figures

Using county-level data and designations, poverty in the U.S. has been systematically tracked and measured since the advent of the official poverty measure (OPM) constructed by Mollie Orshansky, an economist and statistician working for the Social Security Administration in the 1960s. The OPM determines poverty rates for families and individuals on the basis of cash income that falls below thresholds deemed necessary for a minimally adequate standard of living to meet basic subsistence needs. Poverty thresholds are adjusted for age and family size and are updated annually. In 2018, thresholds were approximately $12,000 for a single individual and just under $25,000 for a family of four. The history of the poverty measure is a fascinating story in itself (Fisher, 1992, 2008). For purposes here, its importance is the ability to track changes over time and place in poverty rates. Especially noteworthy, is that according to the OPM, rural poverty has been substantially reduced over time; nevertheless, as seen in Fig. 1, rural poverty remains consistently higher than metro poverty despite a large initial decrease in the gap from the time of its first measurement.

At the time that poverty was first systematically measured and tracked and at the time of the report *The People Left Behind*, rural poverty was noteworthy not only for the extremely high rate of more than twice the level of the metro rate, but also for its demographic characteristics and geographic clusters (Weber & Miller, 2017). Historically, the rural poor were more likely to be white, in married couples, and employed, i.e., members of the working poor. Geographic clusters with high poverty rates included Appalachia, the Southern Blackbelt and Mississippi Delta, native lands and reservations, and borderland portions of the Southwest with a heavy Hispanic presence. The USDA has kept track of persistent poverty counties, defined as counties where at least 20% of residents are poor over multiple decades. The most current map displayed in Fig. 2 looks very much like high poverty areas of the past. Although the number of nonmetro counties classified as persistently poor has diminished, the regions are largely the same. The one area of improvement has been in the Midwest where there has been a decline in nonmetro counties with the highest poverty rates. In basic outlines and contours, the most recent map looks very much like the ones produced in previous decades.

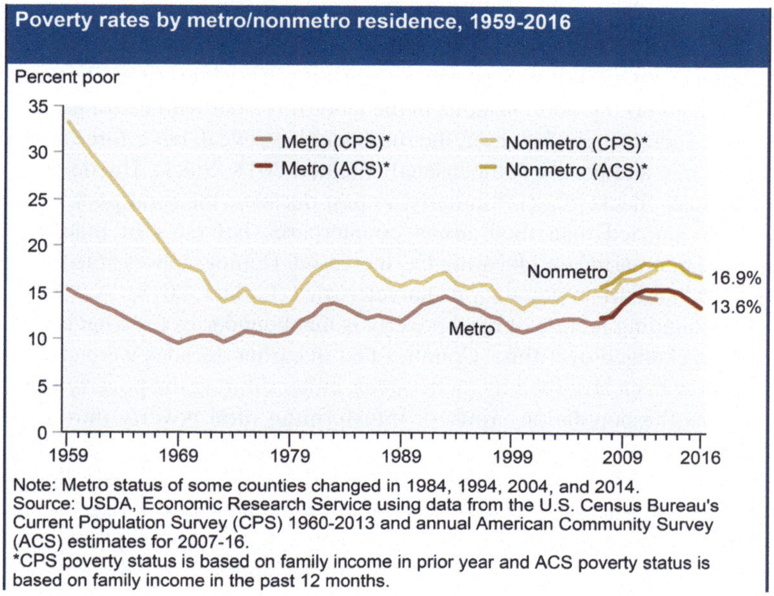

Fig. 1 Official poverty over time by metro/nonmetro classification. Source: USDA, ERS (n.d.-b)

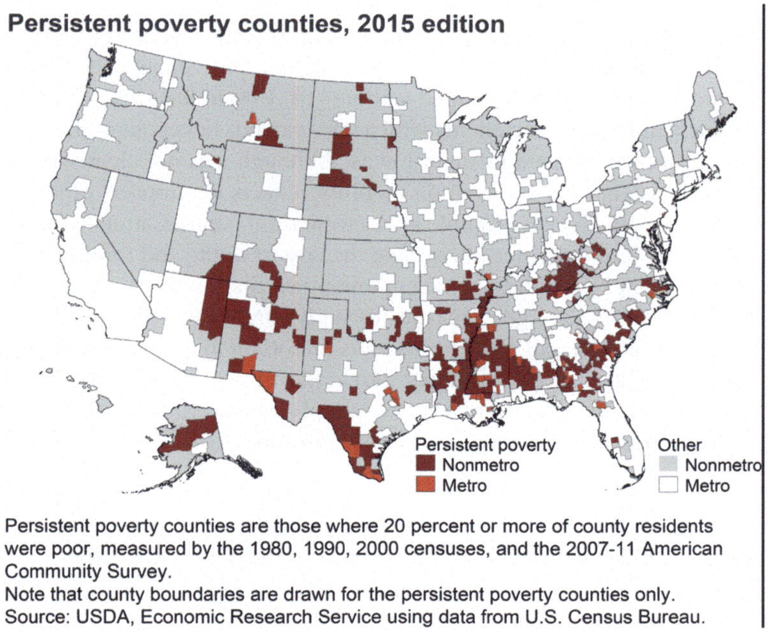

Fig. 2 Persistent poverty counties by metro/nonmetro classification. Source: USDA, ERS (n.d.-b)

Demographically, rural poverty has converged with the rest of the nation. Racial minorities are disproportionally represented as are children, especially those in a female-headed household with no spouse present. For a long time, the rural poor were often the working poor, persons in the labor force but with earnings below the poverty line. Increasingly, however, the rural poor have weak labor force attachment with jobs scarce and poorly compensated (Lichter, 2018; Slack, Thiede, & Jensen, 2018; Thiede & Slack, 2017). Similarly, in past decades, the rural poor were more likely to be married than their urban counterparts, but rates of marriage have declined and nonmarital childbearing has increased. Demographers note the convergence of rural and urban population characteristics (Lichter, 2018).

One confounding feature of rural poverty is that boundaries for what is classified as rural have changed over time. Counties that in earlier decades were classified as rural have now been absorbed by metro areas, either diluting the poverty figures for the county as the population grows or transforming rural poverty into urban and especially suburban poverty. As suburban poverty rates have grown in the most recent U.S. Census figures, one source may be an artifact of reclassification.

Regardless of whether boundary change is implicated in the rise of suburban rates, it is important to recognize that poverty is often linked across space. Population decline in rural areas, a hypothesized "brain drain," and lack of jobs, services, and opportunities will push people from rural locations to urban centers. Indeed, the *People Left Behind* noted the out-migration of the rural poor to urban slums and used that as the basis for arguing the need for coordinated efforts to combat poverty wherever it is found (President's National Advisory, 1967). Conversely, a lower cost of living may lead urban residents to move to or between rural areas. One of the most astute practitioners of rural poverty ethnography, Janet Fitchen (1995), observed the incidence of "Greyhound welfare" (p. 198) in the 1990s. Urban social services provided low-income clients with a one-way bus ticket out of the city (New York in this case) to relocate to small towns. Although it is not clear whether this practice continues, current research on mobility reflects the impacts of geographic mobility. A prominent recent example arises from rural gentrification in rural retirement and amenity communities, increasing the cost of living and forcing poor rural residents to relocate out of their home communities (Sherman, 2017).

In short, there are many good reasons to study rural poverty as a serious social problem in its own right, but also because it is important to understand the linkages across time and space. While in many cases, the rural poor are "the people left behind," who is left and who is not are often deeply connected both at the individual and at the structural levels and require further scrutiny.

Is Rural Poverty Really Different or Worse than Urban Poverty?

In comparing poverty across the rural–urban continuum, it is often asserted that the official poverty measure (OPM) is biased since it does not take into account access to other resources including tax credits, transfers, or cost of living differences. The

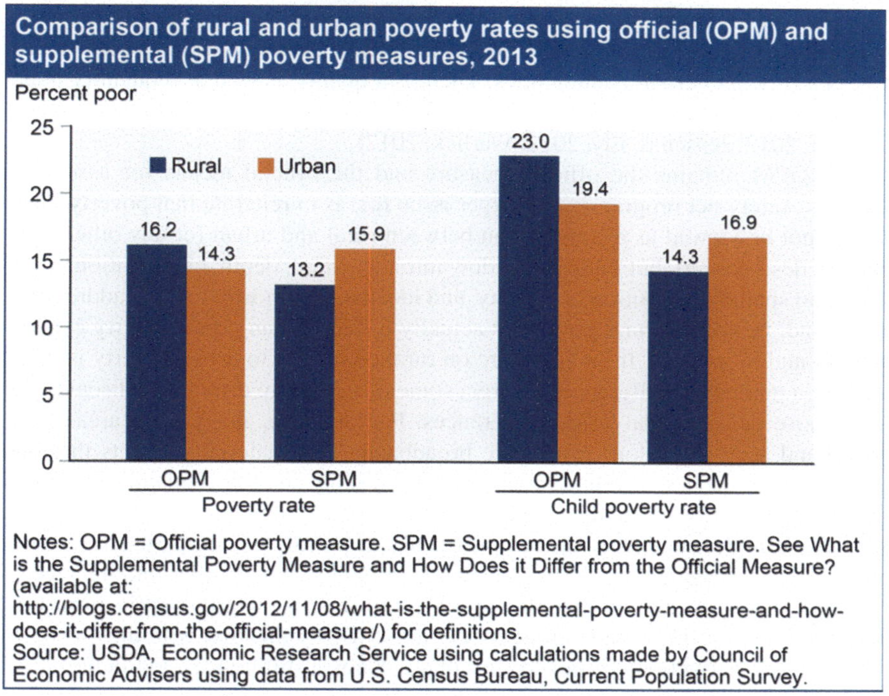

Fig. 3 Comparison of OPM and SPM. Source: USDA, ERS (n.d.-a)

supplemental poverty measure (SPM) was created by a federal government interagency group to address these issues and has been tracked by the U.S. Census Bureau annually since 2011. Interestingly, by this measure, unlike the OPM, nonmetro poverty rates appear to be somewhat better than metro rates by 2000 (Nolan, Waldfogel, & Wimer, 2017; Warlick, 2017; Weber & Miller, 2017; Ziliak, 2019) (Fig. 3).

The SPM corrects for serious problems in the OPM, including adjusting for geographic differences in the cost of living and taking account of cohabiting households whose member resources are viewed as pooled even if the individuals are not legally related. It has a more inclusive definition of families than the OPM which defines families only as those related by blood, marriage, or adoption. The SPM extends the definition to include cohabiting adults and unrelated children in a family's care, a more realistic standard in current times.

Thus, the SPM is more reflective of the totality of resources available to poor persons and families. However, issues remain about how comprehensively it measures the cost of living differences between rural and urban areas, how that affects poverty rates, and more importantly, how it reflects the lived experience of poor people (Warlick, 2017). Poverty thresholds are adjusted based on expenditures for food, clothing, shelter, and utilities (FCSU; Fox, 2017). Housing costs are the only cost of living adjustments between rural and urban areas (B. Weber, personal communication, October 3, 2018). Differences in transportation costs are not included which may be particularly significant in rural areas where long distances are standard for access to employment, social services, groceries, and consumer goods. It is also generally acknowledged that cost is just one factor in assessing housing differences between rural and urban communities. There is a quality as well as a quantity issue with housing (and possibly other items as well) in rural areas (Housing Assistance Council, 2012; Jensen & Ely, 2017; Warlick, 2017).

The OPM remains the official measure and the official means for assessing access to safety net programs. The larger issue first is to reiterate that poverty rates should not be viewed as a competition between rural and urban (or any other geographic designation), but rather a window into the extent, depth, composition, linkages, and spatial distribution of poverty, and ideally a diagnostic tool for addressing it. Second, is whether rural poverty is actually different than urban poverty experientially and in impacts. If the literature on rural compared to urban poverty is marshalled, a number of differences emerge, some of which are difficult to disentangle from more general rural–urban differences. For example, many rural areas lack broadband access let alone affordable broadband. This materially affects the fortunes of everyone in the community as well as possibly creating a qualitative difference for the poorest residents compared to their urban counterparts.

This example illustrates the complexities and pitfalls of comparing rural and urban poverty populations. On the one hand, without getting further into the weeds of defining poverty, all poor people are subject to serious material deprivation. Yet, the experiences, causes, and consequences may vary by location with the outcome of important distinctions in poverty by place. Known differences and deficits for rural residents apart from distance, are the limited or even total lack of availability of public and social services. Access to health care is likely to be limited and insufficient. Food deserts are found in many rural areas, and where grocery stores exist, low volume may mean fewer options, poorer quality, and higher prices. Schools are often inadequate in facilities and curricula, while the frequent solution of consolidation creates excessively long travel times for students and a decline in community support and involvement. Furthermore, there is a lower return to education for rural residents. Some service facilities may be totally absent from rural areas. For example, formal professional child care facilities are nonexistent in many rural communities with care haphazardly dependent on whether there are relatives, friends, or paid unlicensed childminders available, often with few options or ability to evaluate qualifications. Rural economies are less diversified in employment options, and a plant closing or layoff will be devastating to both the community and its residents (Smith & Tickamyer, 2011; Tickamyer et al., 2017).

Finally, it should be noted that the rates of deep poverty, near poverty, and relative poverty are almost universally higher in nonmetro counties than in metro counties. Deep poverty is defined as family income less than half its poverty threshold; near poverty is when income is 150% of its threshold; relative poverty is measured at 50% of median household income (Jensen & Ely, 2017).

These differences suggest that the experience of rural poverty will be qualitatively different for many rural residents, and the ability of a community to marshal resources to assist their poorest residents will be much more limited. Especially in high and persistently poor places, the intersection of poor people and poor places will create a heavy burden that is difficult to escape.

What Are the Causes of Rural Poverty?

If rural poverty is truly different than other forms of poverty, the question arises of whether the causes also vary. Of course, all poverty is caused by a lack of resources, particularly money, but this fails to address why some people in some places experience deprivation. In fact, the issue is complicated due to an immense amount of obfuscating rhetoric about causes that have hindered efforts to address poverty in any location. Before addressing explanations for rural poverty, it is important to examine theories of poverty more generally, starting with two important distinctions: the difference between poverty of people and poverty of place and the difference between individual versus structural explanations.

People Versus Place

Poor people may be found anywhere, but where there are large clusters of impoverished persons, a place, however, defined may be classified as poor. In the U.S. as previously described, there are historical clusters of poor places—nonmetro counties with chronically high poverty rates reaching from the past into the present (Weber & Miller, 2017). Often those places are populated by persons whose demographic characteristics are particularly likely to be poor, racial and ethnic minorities, single- and female-headed households, unemployed, disabled, seniors, and children. At the place level, these are aggregates, and it is important to avoid assumptions about individuals within them. Nevertheless, a spatial perspective is useful in locating sources of poverty.

When considering poor persons, the task is to avoid conflating descriptive and correlational factors with deeper, underlying causal explanations. Demographic characteristics such as those listed above—gender, race/ethnicity, marital status, etc. are correlated with poverty and create a greater likelihood of being poor, but to the extent that they explain poverty, they require identification of underlying mechanisms. For example, the greater representation of women householders with children among the poor may be the result of historical and contemporary divisions of labor, labor market and wage discrimination, gendered family roles that assign women major responsibility for second shift activities (household and family reproduction), and lack of social supports for these tasks. These and related factors combine to constitute the underlying causes of an observed demographic regularity. Similar analyses can (and have) been described for numerous descriptive regularities (Tickamyer & Wornell, 2017).

Individual Versus Structural Explanations

The above description begins to capture an even more fundamental and pervasive distinction in poverty theory: individual versus structural level theories. Individual-level theories look to the individual for causes. Particular behaviors, beliefs, values, practices, motivations, investments, etc. have been argued to be characteristic of poor persons. Culture of poverty, human capital, status attainment, and rational choice theories all focus on individual-level actions by seeing individual decisions and volition as the source of economic outcomes including likelihood of being poor. Alternatively, structural theories locate the sources in larger social organizational and institutional arrangements largely beyond the control of the individual. Thus, the structure of the economy and labor markets, institutional discrimination, historical legacies of disadvantage, domination and subordination shape the opportunities available to individuals and groups, resulting in the greater and lesser propensity to being poor.

Complicating matters, these theories often become mixed up with politics and ideology. Culture of poverty theory makes a prime example. First proposed by an anthropologist to explain why lack of economic opportunity creates disincentives for poor persons to achieve and invest (Lewis, 1959, 1966), the theory has morphed into a focus on negative psychological traits that are attributed to poor persons. The result is a theory that blames the victims for generational poverty based on attributed character flaws and antisocial behaviors. This formulation has huge implications for approaches to policies and programs to assist the poor, often used to justify punitive approaches (Tickamyer & Wornell, 2017). Similarly, structural explanations, while more in accord with the realities of social arrangements that handicap certain individuals and groups, lend themselves to unrealistic prescriptions for social transformation that are unlikely to be implemented or realized in a market economy.

In addition to these overly polarized micro-macro or agency versus structure, explanations are theories that seek to link individual and structural factors and people and places. Theories of social exclusion, social isolation, intersectionality, and forms of capital, represent efforts to seek the linkages between spatial and institutional structures and individual-level outcomes with a focus on the mechanisms that create these relationships. Often persuasive to scholars, the complications entailed in these explanations have little resonance with the larger public or policy makers. More extensive coverage of these and related theoretical perspectives are addressed by Tickamyer (2006) and Tickamyer and Wornell (2017).

Are the Causes of Rural Poverty Different?

These theories apply very generally at least to advanced industrial and postindustrial economies such as the U.S. It is the configuration of factors that will vary by place. Just as students of urban poverty identify a constellation of neighborhood effects that they argue are unique to inner city poverty and residents (Wilson, 1996, 2012), rural poverty can also be characterized by the prevalence of specific configurations of demographic, socioeconomic, and spatial factors. This is easiest to recognize when looking specifically at poor places, but arguments can be made about the larger phenomenon as well.

When *The People Left Behind* was issued in 1967 and for many years subsequently, the rural poor were primarily white, nonfarm, employed, and in traditional married families. As found nationally and in urban areas of the U.S., minority groups were particularly likely to be impoverished, but overall rural poverty presented as described, making its demographic profile different from the urban poor as well as having much higher rates. Fast forward, and the rural population and poor increasingly have converged with urban and national trends so that many of the characteristics and the factors associated with poverty are similar: increasing minority share, weak labor force attachment, under- and unemployment, nonmarital births, cohabitation, and female-headed households (Lichter, 2018; Slack et al., 2018; Weber, Farrigan, Glasmeier, & Gagin, 2018; Ziliak, 2019).

The convergence in the socioeconomic characteristics of the rural poor with urban and national poverty statistics argues for similar sources and explanations for poverty across space, and certainly, the proximal causes will look the same. However, the larger, underlying causes combine to create a profile for rural poverty dissimilar to its urban counterparts. These include the spatial clustering of poor places, the historical legacies of these places and their residents, the economic structure and conditions typical of the rural U.S., particularly deindustrialization, and the sources and impacts of social welfare policies for the rural poor.

The continuing existence of regionally specific high and persistent poverty locations as noted earlier point to unique structural drivers of rural poverty associated with the histories of local development. Thus, high rates of Appalachian poverty speak to a history of resource extraction, underdevelopment, and exploitation in an environment of isolation, lack of infrastructure investment, and political corruption in ways that have been variously explained as "the resource curse" and internal colonialism. The Mississippi Delta and the Southern Black Belt reproduce the legacies of slavery, plantation economies, and Jim Crow segregation and discrimination. Southwest borderlands include the impoverished colonias of Latinx heritage residents and migrants, many of whom work in extremely harsh conditions as agricultural and construction workers. The poverty and social problems found on Indian reservations are the inheritance of centuries of land and livelihood expropriation and oppression (Billings & Blee, 2000; Billings & Tickamyer, 1993; Duncan, 2014; Lyson & Falk, 1993; Harvey, 2011, 2017; Pickering, Harvey, Summers, & Mushinski, 2006; and cf. RSS Task Force, 1993; Tickamyer et al., 2017).

Equally important, the rural U.S. has experienced massive social and economic changes that have reduced opportunities for its residents (Falk, Schulman, & Tickamyer, 2003; Jensen & Jensen, 2011; Smith & Tickamyer, 2011; Thiede & Slack, 2017). Economic restructuring in many rural communities has left empty main streets, few employment opportunities, and lack of social services and health care. Globalization has introduced competition for low-wage labor that even rural labor markets, formerly competitive relative to urban wages, cannot match with the subsequent demise of much rural industry and the decline of labor unions and labor protections. Opportunities for a comfortable living have diminished, reflected in reduction in labor force attachment for men, stagnating wages, and large amounts of under- and unemployment. The Great Recession was particularly brutal for rural economies that lack diversity and jobs, and men's employment has not recovered. Although women have fared a little better, it is not enough to make up for men's loss of wages (Smith, 2011, 2017; Ziliak, 2019). The result is poor economic prospects in rural communities.

In short, the deepest underlying causes of poverty are pretty much the same everywhere, but the specific configuration as well as the size and types of impacts separate rural poverty from other forms. Rural poverty mandates a different understanding and a research and policy agenda of its own, all the while recognizing the diversity of poverty within the rural U.S. as well as across it.

Poverty and Inequality

Across the U.S., growing inequality matches poverty in cause for concern as well as supplying a connection to ongoing poverty that is sometimes hypothesized as causal. It is not entirely clear how rural income and wealth inequality compare nationally and to metro areas. There is some evidence that income inequality as measured by the Gini coefficient is somewhat lower in rural than urban areas (Bishaw & Posey, 2016). Higher levels of parent-to-child income mobility in rural commuting zones have been reported (Chetty, Hendren, Kline, & Saez, 2014). There is also a substantial amount of variation within nonmetro counties with higher levels of income inequality associated with lower levels of parent-to-child income mobility (Krause & Reeves, 2017), and distance from metro areas predictive of higher upward mobility (Weber, Fannin, Miller, & Goetz, 2018). To the extent that aggregate income inequality is lower within nonmetro counties, it may be a function of overall lower average incomes, or alternatively, reflect that the richest persons in the U.S. live in urban areas, so that the gap between the highest and the lowest incomes are the same across rural and urban areas (B. Weber, personal communication, October 3, 2018). Nevertheless, inequality has increased over time in nonmetro and urban locations for both income and wealth, and this in turn has been linked to increases in poverty.

Policy and Programs

If the causes, profiles, and consequences of rural poverty vary substantially from poverty in other locations, are different solutions, policies, and programs needed to address particular manifestations? Policy and consequent programs have distinct impacts and implications for particular populations and places. Here too, prescriptions for how to address rural poverty run into interference from adherence to different theoretical perspectives, political and ideological viewpoints, and perhaps most importantly, the availability (or lack) of research evidence. If the sources of poverty are conceived to lie primarily in the individual, then mitigation efforts will be directed toward dealing with individual deficits, providing incentives and sanctions for designated behaviors. Alternatively, if a structural perspective prevails, efforts are more likely to be directed at the organizations and institutions that foster opportunity along with redistributive programs to assist the poor. In fact, both types and many mixed versions can be found, although often with little real understanding of their underlying assumptions and both direct and indirect consequences.

Efforts to provide assistance to poor individuals and families take multiple forms, including some that directly target poor persons, others that are designed to create incentives and support to avoid or lift persons out of poverty, and still others that operate indirectly to assist either poor people or places. At the policy level, several facts should be noted. First, U.S. social policy is notably less redistributive and less generous than correspondingly affluent societies. Thus, the U.S. compares unfavorably with OECD (Organisation for Economic Co-operation and Development) nations in its numbers and forms of assistance available to the lowest and poorest members (Maldonado & Nieuwenhuis, 2015).

Second, U.S. social welfare is roughly divided between universal benefits available to all eligible members of society regardless of income (e.g., social security for the elderly with qualifying records of employment, unemployment insurance for workers who lose their jobs for reasons beyond their control) versus means-tested programs for which income and asset requirements must be met for eligibility. Even universal programs are highly restricted in many cases. For example, social security requires a sustained work history of at least 40 quarters; unemployment insurance is time limited and depends on the reason for job loss and time employed.

Third, it is possible to have policies that target specific areas or regions. Place-based policies have a mixed history but rarely target rural places. In fact, although there is a great deal of policy that affects the rural U.S. and its dominant industries such as agricultural supports and environmental controls, there is little that is directed specifically to rural communities and residents (Tickamyer & Smith, 2011).

Finally, in a federal system, policies and programs exist at multiple spatial scales from the federal government to the most local jurisdiction and everything in between. Some programs are designed to combine multiple overlapping responsible jurisdictions, including national, state, and local government. A prime example currently popular among legislators is block grants to the states for cost sharing, program design, administration, and implementation. Within certain guidelines, states are free to use federal funds as they see fit. At least since the advent of the redesign of poverty programs in the 1990s known as welfare reform, there has been a push for devolution and decentralization of welfare programs from the federal government to the states, and in a number of states, further down to the county. The multiplicity of policies, programs, and jurisdictions makes it difficult to make comparisons across space and place.

PRWORA and TANF

Given these complexities, there are notable differences in how programs are implemented and affect rural areas. It is not possible in limited space to discuss all programs that are relevant. Rather, selected major programs and issues will be highlighted, starting with the safety net program embedded in the Personal Responsibility and Work Opportunity Reconciliation Act (PRWORA) of 1996 and implemented in subsequent years. The authorizing language of PRWORA stated the goals of restoring the American family, reducing illegitimacy, controlling welfare spending, and reducing welfare dependency. These goals demonstrate the underlying philosophy of the policy, i.e., a combination of belief in individual responsibility and neoliberal curbs on spending (Warlick, 2017). PRWORA created legislation to replace the existing primary means tested program, Aid to Families with Dependent Children (AFDC), that provided cash assistance, with Temporary Assistance to Needy Families (TANF). Multiple differences in the intent and implementation of the programs have resulted in a much less generous package of benefits. Compared to AFDC, TANF includes stringent time limits for cash assistance (that vary by state), work requirements, sanctions for compliance failures, and notably, devolution to the states as block grants for meeting legislation goals, program design, administration, and funding. This last component has resulted in diversion of funds to pet programs such as premarital counseling with limited utility for the majority of poor families (Schott, Pavetti, & Floyd, 2015).

In fact, PRWORA has succeeded in meeting its goal of reducing spending (at least per capita) while failing miserably in its assistance to poor families. Spending is down, take-up rates are down, and numbers of families benefiting are greatly reduced without corresponding reductions in poverty rates. Between 1979 and 1996, 82% of families with children in poverty received cash assistance from AFDC. In 1996, with the transition to TANF, it dropped to 68% and by 2010 it was 27%. During the same period, the purchasing power of TANF benefits decreased by 20% because of states' failure to adjust for cost of living increases (Warlick, 2017).

The specific impacts of PROWRA and related programs in rural areas are contradictory. There is evidence that take-up rates are even lower as is ability to serve clientele. At the same time, however, there is clear evidence that in aggregate, rural users benefit more. There have been few studies of the specifically rural impacts of welfare reform at the national level (Lichter & Jensen, 2002; Weber, Duncan, & Whitener, 2002). Local case and case comparative studies suggest large challenges in meeting expectations or effective implementation of welfare reform due to the limits of rural communities' capacities to deliver programs, the lack of both jobs and services, including those that would assist in gaining and keeping employment such as child care, and the long travel distances in the absence of good transportation options for recipients (Tickamyer & Henderson, 2010, 2011; Tickamyer, White, Tadlock, & Henderson, 2007).

Other Family Assistance Programs

Numerous other programs targeted to poor and near poor families, and especially children, range from Supplemental Nutrition Assistance Program (SNAP, formerly Food Stamps and still popularly referred to that way), tax credits such as the Earned Income Tax Credit (EITC) and Additional Child Tax Credit (ACTC), universally available programs such as Social Security and Unemployment Compensation for those who qualify, and a hodgepodge of other programs targeted at specific populations such as supplemental nutrition for Women, Infants, and Children (WIC), Supplemental Security Income (SSI), and Social Security Disability Insurance (SSDI) for the disabled, free and subsidized lunch and breakfasts in many schools, and various (and changing) medical benefits available for children and in some cases their parents, depending on the state. SNAP became one of the largest sources of assistance to all low-income families, especially during the Great Recession. As with other programs viewed as welfare, there is stigma and reluctance to use in rural communities, especially where recipients are likely to be known by their neighbors (Sherman, 2009a, 2009b, 2017). Nevertheless, it is the second largest program lifting children out of poverty (Warlick, 2017). Bartering SNAP benefits for cash is illegal, but it is sometimes a rare source of cash in the underground economy for families experiencing deep poverty with little access to cash money (Edin & Schaefer, 2015). How much this practice occurs in rural areas is unknown.

A thorough account, let alone a spatial analysis of the relative effectiveness of the patchwork of programs, requires a much larger study, most of which remains to be done (see Warlick, 2017 ; Ziliak, 2019). It can safely be said that rural residents face greater obstacles to access and successful use of many different programs for all the reasons that rural poverty presents unique challenges as described throughout. At the same time, there is some evidence that safety net programs have been more effective in assisting low-income rural residents, in part because of the prominent role of tax credits to workers as a poverty alleviation mechanism (Warlick, 2017; Ziliak, 2019).

Structural Level Approaches

These vary from programs that have indirect effects spatially to those that are specifically place-based and even target rural areas. For example, school funding formulas which are primarily state and local often disadvantage rural districts, especially poor ones, because the districts do not have the tax base or the support to supplement state funds (Biddle & Mette, 2017). Jobs programs and employment supports may not be effective in rural communities with few industries and employers (Thiede & Slack, 2017) and that need to serve both private and public means and ends (Green, 2017). Furthermore, they are subject to being used as an employer subsidy that operates more as corporate welfare than as help for poor families

(White, Tickamyer, Henderson, & Tadlock, 2003). The historical model of rural electrification which specifically assisted rural areas to electrify, so far has not been replicated for broadband access, and large swathes of the rural U.S. are unable to use high-speed Internet and web services, increasingly a necessity in a high-tech information society (FCC, 2018).

Large-scale place-based programs have a mixed record. Examples such as the Tennessee Valley Authority (TVA) and the Appalachian Regional Commission (ARC) historically had a huge impact in improving the infrastructure of formerly remote rural places, and there have been substantial gains in access, urbanization, and poverty reduction. However, disentangling the extent of poverty reduction from these programs is not totally transparent or readily estimated. Large-scale place-based programs are few and far between and often immersed in much politicking. More recent examples include enterprise zones and industrial cluster policies (Neumark & Simpson, 2014). More generally, there is some evidence to support the need and value for place-based policy to address rural poverty, but there has been little support for this approach (Partridge & Rickman, 2008) and some evidence that they face serious obstacles (Reimer & Markey, 2008).

Impediments to Effective Policy and Programs

In general, effective programs to address poverty are expensive and require political will and resources in short supply in the current policy environment. One problem is that many social welfare programs are designed and implemented in response to popular theories, opinions, and political calculations rather than evidence. For example, PRWORA and TANF, although originally designed to provide incentives for employment ended up reflecting policy and popular beliefs about the dysfunctional lives of the poor and emphasized limits to "dependency" often with severe sanctions that hurt the clients they were to serve (Schram, Soss, Fording, & Houser, 2009; Soss, Fording, & Schram, 2011; Tickamyer, Henderson, White, & Tadlock, 2000). Placing work requirements for assistance has been an increasingly popular approach to means-tested programs with little recognition of the lack of jobs, especially in rural areas with the advent of the Great Recession. Yet, current proposals would extend work requirements to programs such as SNAP that previously were exempt.

Designing evidence-based programs creates its own challenges, also requiring substantial funding and resources and subject to all the restrictions necessitated by ethical concerns and human subject protections. Thus, large-scale social experiments such as the negative income tax (essentially designed to provide a living wage) in the 1970s during the Nixon administration have been rare and have floundered from negative publicity and misinterpretation (Widerquist, 2005). Other experiments such as the Moving to Opportunity (MTO) program require a very long-time frame and have had mixed results. (Chetty, Hendren, & Katz, 2016; Clampet-Lundquist & Massey, 2008; Clark, 2008; Ludwig et al., 2013). Furthermore, the experiment, like most such efforts including household surveys, is focused on urban and central city poverty. In the rare cases where rural communities are included, they have inadequate numbers of rural persons or communities to reliably assess the effects.

Research and Policy Agendas Going Forward: What Do We Need to Do?

The amount of research that has accumulated on rural poverty is impressive. As this brief review and numerous cited sources demonstrate, the research enterprise on rural poverty is quite robust. Nevertheless, the topic is still a stepchild of poverty research and policy agendas. It primarily takes place in fits and starts through concerted initiatives of concerned individuals and organizations, rather than being institutionalized in ongoing organizations and programs. Rural poverty research is often disconnected from other poverty research conducted at urban and national levels, and much of the necessary data for ongoing work is limited or unavailable. A productive agenda for going forward would include research on the following:

1. **Links across space and place:** The Commission's report, *The People Left Behind,* smartly recognized the connections between rural and urban poverty. More recent work demonstrates at length the connections across rural and urban space and place and convincingly argues for their growing integration (Lichter & Ziliak, 2017). It is important not to silo rural poverty and continue to investigate the linkages across space and place. As interest in the rise of suburban poverty has grown, it becomes increasingly necessary to incorporate it into our comparative research on poverty and understand how it relates to rural poverty. Similarly, in a global economy, the connections across national boundaries must be recognized. It is well-known that rural industry and employment have been the victim of increasing competition from globalization and lower labor costs overseas. Yet, poverty is often treated as a problem that is localized in individuals, groups, and places.
2. **Policy and public opinion:** Although there is a vast literature on poverty policy and programs, two gaps remain: comprehensive rural coverage and deeper analysis of drivers of public opinion about poverty causes and solutions. Compendiums and discussion of policy and programs are particularly likely to consider national analyses or focus on urban and metro issues. Much more attention needs to be paid to the challenges of rural poverty and policy.

   The second issue is perhaps more vexing and also more universal. Despite a vibrant poverty policy industry, we have inadequate knowledge of why the public and policy makers cling unyieldingly to outdated and pejorative views about who is poor and what should be done about it. Our wealth of research findings does not translate into good and effective policy. Rather we see popular and policy discussions driven by the same old tired and offensive but nevertheless politically animating issues. These include:

- Underlying assumptions about who is deserving and who is not, with the undeserving predictably falling into categories of the "other" (i.e., minorities based on race, ethnicity, nationality, and nonconforming sex, gender, and family structure).
- Efforts to impose sanctions and proposals for the kinds of "sticks" we must use to make "them" share "our values" (e.g., the beliefs that poor people are lazy so we must tie benefits to work effort, or poor people do not value family so we must tie benefits to those who somehow demonstrate "family values" or appear to be "truly deserving" as deemed by the fickle public). Work requirements where they make little sense are ever popular and are central to new efforts to limit public assistance.
- Failure to recognize the diversity among rural poor peoples and places.
- Efforts to create a competitive notion of whose poverty is the worst and who needs the most attention—rural, urban, and most recently, suburban.

All of these represent either the continuous efforts to demonize the poor and make welfare receipt difficult, stigmatizing, and even impossible or the well-intentioned but misguided efforts to prioritize particular groups, places, problems, and populations. With few exceptions (Rose & Baumgartner, 2013), there is insufficient research that studies why poverty policy is so impervious to evidence. Why are all those tired old tropes still the dominant frames for poverty, whether rural or otherwise? Research on communication, the drivers of public opinion, and how we translate and deliver our findings is critical.

3. **Links between macro and microlevels or structure, culture, and action:** The need to pay more attention to neglected topics that link the larger social structure with practice and behavior. In other words, what are the intermediate institutions and organizations that link the macro structural constraints on behavior with the microlevel actions and decisions of individuals and families? For example, we hear all the time that politics and policy are driven by religious beliefs and practices. Where is this in our research? What other cultural factors (and this does not mean the culture of poverty) are important in shaping poverty outcomes, opinions, attitudes, and practices? Where are the intermediate institutions? The numerous reports on child poverty are not matched adequately with corresponding research on family processes in the rural U.S. We hear about the disappearance of men's jobs but not about the gender identities, roles, and relations that turn that result into failure to cope and exit from the labor force. Other chapters in this volume attend to these but they are the exception rather than the rule and we can do more, especially when it comes to incorporating family processes into policy for rural areas.
4. **Diversity and intersectionality:** The importance of continuing to probe the diversity of rural peoples and places—whether race and ethnicity, age, gender and sexuality, geographic location, or forms of economic development. How do these intersect and interact with each other and how do they vary across place? What are the consequences for rural peoples? Much research focuses on various poor populations including African Americans, Latinx, residents of persistent

poverty locations such as Appalachia, the Delta, and "Black Belt," immigrants, and children. These groups are extremely vulnerable to poverty, and it goes without saying that their circumstances require focused and ongoing attention. However, the need for analytic clarity should not preclude investigation of intersectional complexity across different groups and identities, nor should attention be limited only to the most visible populations.

5. **Methods and data:** More qualitative and mixed methods research and new sources of information. Some of the most revealing work on rural poverty comes from rigorously conducted deep ethnography and case studies such as those by Sherman (2009a, 2009b, 2017) and Duncan (2014). Especially important are mixed-methods approaches that link quantitative and qualitative methods to address issues that cannot be understood with only one tool. To reiterate a previous point, this requires coming down from the loftiest view to connect how structure shapes behavior on the ground. Similarly, we need more efforts to grapple with new sources of data and new ways to collect it. This includes Big data but goes beyond. Our tried and true survey methods are faltering. What will replace them? How will we train our students to use them? That said, where are the large-scale rural household surveys (and especially longitudinal and panel rural studies) that supply adequate numbers of cases for reliable analysis? These are in notably short supply, although, there are promising new plans in development for longitudinal studies that include rural communities (Alexander et al., 2017). Finally, can we agree on the appropriate ways to measure poverty in the next 50 years and then pursue efforts to realize that goal? It is not enough to look at poverty but we also need linked data on wealth and inequality to understand the economic fortunes of the poor.
6. **Future visioning**: Numerous current trends need ongoing analysis with a rural focus to anticipate what are the rising issues for study. These include:

   - What do current employment trends mean for rural poverty, especially the growth of labor market dislocation, underemployment, and dropping out of the labor force? How will the increasing casualization of labor, its feminization, the relentless move to service sector positions, the disassociation of benefits from jobs, and the impacts of the growth of automation and artificial intelligence affect poor people and places?
   - Where will family supports come from? Studies of child poverty must be matched with knowledge of important services such as child care to promote child and family well-being. It is well-documented that child care is a major issue for most families, let alone poor rural women where child care services are scarce to nonexistent.
   - More generally, what are the social service needs across space and place? How do rural places fare in access to services and benefits?
   - On a larger scale: What does increasing globalization mean for rural poverty in the U.S.?
   - What about the reverse trend—the current effort toward protectionism, isolationism, and anti-immigration sentiment?

- Rural places are already behind in the digital world with limited access to broadband and related services. Will this gap be addressed or will it accelerate with the ever-increasing pace of change?
- What are the consequences of devolution for poor peoples and places? What are the limits of this trend?
- What are the connections and implications between rising inequality in the U.S. and globally for rural poverty?
- How has a global and local neoliberal agenda influenced poverty policy and outcomes?

Conclusion: Trouble in the Heartland

Rural poverty is just one indicator, although a deeply troubling one, of the problems and challenges facing rural families and communities. As discussed in this chapter, however, the rural U.S. does not stand alone. Neglect of rural poverty has profound implications for the well-being of the entire nation. Numerous observers have pointed out that it is no accident that the most recent presidential election revolved in part around feelings of rage and despondency over the neglect and disrespect for large swathes of rural residents. They were certainly not alone, but their presence and votes cannot be ignored. Neither can the existence, persistence, causes, and consequences of rural poverty in a nation of affluence. The contradictions raised by poverty and inequality amidst affluence rankle. Fifty years after the report of *The People Left Behind* by the President's National Advisory Commission on Rural Poverty, the issues and recommendations made there remain relevant today. It should not take another 50 years to address them.

Acknowledgments This work was supported by the USDA National Institute of Food and Agriculture Multistate Research Project PEN04623 (Accession#1013257): *Social, economic and environmental causes and consequences of demographic change in rural America.*

References

Alexander, J. T., Andersen, R., Cookson, P. W., Jr., Edin, K., Fisher, J., Grusky, D. B., ... Varner, C. (2017). A qualitative census of rural and urban poverty. *The Annals of the American Academy of Political and Social Science, 672*(1), 143–161. https://doi.org/10.1177/0002716217714156

Biddle, C., & Mette, I. (2017). Education and information. In A. R. Tickamyer, J. Sherman, & J. Warlick (Eds.), *Rural poverty in the United States* (pp. 322–338). New York, NY: Columbia University Press.

Billings, D. B., & Blee, K. M. (2000). *The road to poverty: The making of wealth and hardship in Appalachia*. New York, NY: Cambridge University Press.

Billings, D. B., & Tickamyer, A. R. (1993). Uneven development in Appalachia. In T. Lyson & W. Falk (Eds.), *Forgotten places: Uneven development in rural America* (pp. 7–29). Lawrence, KS: Kansas University Press.

Bishaw, A., & Posey, K. G. (2016). Comparison of rural and urban America: Household income and poverty. *Census Blogs*. Retrieved from https://www.census.gov/newsroom/blogs/random-samplings/2016/12/a_comparison_of_rura.html

Chetty, R., Hendren, N., & Katz, L. F. (2016). The effects of exposure to better neighborhoods on children: New evidence from the moving to opportunity experiment. *American Economic Review, 106*(4), 855–902.

Chetty, R., Hendren, N., Kline, P., & Saez, E. (2014, November). Where is the land of opportunity? The geography of intergenerational mobility in the United States. *The Quarterly Journal of Economics, 129*, 1553–1623.

Clampet-Lundquist, S., & Massey, D. S. (2008). Neighborhood effects on economic self-sufficiency: A reconsideration of the moving to opportunity experiment. *American Journal of Sociology, 114*(1), 107–143.

Clark, W. A. V. (2008). Reexamining the Moving to Opportunity study and its contribution to changing the distribution of poverty and ethnic concentration. *Demography, 45*(3), 515–535.

Duncan, C. M. (2014). *Worlds apart: Poverty and politics in rural America* (2nd ed.). New Haven, CT: Yale University Press.

Edin, K., & Schaefer, H. L. (2015). *$2.00 a day: Living on almost nothing in America*. Boston, MA: Houghton Mifflin Harcourt.

Falk, W. W., Schulman, M. D., & Tickamyer, A. R. (2003). *Communities of work: Rural restructuring in local and global contexts*. Athens, OH: Ohio University Press.

Federal Communications Commission (FCC). (2018). *2018 Broadband deployment report*. Retrieved from https://www.fcc.gov/reports-research/reports/broadband-progress-reports/2018-broadband-deployment-report

Fisher, G. M. (1992). The development and history of the poverty thresholds. *Social Security Bulletin, 55*(4), 3–14. Retrieved from http://www.socialsecurity.gov/history/fisheronpoverty.html

Fisher, G. M. (2008). Remembering Mollie Orshansky—The developer of the poverty thresholds. *Social Security Bulletin, 68*(3). Retrieved from https://www.ssa.gov/policy/docs/ssb/v68n3/v68n3p79.html

Fitchen, J. (1995). Spatial redistribution of poverty through migration of poor people to depressed rural communities. *Rural Sociology, 60*(2), 181–201.

Fox, L. (2017). *The supplemental poverty measure: 2016* (Report No. P60-261). U.S. Census Bureau. https://www.census.gov/library/publications/2017/demo/p60-261.html

Green, G. P. (2017). The opportunities and limits of economic growth. In A. R. Tickamyer, J. Sherman, & J. Warlick (Eds.), *Rural poverty in the United States* (pp. 416–438). New York, NY: Columbia University Press.

Harvey, M. (2011). Welfare reform and household survival: The interaction of structure and network in the Rio Grande Valley, Texas. *Journal of Poverty, 15*(1), 43–64.

Harvey, M. (2017). Racial inequalities and poverty in rural America. In A. R. Tickamyer, J. Sherman, & J. Warlick (Eds.), *Rural poverty in the United States* (pp. 141–162). New York, NY: Columbia University.

Housing Assistance Council. (2012). *Taking stock: Rural people, poverty, and housing in the 21st Century*. Washington, DC: Housing Assistance Council. http://www.ruralhome.org/storage/documents/ts2010/ts_full_report.pdf

Jensen, L., & Ely, D. (2017). Measures of poverty and implications for portraits of rural hardship. In A. R. Tickamyer, J. Sherman, & J. Warlick (Eds.), *Rural poverty in the United States* (pp. 67–83). New York, NY: Columbia University Press.

Jensen, L., & Jensen, E. B. (2011). Employment hardship among rural men. In K. E. Smith & A. R. Tickamyer (Eds.), *Economic restructuring and family well-being in rural America* (pp. 40–59). University Park, PA: The Pennsylvania State University Press.

Johnson, K. (2017). Where is rural America and who lives there? In A. R. Tickamyer, J. Sherman, & J. Warlick (Eds.), *Rural poverty in the United States* (pp. 3–27). New York, NY: Columbia University Press.

Krause, E., & Reeves, R. V. (2017). *Rural dreams: Upward mobility in America's countryside*. Washington, DC: Center on Children and Families at Brookings. Retrieved from https://www.brookings.edu/wp-content/uploads/2017/08/es_20170905_ruralmobility.pdf

Lewis, O. (1959). *Five families: Mexican case studies in the culture of poverty*. New York: Basic Books.

Lewis, O. (1966). The culture of poverty. *Scientific American, 215*(4), 19–25.

Lichter, D. T. (2018, March 21). *The demography of rural poverty since the people left behind*. Washington, DC: Presentation at the Rural Policy Research Institute 2018 Rural Poverty Research Conference.

Lichter, D. T., & Jensen, L. (2002). Rural America in transition: Poverty and welfare at the turn of the 21st century. In B. A. Weber, G. J. Duncan, & L. A. Whitener (Eds.), *Rural dimensions of welfare reform* (pp. 77–112). Kalamazoo, MI: Upjohn Institute Press.

Lichter, D. T., & Ziliak, J. P. (2017, July). The rural-urban interface: New patterns of spatial interdependence and inequality in America. *The Annals of the American Academy of Political and Social Science, 672*, 6–25.

Ludwig, J., Duncan, G. J., Gennetian, L. A., Katz, L. F., Kessler, R. C., Kling, J. R., & Sanbonmatsu, L. (2013). Long-term neighborhood effects on low-income families: Evidence from moving to opportunity. *American Economic Review, 103*(3), 226–231.

Lyson, T. A., & Falk, W. W. (Eds.). (1993). *Forgotten places: Uneven development in rural America*. Lawrence, KS: University Press of Kansas.

Maldonado, L. C., & Nieuwenhuis, R. (2015). Family policies and single parent poverty in 18 OECD countries, 1978–2008. *Community, Work & Family, 18*(4), 395–415.

Neumark, D., & Simpson, H. (2014). *Place-based policies* (Working Paper 20049). Cambridge, MA: National Bureau of Economic Research. https://www.nber.org/papers/w20049.

Nolan, L., Waldfogel, J., & Wimer, C. (2017). Long-term trends in rural and urban poverty: New insights using a historical supplemental poverty measure. *The Annals of the American Academy of Political and Social Science, 672*(1), 123–142.

Partridge, M. D., & Rickman, D. S. (2008). Place-based policy and rural poverty: Insights from the urban spatial mismatch literature. *Cambridge Journal of Regions, Economy and Society, 1*(1), 131–156.

Pickering, K., Harvey, M. H., Summers, G. F., & Mushinski, D. (2006). *Welfare reform in persistent rural poverty: Dreams, disenchantments and diversity*. University Park, PA: The Pennsylvania State University Press.

President's National Advisory Commission on Rural Poverty. (1967). *The people left behind*. Washington, DC: Government Printing Office. Retrieved from https://files.eric.ed.gov/fulltext/ED016543.pdf

Reimer, B., & Markey, S. (2008). *Place-based policy: A rural perspective*. Canada: Human Resources and Social Development Canada. Retrieved from https://www.crcresearch.org/files-crcresearch_v2/ReimerMarkeyRuralPlaceBasedPolicySummaryPaper20081107.pdf

Rose, M., & Baumgartner, F. R. (2013). Framing the poor: Media coverage and U.S. poverty policy, 1960–2008. *Policy Studies Journal, 41*, 22–53.

Rural Sociological Society (RSS) Task Force on Persistent Rural Poverty. (1993). *Persistent poverty in rural America*. Boulder, CO: Westview Press.

Schott, L., Pavetti, L., & Floyd, I. (2015). *How states use federal and state funds under the TANF block grant*. Washington DC: Center on Budget and Policy Priorities. Retrieved from https://www.cbpp.org/research/family-income-support/how-states-use-federal-and-state-funds-under-the-tanf-block-grant

Schram, S. E., Soss, J., Fording, R. C., & Houser, L. (2009). Deciding to discipline: Race, choice, and punishment at the frontlines of welfare reform. *American Sociological Review, 74*(3), 398–422.

Sherman, J. (2009a). Bend to avoid breaking: Job loss, gender norms, and family stability in rural America. *Social Problems, 56*(4), 599–620.

Sherman, J. (2009b). *Those who work, those who don't: Poverty, morality, and family in rural America*. Minneapolis, MN: University of Minnesota Press.

Sherman, J. (2017). Rural poverty and symbolic capital: A tale of two valleys. In A. R. Tickamyer, J. Sherman, & J. Warlick (Eds.), *Rural poverty in the United States* (pp. 205–230). New York, NY: Columbia University.

Slack, T., Thiede, B., & Jensen, L. (2018, March). *Race, residence and underemployment: 50 Years in comparative perspective, 1964–2017*. Presented at RUPRI conference: Rural Poverty, Fifty Years After The People Left Behind—A Research Conference. Looking Backward and Forward, Washington, DC. www.rupri.org/wp-content/uploads/slack-thiede-and-jensen.-RACE-RESIDENCE-AND-UNDEREMPLOYMENT-50-YEARS-IN-COMPARATIVE-PERSPECTIVE-1964-2017-.pdf

Smith, K. E. (2011). Changing roles: Women and work in rural America. In K. E. Smith & A. R. Tickamyer (Eds.), *Economic restructuring and family well-being* (pp. 60–81). University Park, PA: The Pennsylvania State University Press.

Smith, K. E. (2017). Changing gender roles and rural poverty. In A. R. Tickamyer, J. Sherman, & J. Warlick (Eds.), *Rural poverty in the United States* (pp. 117–132). New York, NY: Columbia University Press.

Smith, K. E., & Tickamyer, A. R. (Eds.). (2011). *Economic restructuring and family well-being in rural America*. University Park, PA: The Pennsylvania State University Press.

Soss, J., Fording, R. C., & Schram, S. F. (2011). *Disciplining the poor: Neoliberal paternalism and the persistent power of race*. Chicago, IL: University of Chicago Press.

Thiede, B., & Slack, T. (2017). The *old* versus the *new* economies and their impacts. In A. R. Tickamyer, J. Sherman, & J. Warlick (Eds.), *Rural poverty in the United States* (pp. 231–249). New York, NY: Columbia University.

Tickamyer, A. R. (2006). Rural poverty. In P. Cloke, T. Marsden, & P. Mooney (Eds.), *Handbook of rural studies* (pp. 411–426). London: Sage Publications.

Tickamyer, A. R., & Henderson, D. A. (2010). Devolution, social exclusion, and spatial inequality in U.S. welfare provision. In P. Milbourne (Ed.), *Welfare reform in rural places: Comparative perspectives, research in rural sociology and development* (Vol. Vol. 15, pp. 41–59). Bingley: Emerald Publishing Group.

Tickamyer, A. R., & Henderson, D. A. (2011). Livelihood practices in the shadow of welfare reform. In K. Smith & A. Tickamyer (Eds.), *Economic restructuring and family well-being in rural America* (pp. 294–319). University Park, PA: The Pennsylvania State University Press.

Tickamyer, A. R., Henderson, D. A., White, J. A., & Tadlock, B. (2000). Voices of welfare reform: Bureaucratic rationality vs. participant perceptions. *Affilia, 15*(2), 173–192.

Tickamyer, A. R., Sherman, J., & Warlick, J. (Eds.). (2017). *Rural poverty in the United States*. New York, NY: Columbia University Press.

Tickamyer, A. R., & Smith, K. E. (2011). Conclusions. In K. E. Smith & A. R. Tickamyer (Eds.), *Economic restructuring and family well-being in rural America* (pp. 226–346). University Park, PA: The Pennsylvania State University Press.

Tickamyer, A. R., White, J., Tadlock, B., & Henderson, D. (2007). Spatial politics of public policy. In L. Lobao, G. Hooks, & A. R. Tickamyer (Eds.), *The sociology of spatial inequality* (pp. 113–139). New York, NY: SUNY.

Tickamyer, A. R., & Wornell, E. J. (2017). How to explain poverty? In A. R. Tickamyer, J. Sherman, & J. Warlick (Eds.), *Rural poverty in the United States* (pp. 84–114). New York, NY: Columbia University.

U.S. Department of Agriculture (USDA) Economic Research Service (ERS). (n.d.-a). *Comparison of rural and urban poverty rates using official (OPM) and supplemental poverty measures (SPM), 2013*. Retrieved from https://www.ers.usda.gov/data-products/chart-gallery/gallery/chart-detail/?chartId=82270

USDA Economic Research Service (ERS). (n.d.-b). *Rural poverty & well-being*. Retrieved from https://www.ers.usda.gov/topics/rural-economy-population/rural-poverty-well-being/

USDA Economic Research Service (ERS). (n.d.-c). *Rural-urban continuum codes*. Retrieved from https://www.ers.usda.gov/data-products/rural-urban-continuum-codes/

USDA Economic Research Service (ERS). (n.d.-d). *What is rural?* Retrieved from https://www.ers.usda.gov/topics/rural-economy-population/rural-classifications/what-is-rural.aspx

Warlick, J. (2017). The safety net in rural America. In A. R. Tickamyer, J. Sherman, & J. Warlick (Eds.), *Rural poverty in the United States* (pp. 389–415). New York, NY: Columbia University.

Weber, B., Duncan, G., & Whitener, L. (Eds.). (2002). *Rural dimensions of welfare reform*. Kalamazoo, MI: W. E. Upjohn Institute.

Weber, B., Fannin, J. M., Miller, K., & Goetz, S. (2018, June). Intergenerational mobility of low-income youth in metropolitan and nonmetropolitan America: A spatial analysis. *Regional Science Policy and Practice, 10*, 87–101.

Weber, B., Farrigan, T., Glasmeier, A., & Gagin, C. (2018, March). *Rural poverty fifty years after The People Left Beind: An unfinished legacy* [PowerPoint slides]. Presented at RUPRI conference: Rural poverty, fifty years after *The People Left Behind*—A research conference. Looking backward and forward, Washington, DC. Retrieved from http://www.rupri.org/wp-content/uploads/Overview_Unfinished_Legacy.final_.pptx

Weber, B., & Miller, K. (2017). Poverty in rural America then and now. In A. R. Tickamyer, J. Sherman, & J. Warlick (Eds.), *Rural poverty in the United States* (pp. 84–114). New York, NY: Columbia University.

White, J., Tickamyer, A. R., Henderson, D., & Tadlock, B. (2003). Does Welfare-to-Work work? Rural employers comment. In W. W. Falk, M. D. Schulman, & A. R. Tickamyer (Eds.), *Communities of work: Rural restructuring in local and global context* (pp. 240–264). Athens, OH: Ohio University Press.

Widerquist, K. (2005). A failure to communicate: What (if anything) can we learn from the negative income tax experiments? *The Journal of Socio-Economics, 34*(1), 49–81.

Wilson, W. J. (1996). *When work disappears: The world of the new urban poor*. New York: Alfred A. Knopf.

Wilson, W. J. (2012). *The truly disadvantaged: The inner city, the underclass, and public policy* (2nd ed.). Chicago, IL: University of Chicago Press.

Ziliak, J. P. (2019). *Economic change and the social safety net: Are rural Americans still behind?* (Working paper). Washington, DC: Washington Center for Equitable Growth. https://equitablegrowth.org/working-papers/economic-change-and-the-social-safety-net-are-rural-americans-still-behind/

Changes in Work and Family Across the Rural U.S.

Marybeth J. Mattingly

Perceptions of the rural U.S. often evoke pastoral images of an idyllic landscape of rolling hills and hayfields peppered with farmhouses, barns, and livestock. Taken further, our collective imagination may conjure farm families growing food and maintaining the land. Dad, up at dawn, feeding the cattle, sheep, horses, pigs, and chickens. Mom, up even earlier preparing a rich breakfast of fried eggs, bacon, toast, and orange juice to fuel the day. The kids romping around, helping with farm chores before going off to school. But to what extent is this imagery a relic of the past, and to what extent does it survive in the contemporary era?

Although rural places may be seen as slow to change, considerable changes in population structure, work opportunities, and family life that affected rural and urban places alike were already unfolding by the middle of the last century. First, while the population density of the U.S. was 7.9 persons per square mile in 1850, by 1960 it had risen to 50.6. Second, in 1850, the majority of workers in the U.S. were employed in agriculture (54.8% of U.S. workers across place types; breakdowns are not available by rural/urban status; Lebergott, 1966). However, by 1960 work opportunities had diversified, and agriculture employed an average of just 6.9% of workers nationwide (The breakout between rural and

Note: This chapter was completed in Dr. Mattingly's capacity as Director of Research on Vulnerable Families at the Carsey School of Public Policy, University of New Hampshire.
The views expressed are the author's own and not those of the Federal Reserve Bank of Boston or the Federal Reserve System.

M. J. Mattingly (✉)
Federal Reserve Bank of Boston, Boston, MA, USA
e-mail: Beth.Mattingly@bos.frb.org

J. E. Glick et al. (eds.), *Rural Families and Communities in the United States*,
National Symposium on Family Issues 10, https://doi.org/10.1007/978-3-030-37689-5_2

urban places was 15.4% versus 1.9%, respectively; Carsey School analysis of Decennial Census data; Ruggles et al., 2018).[1] Third, in 1850 the average household size was just over 6 members, including 2.7 children. By 1960, household size had shrunk dramatically to 3.7 members on average, 1.3 of whom were children (Carsey School analysis of Decennial Census data). Fourth, traditionally, U.S. families were overwhelmingly nuclear in structure due to strict social and legal norms around relationships and childrearing. According to U.S. Census and ACS data, in 1960, 8.0% of children lived in single-mother families and 3.2% lived in single-father families. By 2016, 23% of children lived in single-mother families and 4% lived in single-father families (Census Bureau, 2016). Taken together, these patterns suggest dramatic change even prior to the middle of the twentieth century.

To what extent has the rural U.S. further changed since 1960? Has a true convergence with urban areas in the U.S. occurred? In this chapter, I examine the intersection of changes in the nature and substance of work in the rural U.S. with changes in rural family life over the past 50 years. Throughout I make comparisons to urban U.S. areas and discuss persistent differences that distinguish rural U.S. areas. I conclude by discussing the consequences of these intersecting changes for rural families and consider the policy implications of changes to work and family life in rural areas of the U.S.

Rural Employment Then and Now

Labor Force Attachment

Two of the most profound societal changes over the past 50 years are the dramatic increase in women's labor force participation and the racial-ethnic diversification of the workforce, changes that are evident in both rural and urban parts of the U.S. In this section, I explore how labor force attachment, the extent to which individuals work, varies by gender and race-ethnicity over time and across place, documenting where these intersecting changes have converged in rural and urban places.

In 1960, 86.3% of working-age rural men and 35.2% of rural women were employed at least part time. By 2016, those numbers had shifted to 68.7% of men and 63.2% of women in the rural U.S., mirroring trends in urban places (Carsey School analyses of Decennial Census and American Community Survey data). It is estimated that fewer than 40% of women across all place types were working or seeking work in 1960 (Toossi & Morisi, 2017). Across

---

[1] Analyses performed by the Carsey School for this chapter use data from IPUMS (Ruggles et al., 2018).

rural places, women's employment grew from 57% in 1970 to 71% in 2007, though it had peaked at 74% in 2001 (Smith, 2011). A similar trend is evident for women in urban places. Within rural places, the share of women working is further stratified by marital status: married women in the rural U.S. are slightly more likely to be working than their urban counterparts. Single women in the rural U.S. are somewhat less often employed than their urban counterparts (Smith, 2011).

In addition to shifts in married women's labor force participation, employed women have experienced changes in their hours worked over time (Mattingly & Smith, 2010). Between 1980 and 2007, increases in annual hours are evident across place type and family structure. The most dramatic increases though were seen for married women with young children, whose average annual hours jumped by more than the equivalent of 10 weeks of full-time employment in both rural and urban places (Smith, 2011). Though it may be tempting to interpret this as evidence that women are increasingly working full-time, the Bureau of Labor Statistics (2017) reports that the same share (24.9%) of women were working full-time in 2016 as in 1969, suggesting instead that part-time workers are working more hours, although not enough to be considered employed full time. An opposite trend was observed for men: In both rural and urban places, 92% of men were employed in 1970. By 2007, this fell to 80% in rural places and 83% in urban places, with the largest declines occurring since 2000 (Smith, 2011).

Employment, like many economic and social characteristics, is shaped not only by gender and family structure but also by race-ethnicity, education, and family income (The latter are beyond the scope of this chapter). The most recent research has shown little difference in rural employment rates by race (Slack & Jensen, 2002). Though blacks and Hispanics are not less likely to be working, they are both more likely to be underemployed than their white counterparts in rural America. (Underemployed being broadly defined to include discouraged workers, the unemployed, involuntary part-time workers, and the working poor.) Although rural black and Hispanic underemployment has decreased since 1968, it remained high in rural America near the turn of the millennium (Slack & Jensen, 2002). In 1998, more than one-quarter of blacks and Hispanics were underemployed (28 and 27%, respectively), as were nearly 18% of rural whites. By 2012, 21.8% of the rural black labor force was unemployed or underemployed, compared with 18.1% of Hispanics and 11.4% of the white workforce (Young, 2012). Despite these high rates, there is little evidence that this is a distinctly rural concern. Researchers have documented that trends in involuntary part-time work, a small subset of underemployment, are not higher for rural residents in general. Indeed, race-ethnicity and education, among other characteristics, are more important than place of residence when predicting the desire to work more hours than one is able to get (see Young, 2012; Young & Mattingly, 2016).

Changing Nature of Work

The transition to a service-based economy in rural places represents a shift from one driven largely by agriculture and manufacturing. Indeed, in 1960, agriculture was the top industry in nonmetropolitan places, employing 15.4% of rural workers. By 2016, only 4.6% of rural workers were employed in agriculture (Carsey School analyses of Decennial Census and American Community Survey data). A large share of jobs persists in construction, but employment in the service sectors such as education, food service, and health care was more prominent in 2016. Further, the share of the non-metropolitan population employed in manufacturing industries fell from 26.0% in 1960 to 6.6% in 2016 (Carsey School analyses of Decennial Census and American Community Survey data). These changes in the composition of rural work have resulted in a restructuring of skills required to obtain and retain those jobs. In many rural places in the past, individuals could be assured of good jobs with decent consistent earnings and benefits without even so much as a high school degree (e.g., Duncan, 2015). However, with declines in agriculture and manufacturing, that is largely no longer possible. Historically low demand for formal education has led to underinvestment in rural schools, which has implications today as many communities struggle with an educational infrastructure that is inadequate for developing twenty-first-century skills (Duncan, 2015).

In the past, many rural counties were attractive to businesses seeking a location at least in part because of plentiful land and relatively cheap nonunionized labor (Nelson, 2011). Union membership has declined sharply over the past half-century, and currently only 8.8% of rural workers and 11.6% of urban workers are union members (Carsey School analyses of 2016 Current Population Survey Data). While being able to offer lower wages to nonunion workers is an advantage for businesses, workers may suffer not only with low wages but with worse working conditions as well. In spite of decreased demand by union workers for higher wages, businesses are often able to obtain lower priced labor overseas (see Bell & York, 2010).

The transition from an agricultural- and manufacturing-based economy to a service-based economy has brought about dramatic changes in the nature of work. Two of the most important changes are the increase of on-demand work scheduling and the transition to a 24-hour economy. The service sector is not typically unionized, relies on low-wage labor, and offers limited employment benefits. As such, workers often face unpredictable schedules, work outside of traditional business hours, and struggle to make ends meet. These trends are evident across rural America and are sometimes even more apparent there than in cities and suburbs (see Snyder, 2011). For example, rural workers, especially men, are more likely to face variable weekly work hours than their urban counterparts (McCrate, 2011). Indeed, more than one in ten rural workers face such instability and do not control their work hours. Only one in ten has flexibility that they control. They are more often in jobs with fixed start and end times that offer very little flexibility. Rural blacks and Hispanics disproportionately hold jobs with variable work hours and limited flexibility, having less control over their work hours compared to their white counterparts (McCrate, 2011). Variable work hours make it difficult to predict income and maintain the ability to pay bills week-to-week. Additionally, this kind of work may make securing adequate and high-quality child care especially difficult, as providers typically require consistent and predictable schedules for their own planning purposes.

Coupled with changes in the nature and timing of work is a rural disadvantage in earnings. Relative to their peers in urban parts of the country, rural workers earn less for each hour of work. While in 1979, rural workers' real hourly wages averaged $14.77, workers in central cities earned 11% more at $16.44. By 2007, rural workers' wages had increased to only $15.87 while urban workers earned $19.50, or 22% more, doubling their advantage. Meanwhile, suburban workers had the highest wages and also increased their advantage vis-a-vis both rural and urban workers over time (Smith & Tickamyer, 2011). This earnings disadvantage holds especially true for rural women, who consistently make less than their urban peers (Smith, 2011). Of course, overall earnings are driven by wages and hours worked, and vary dramatically by region, occupation, education, gender, race-ethnicity, and a host of other factors. For example, rural married mothers increased their median earnings from just over $11,000 (2006 dollars) in 1969 to over $21,000 in 2006, but this reflects dramatically higher levels of labor force engagement. Rural married fathers, on the other hand, saw their earnings decline slightly over this time period, from under $41,000 to $38,000 while urban married fathers had more stable earnings over the period (Smith, 2011).

In this section, I have discussed broad-scale changes to the employment patterns in rural places in the U.S. In sum, although most in rural areas are working, their jobs are often not good jobs (Smith, 2011). Employment is too often characterized by low wages and a lack of benefits. Complicating this in many areas is the seasonality of work and the need for labor on demand, often outside traditional work hours and with hours that may vary from week to week, making it difficult to maintain economic stability.

In addition to changes to the type and quality of work, it is important to consider how the context of living in rural or urban areas may shape the opportunities for engaging in work. For individuals to participate fully in the labor market, they need first and foremost to have good job options within a reasonable distance. For many rural residents, such jobs simply do not exist, especially for workers who may lack advanced education and training. The issue is compounded by the fact that opportunities for advanced education and job training may be more limited in rural places. Workers also need to have means of getting to work and adequate care for their children. Researchers have long documented transportation challenges across the rural U.S. where public transit is severely lacking and a personal vehicle is typically essential for getting around. Finally, though access to child care is a challenge for families across geography, rural workers face the added challenge of distance. Finding child care on the route between home and work is difficult and can mean longer commute times resulting in the need for more gas and more hours of care.

Rural Families Then and Now

Historically, rural families were much different than their urban counterparts. They had higher marriage rates, higher fertility and were more traditionally structured (e.g., with a male sole breadwinner). Rural families were less racially and ethnically diverse, and fewer immigrants resided in rural America (Lichter, 2012). However, by the end of the nineteenth century, rural family patterns started converging with urban ones and today, the differences are far less dramatic (Carson & Mattingly, 2014).

Age and Racial-Ethnic Structure

Constituting part of the change in rural families are shifts in both their age structure and racial-ethnic composition. To understand changes in the share of households with children, it is critical to consider the aging of the population (see Glasgow & Berry, 2012; Nelson, 2014; Smith & Mattingly, 2012). It is also important to understand how Hispanic populations are shaping rural places in the U.S., given that their families are often a lot different—typically younger and larger—than their non-Hispanic white counterparts.

Demographers frequently use population pyramids to display the age structure of a population. Conventionally, the male population is plotted on one side of the *X*-axis while the female is on the other. To demonstrate the changes in population by race ethnicity, I have altered this format to show the white population age structure on the right and the minority age structure on the left. Figure 1 shows the population age structure in the rural U.S. in 1960 and Fig. 2 shows that of 2016. Figures 3 and 4 display the population age structure for the urban U.S. for 1960 and 2016. Each of these pyramids sums to 100% to show comparisons in the age structure. Note however, that this masks changes in the total size of the population. What is not shown is that the urban U.S. population of 272.5 million was 5.9 times the rural population of 46.1 million in 2016 (Carsey School analysis of American Community Survey data). This difference increased since 1960 when urban areas, with a population of 125.3 million, constituted only 2.32 times the population of the rural U.S. where the population was 54.1 million (U.S. Census Bureau, 1995).

Several trends are evident from the population pyramids. First, the white population is aging rapidly and this phenomenon is more dramatic in rural parts of the U.S. Research shows that this is driven by two primary factors: outmigration of youth and young adults and low fertility (Johnson & Lichter, 2010, 2012). Taken together, these changes have implications for household structure in rural areas of the U.S. and will shape both community needs and the workforce in rural places for the coming decades.

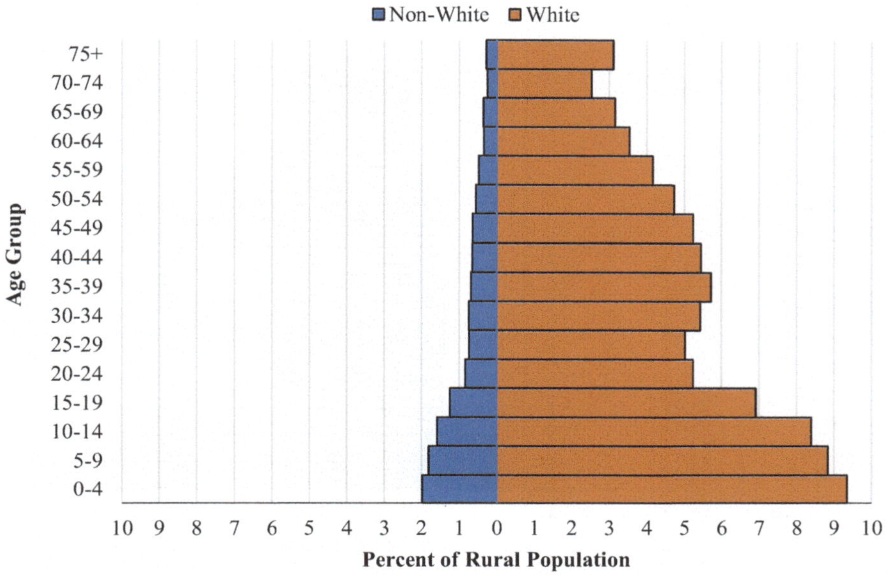

Fig. 1 1960 Rural U.S. population pyramid: White and non-white. Source: Carsey School analysis of 1960 Decennial Census. Note: Rural includes those counties designated nonmetropolitan at the time of the 2010 Census

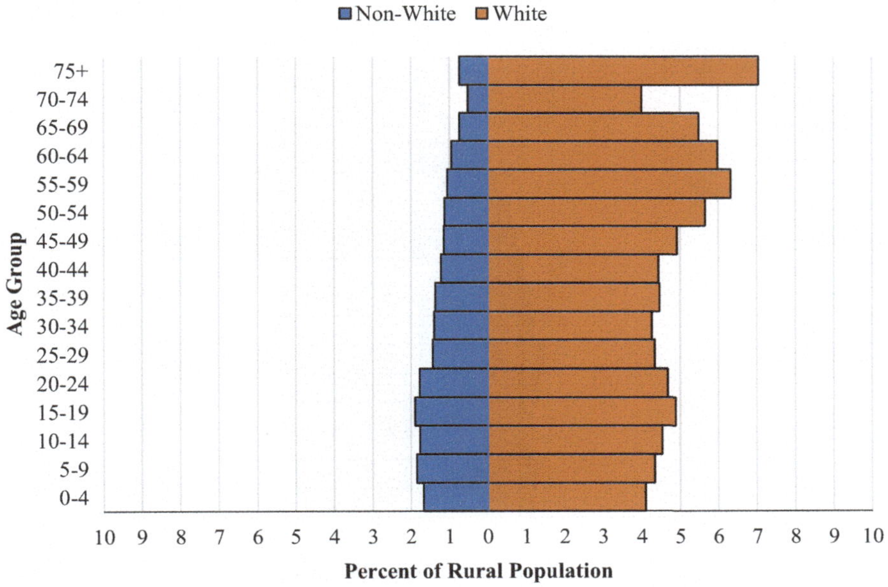

Fig. 2 2016 Rural U.S. population pyramid: White and non-white. Source: Carsey School analysis of 2016 ACS data, 1-year estimates. Note: Rural includes those counties designated nonmetropolitan at the time of the 2010 Census

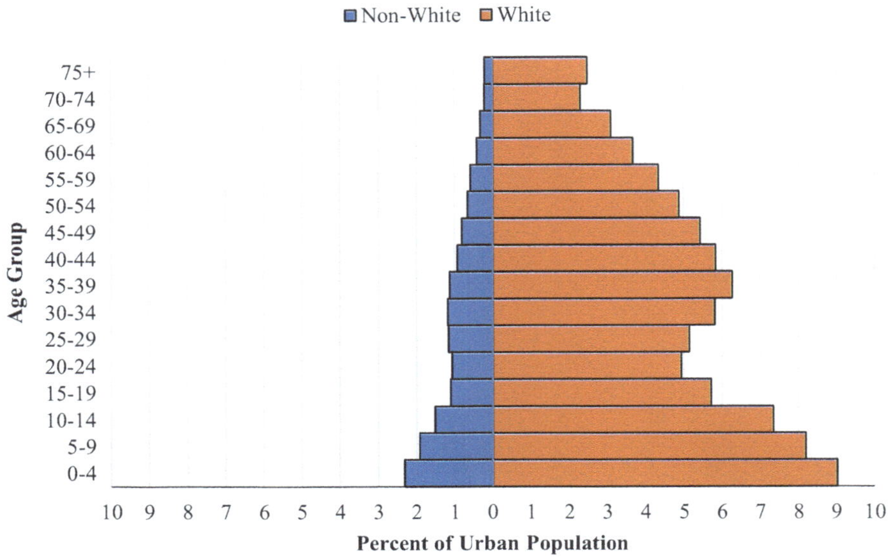

Fig. 3 1960 Urban U.S. population pyramid: White and non-white. Source: Carsey School analysis of 1960 Decennial Census. Note: Rural includes those counties designated metropolitan at the time of the 2010 Census

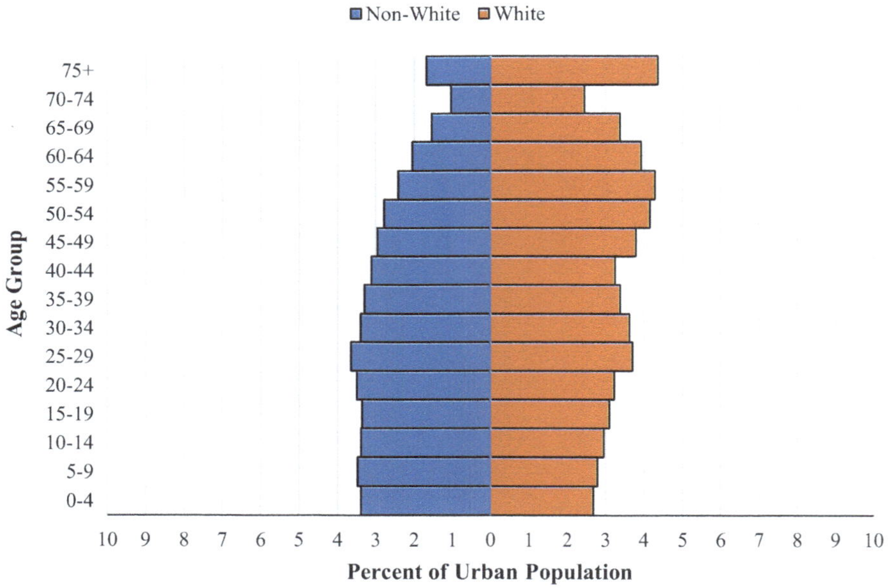

Fig. 4 2016 Urban U.S. population pyramid: White and non-white. Source: Carsey School analysis of 2016 ACS data, 1-year estimates. Note: Rural includes those counties designated metropolitan at the time of the 2010 Census

Second, the urban U.S. was more diverse than the rural U.S. in 1960, and growth in the minority population has been much faster in urban places. Across all ages, urban places were 16% minority in 1960, a share that grew to 42% in 2016. Thus, the share of the urban population that is racial-ethnic minority grew by more than 250% between 1960 and 2016. Though still whiter than urban places today, the rural U.S. is indeed diversifying, with 46% growth in minority populations since 1960 (from 13 to 19%), largely driven by Hispanic populations (Johnson & Lichter, 2008). The share of rural populations that is Hispanic is nearly 2.5 times as large in 2016 as in 1960. This is driven by higher birthrates and a younger age structure among Hispanics than among the white population. Note, however, the share of the total population that is young minority is small and relatively unchanged given the dominance of the entire population by an aging white majority.

Findings regarding rural growth in the Hispanic population are widely documented. Between 2000 and 2010, 56% of rural population growth was among Hispanics, representing nearly 1.2 million people (Lichter, 2017). As a result of this growth, the Hispanic share of the total nonmetropolitan population grew to 7% (Lichter, 2012). This is due to both higher birth rates and in-migration (Johnson & Lichter, 2008). Growth is also evident among other racial-ethnic groups though the share of the rural population that is black declined (data available upon request). Such growth—from the "bottom up"—will fuel increases in the share of the population that is racial-ethnic minority for years to come. Additional growth will persist as a larger cohort of minority children enters the childbearing years, and will be amplified if higher birth rates are sustained. These patterns have important implications for both rural and urban families and workforces in the coming decades.

Finally, the graphs do not show the sex distribution which would reveal that women are overrepresented at the oldest ages due to longer life expectancy. Indeed, according to Carsey School analyses of American Community Survey data, women outnumber men at a slightly higher rate in rural than urban places, although the pattern of older women outliving men is the same in both places. That is, 9% of rural females are age 75 years or older, while only 3% of rural men are. Across urban places in the U.S., 7% of females are age 75 years or older, while 2% of men are. This is important as women are increasingly living alone in their oldest years and often face greater financial insecurity and hardship than men (Brown & Dynan, 2017; Meschede, Cronin, Sullivan, & Shapiro, 2011).

Although rural areas represent 72% of the land in the U.S., only 15% of the total population lives there (Resources & Administration, 2018). Research shows that young people are moving away from the rural U.S. in search of better opportunities in more populated places (e.g., Carr & Kefalas, 2009). For many, this means leaving a beloved place and family connections, but is seen as a necessity due to lack of opportunity near home. During a Carsey School interview on making ends meet in rural New England, as part of the Carsey Study of Community and Opportunity, one young woman explained her struggle to our research team, saying:

> I don't want to go too far away. I want to go far enough that, you know, I can make money and be on my own and do my own thing. But I don't want to be far enough that I can't come home. I want to be close enough that I can come home if I need to because everybody's here.

If those who are best able to leave do so (e.g., those with resources, talents, and limited barriers), what are the implications for rural places with vibrant histories and how can these be best preserved? This is a central question that rural policy makers, advocates, service providers, and citizens will need to address.

Family Composition

The age and racial-ethnic profiles of the rural U.S. are changing in ways that have implications for the structure of rural families and households. On the one hand, minority families have relatively high fertility rates, and increasingly account for rural households with children. However, o verall, rural areas in the U.S. face an aging population, and fewer rural households include children. Not surprisingly, given the trends discussed, elderly households are becoming increasingly dominant across rural places in the U.S. and many older adults live alone. While in 1960, elderly only households, where all residents were at least age 65 years, represented only 12.1% of all households in rural places (and 9.7% in urban places), today that number is 22.1% (16.9% in urban places; see Fig. 5). Of those

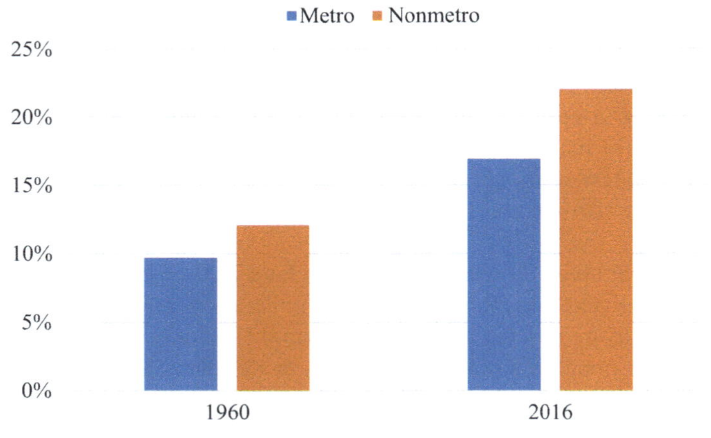

Fig. 5 Share of households that are elderly only by place type, 1960 and 2016. Source: Carsey School analyses of Decennial Census, 1960 and 2016 ACS data, 5-year estimates

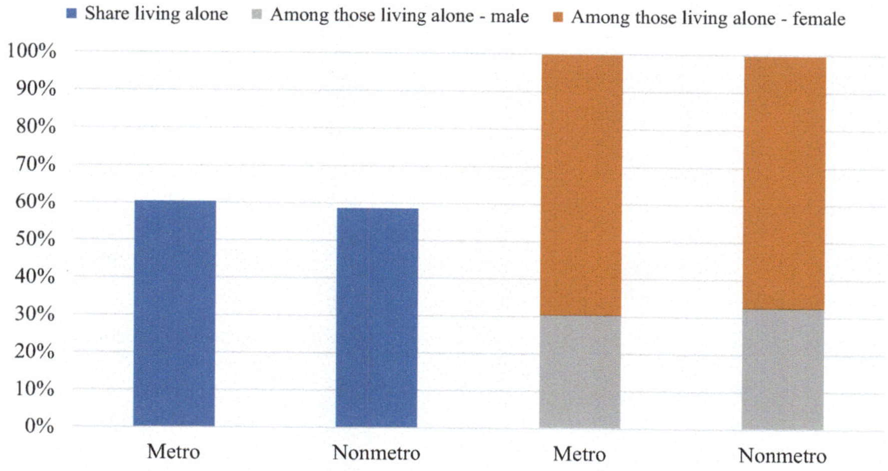

Fig. 6 Sex distribution of elderly only households by place type, 2016. Source: Carsey School analyses of 2016 ACS data, 5-year estimates

in elderly only households, the majority live alone in both rural and urban areas, with 67.4% of those households in rural areas headed by senior women (69.6% in urban places; see Fig. 6).

Coupled with the increasing share of households headed by seniors is fewer households with children, as shown in Fig. 7. In 1960, 49.2% of all rural households included at least one child, but by 2016, this fell to 26.7%. While in 1960, the share of rural households that included a child was 1.05 times the share of urban households, by 2016 the share of rural households dropped to 0.87 times urban households (Carsey School analyses of Decennial Census and American Community Survey data). This is echoed in findings that in 1970 almost 55% of all rural adults lived with at least one child. That share fell to 41% by 2009 (Smith & Mattingly, 2012). In addition, the size of families with children declined over the same time period, from a mean of 2.4 children in 1970 to 1.9 in 2009.

Rural places are also home to a declining share of married couple families. Partly, this reflects declines in marriage. In 1960, 72.2% of adult rural women were married compared to 67.9% of urban women. By 2016, the number declined to 52.1% of rural women and 47.5% of urban women (Carsey School analysis of Decennial Census and American Community Survey data). It is also noteworthy that women everywhere were less likely to have been married more than once in 1960 (12.0% in nonmetropolitan places, 12.6% in metropolitan places) than in 2016 when remarriages in rural U.S. areas were far more common. In 2016, more than one in five (22.4%) rural adults had been married at least twice, while only 16.1% of adults in cities and suburbs had been married at least two times (Carsey School analyses of American Community Survey data). Following this trend, we

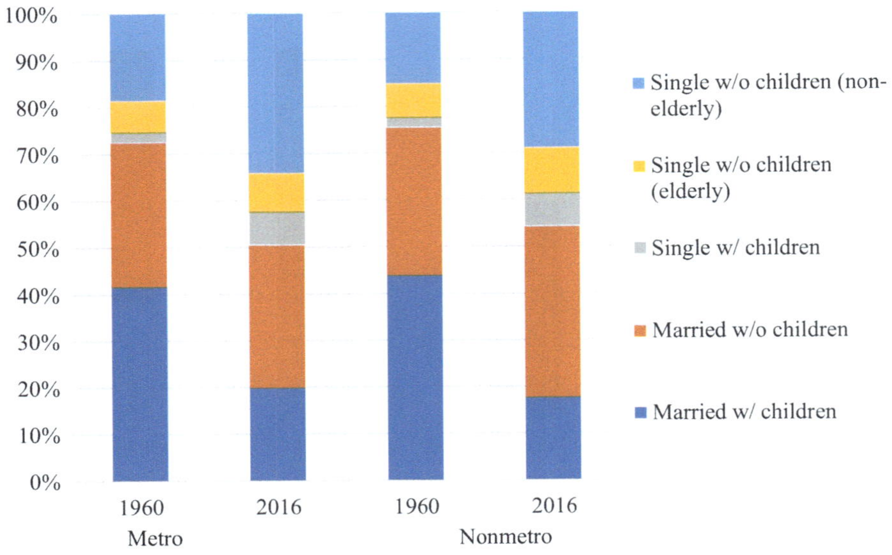

Fig. 7 Metro and nonmetro adult population composition by marital and fertility status, 1960 and 2016. Note: Population age 18 years and older. Source: Carsey School analysis of 1960 Decennial Census and 2016 ACS data, 5-year estimates

see that fewer children lived with both parents. Between 1990 and 2008, the share of children residing with both parents declined from 76% to 68% (O'Hare & Churilla, 2008).

Finally, even though the share of rural married couples living with children declined dramatically, the share of households that are traditional, with a male breadwinner and female caregiver has declined even more precipitously. In 1969, 48% of rural married couples with children had a husband as the sole provider, but by 2006, only 22% of these families had a male sole provider (Smith, 2011). Similar declines are evident across the urban U.S. In both places, these shifts are largely driven by the increased share of women in the labor force even in married couple families.

Data Limitations

The data for this project is drawn from the American Community Survey, Decennial Census, and Current Population Survey microdata, as indicated. Except in the population pyramids, where we overlay the populations of the same county groupings, rural status is determined based on the county classification at the time of the survey. Therefore, those surveyed in the 1960s are classified based on the 1960 Census classifications of metropolitan/nonmetropolitan status, and those surveyed after

2010 are classified based on 2010 Census classifications. While this provides a portrait of the rural U.S. then and now, it obfuscates important changes in the county classifications. Indeed, many counties that became much more populous over the fifty-year window were reclassified as metropolitan. However, it remains a question whether the places that have changed from rural to urban classification over time are more like rural or urban places today based on the characteristics studied here (e.g., family structure, educational attainment, and economic characteristics). Importantly, the data presented in the population pyramids do not follow this classification structure. Rural places in these data are classified based on the post-2010 definition of rurality. An interesting avenue of further research is to use consistent 1960s or 2010 classifications to compare the same counties over time. Perhaps more interesting is to tease out counties that have changed designation to see if they are indeed more reflective of rural or urban patterns.

Discussion

At the outset I posed two questions: To what extent have work and family life in rural places changed in the U.S. over the past fifty years? Has a true convergence with urban places occurred?

In response to the first question, this chapter has documented dramatic changes in rural U.S. since 1960. Changes in the nature, timing, and availability of work coupled with changes in the family have brought about dramatic shifts in the lives of rural persons. Though no doubt some have benefited, particularly those who can work remotely in professional jobs, for too many the intersecting work and family changes have made it difficult to make ends meet in rural areas. However, supplemental poverty measurement data computed by researchers at Columbia University (Wimer et al. 2017), which account for income, expenses, and safety net benefits, reveal that poverty actually fell dramatically over the near 50-year period, as shown in Fig. 8. In 1967, the first year for which these data are available from Columbia University, one in four rural residents were poor. By 2016, this had fallen to fewer than one in seven or 15%, with changes in social safety net programs likely accounting for much of these differences. We also see that declining poverty rates reversed by the Great Recession in December, 2007–June, 2009 (NBER, 2012) and have remained largely stagnant since.

Declines in key rural industries like agriculture and manufacturing mean that attaining a middle-class lifestyle without higher education is now generally out of reach. High rates of divorce and out-of-wedlock child-bearing mean single parents are the sole providers of both care and financial support for their children. These changes, coupled with challenges finding quality affordable child care while working jobs that are often unpredictable and during nonstandard hours means families are under a lot of stress to put food on the table and afford shelter. Family life is complicated in many places today by the opioid crises and legacies of poverty.

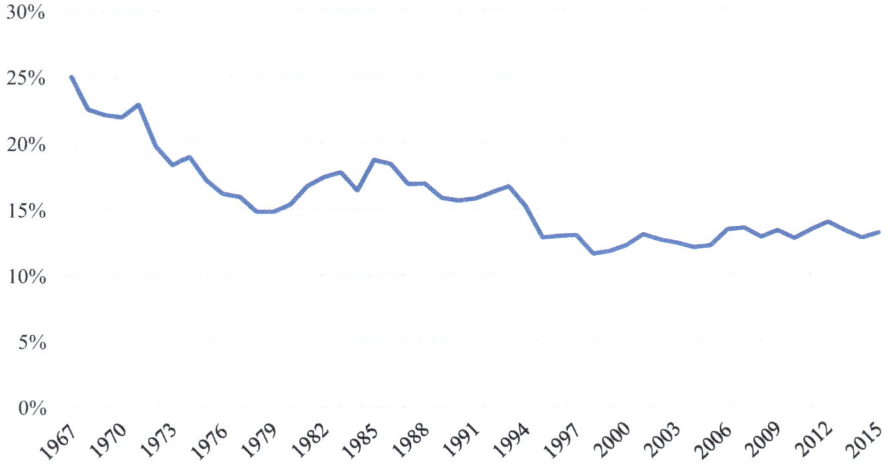

Fig. 8 Poverty across nonmetropolitan places, supplemental poverty measure 1967–2015. Source: Carsey School Analyses of Annual Social and Economic Supplement, Current Population Survey 1968 and 2016; Columbia Population Research Center, 2017

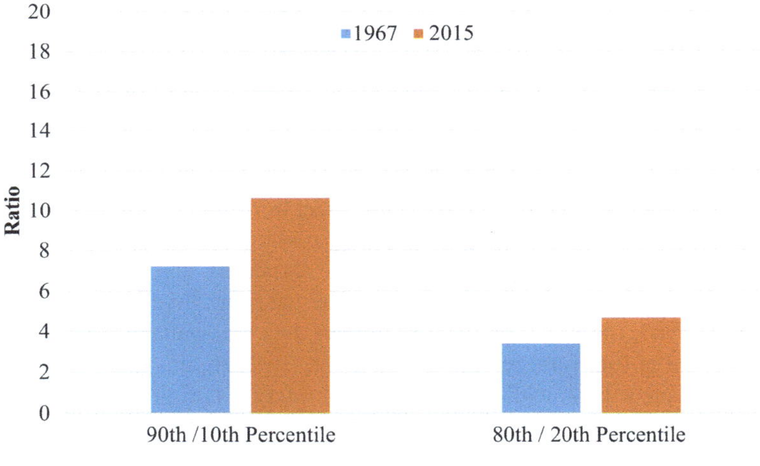

Fig. 9 Ratio of median family income at respective percentiles, 1967 and 2015. Source: Carsey School analyses of Annual Social and Economic Supplement, Current Population Survey 1968 and 2016. Note: Among families with any income

Without significant policy change and support, many families in rural areas may continue to be left behind as jobs become more urbanized.

Concurrently, and in large part resulting from many of the aforementioned changes and challenges, inequality has increased dramatically as shown in Fig. 9. Rural families with incomes at the 90th percentile now have more than ten times the income of those at the 10th percentile. The change represents an increase of nearly 50% since 1967, when they had roughly 7.2 times the income of the lowest income families. The difference is less dramatic when we compare families at the 20th percentile of family income with the 80th percentile percent. The growth is still staggering, and families at the 80th percentile now earn about 4.7 times the income of those at the 20th percentile. Note that both ratios displayed grew more dramatically in rural than in urban U.S., where inequality also rose substantially (not shown). Such dramatic inequality has broad implications for social mobility, youth opportunity, and the ability to work hard and achieve the American Dream.

As previously mentioned, there is an increase in seniors, particularly women, living alone in rural U.S. What does this mean for rural communities? There are several potential implications. First, women living alone may face challenges in meeting their expenses. This may be compounded by old housing and the desire to age in place rather than downsize or move to a communal living arrangement. Second, a growing elderly population creates demand for specialized medical care as well as lower wage caregiving. Finally, an aging population in rural U.S. areas may be very isolated, particularly if they lose the ability to drive. Loneliness and isolation may lead to or compound mental and physical health problems.

The aging of the white population coupled with growth in minority populations across rural areas has implications for the future of rural communities. Schools, service providers, and others must become culturally competent to understand diverse populations and understand their cultures, histories, and to best support their full potential. Increasingly the workforce may be comprised of younger racial-ethnic minorities reporting to older, white employers, or managers. How can communities prepare for inclusivity, and what steps can be taken to ensure that voices are heard across all levels and powerful positions are not reserved for the "old elite"?

In effect, I have answered the question of whether a true convergence with urban U.S. has occurred. Rural families are increasingly similar to urban ones, but the uniqueness of their geography may pose special challenges to finding and maintaining work and accessing critical supports.

Though this chapter has discussed broad differences between rural and urban communities in the U.S. It is critical to remember that this birds' eye view fails to consider the nuance and heterogeneity across rural areas in the U.S. We know well that there is no single *rural America* and that communities vary dramatically based on local history and culture, amenities and resources, and the people who live there. While rural places that are resource- or amenity-rich may be thriving, those plagued by decades of poverty will have a much harder time catching up and thriving in the new economy (Colocousis, Hamilton, & Hamilton, 2008; Ulrich-Schad & Duncan, 2018). By necessity, a short overview could not tackle all these distinctions, although in thinking about rural places, it is important to consider how the trends captured here on average, play out differently on the ground and what implications that has for local economies, development, growth, and future plans.

Policy Implications

Persistent differences between rural and urban areas of the U.S., in conjunction with dramatic changes in the structure of rural economies and the composition of families there, have implications for policy development. Specifically, many of the safety net policies designed closer to 1960 than 2016 no longer work as well in rural places. Deepening work requirements for social service receipts will pose unique challenges in rural places where jobs are often scarcer, work supports like transportation and child care more difficult to obtain, and wages are lower. Given these constraints, poverty alleviation strategies that address the needs of the working poor are essential. Further, the small nature of rural communities, where "everyone knows everybody" often means that the stigma associated with some safety net benefits precludes participation. This is nicely documented by Sherman (2009) who shows that in one rural community, safety net programs linked to work, such as disability and unemployment compensation, are socially acceptable. Programs that are means tested alone (e.g., Supplemental Nutrition Assistance Program or SNAP) and cash assistance (e.g., Temporary Assistance to Needy Families or TANF) are highly stigmatized, and those who participate in these programs are often viewed as lazy or inadequate. Such harsh judgments mean that participation is often much lower than eligibility allows or that people go to lengths to avoid detection of their participation, such as driving several towns away to buy groceries with SNAP (Sherman, 2009). This, of course, imposes additional costs in terms of both time and transportation expenses. In contrast, programs such as the Earned Income Tax Credit (EITC) provide a model for delivering social programs with dignity (Edin, Shaefer, & Tach, 2017). Delivered through the income tax system, recipients cannot easily be discerned. This model may prove valuable in developing or altering our existing social programs in ways that may increase uptake, particularly in rural places.

Much could be improved by considering the circumstances of rural families when developing safety net programs. By thinking through remoteness, transportation issues, and community structure, programs could be designed to allow better coordination among local providers and have flexibility in how and where programs are delivered.

Additionally, we know that much of the persistent, or generational poverty is in rural places. While 63% of U.S. counties are nonmetropolitan, they comprise 77% of the nation's counties where child poverty is persistently high (Schaefer, Mattingly, & Johnson, 2016). As such, efforts that span multiple generations may be most promising at improving the economic situation in rural places. By helping parents with job training, parenting skills, and relationship supports, children will benefit and the foundation may be laid for later life economic gains. At the same time, the children need high-quality early environments, adequate nutrition, and safe places to live. By taking a multigenerational lens, investments today can have a large return down the road. Unfortunately, the returns on such investments do not align with political timelines that often favor immediate results, rather than improvements that accumulate over the long term, and are thus not always popular. If given time, longer term investments do have the potential to dramatically improve the economic circumstances of many rural (and urban) families as well as to build communities through developing a qualified workforce and ensuring a positive future for coming generations.

Acknowledgments I gratefully acknowledge research assistance from Sarah Leonard and Anita Mathur, and analytic support from Jessica Carson and Andrew Schaefer, at the Carsey School of Public Policy. This research was supported, in part, by a grant from anonymous donors and by Grant Number 90PD0275 from the Office of Planning, Research, and Evaluation, Administration for Children and Families, U.S. Department of Health and Human Services. Its contents are solely the responsibility of the authors and do not necessarily represent the official views of the Office of Planning, Research, and Evaluation, the Administration for Children and Families, or the U.S. Department of Health and Human Services.

References

Bell, S. E., & York, R. (2010). Community economic identity: The coal industry and ideology construction in West Virginia. *Rural Sociology, 75*(1), 111–143.

Brown, J., & Dynan, K. (2017). Increasing the economic security of older women. In D. W. Schanzenbach & R. Nunn (Eds.), *The 51%: Driving economic growth through women's participation*. Washington, DC: The Hamilton Project, Brookings Institution Press. https://www.brookings.edu/research/increasing-the-economic-security-of-older-women/

Bureau of Labor Statistics, United States Department of Labor. (2017). *Percentage of employed women working full time little changed over past 5 decades*. Retrieved from https://www.bls.gov/opub/ted/2017/percentage-of-employed-women-working-full-time-little-changed-over-past-5-decades.htm?view_full

Carr, P. J., & Kefalas, M. J. (2009). *Hollowing out the middle: The rural brain drain and what it means for America*. Boston, MA: Beacon Press.

Carson, J. A., & Mattingly, M. J. (2014). Rural families and households and the decline of traditional structure. In C. Bailey, L. Jensen, & E. Ransom (Eds.), *Rural America in a globalizing world* (pp. 347–364). Morgantown, WV: West Virginia University Press.

Colocousis, C., Hamilton, L., & Hamilton, L. (2008). Place matters: Challenges and opportunities in four rural Americas. Reports on Rural America 1(4). Durham, NH: Carsey School of Public Policy.

Duncan, C. M. (2015). *Worlds apart: Poverty and politics in rural America* (2nd ed.). New Haven, CT: Yale University Press.

Edin, K., Shaefer, H. L., & Tach, L. (2017). A new anti-poverty policy litmus test. In *Pathways Magazine*. Stanford, CA: Stanford Center on Poverty & Inequality.

Glasgow, N., & Berry, H. E. (2012). Introduction to rural aging in twenty-first century America. In N. Glasgow & E. H. Berry (Eds.), *Rural aging in 21st century America* (pp. 1–13). New York: Springer.

Health Resources and Services Administration. (2018). *Defining rural population*. Washington, DC: U.S. Department of Health and Human Services. Retrieved from https://www.hrsa.gov/rural-health/about-us/definition/index.html

Johnson, K. M., & Lichter, D. T. (2008). Natural increase: A new source of population growth in emerging Hispanic destinations in the United States. *Population and Development Review, 34*(2), 327–346.

Johnson, K. M., & Lichter, D. T. (2010). Growing diversity among America's children and youth: Spatial and temporal dimensions. *Population and Development Review, 36*(1), 151–176.

Johnson, K. M., & Lichter, D. T. (2012). Rural retirement destinations: Natural decrease and the shared demographic destinies of elderly and Hispanics. In N. Glasgow & E. H. Berry (Eds.), *Rural aging in the 21st century* (pp. 275–294). New York: Springer.
Lebergott, S. (1966). Labor force and employment, 1800–1960. In D. S. Brady (Ed.), *Output, employment, and productivity in the United States after 1800* (pp. 117–204). Cambridge, MA: National Bureau of Economic Research.
Lichter, D. T. (2012). Immigration and the new racial diversity in rural America. *Rural Sociology, 77*(1), 3–35.
Lichter, D. T. (2017). *Rural population change [PowerPoint slides]*. Retrieved from http://www.populationassociation.org/wp-content/uploads/Lichter_Rural-Population-Change.pdf
Mattingly, M. J., & Smith, K. E. (2010). Changes in wives' employment when husbands stop working: A recession-prosperity comparison. *Family Relations, 59*(4), 343–357.
McCrate, E. (2011). Parents' work time in rural America: The growth of irregular schedules. In K. E. Smith & A. R. Tickamyer (Eds.), *Economic restructuring and family well-being in rural America* (pp. 177–193). University Park, PA: The Pennsylvania State University Press.
Meschede, T., Cronin, M., Sullivan, L., & Shapiro, T. (2011, October). *Rising economic insecurity among senior single women (Research and Policy Brief)*. Waltham, MA: Institute on Assets and Social Policy.
National Bureau of Economic Research (NBER). (2012). *US business cycle expansions and contraction*. Retrieved from https://www.nber.org/cycles/US_Business_Cycle_Expansions_and_Contractions_20120423.pdf
Nelson, K. M. (2011). Job characteristics and economic survival strategies: The effect of economic restructuring and marital status in a rural county. In K. E. Smith & A. R. Tickamyer (Eds.), *Economic restructuring and family well-being in rural America* (pp. 136–157). University Park, PA: The Pennsylvania State University Press.
Nelson, P. B. (2014). Concentrations of the elderly in rural America: Patterns, processes, and outcomes in a neoliberal world. In C. Bailey, L. Jensen, & E. Ransom (Eds.), *Rural America in a globalizing world* (pp. 347–364). Morgantown, WV: West Virginia University Press.
O'Hare, W. P., & Churilla, A. (2008). *Rural children now less likely to live in married-couple families* (Carsey Institute Fact Sheet 13). Durham, NH: Carsey School of Public Policy. https://scholars.unh.edu/cgi/viewcontent.cgi?referer=&httpsredir=1&article=1055&context=carsey
Ruggles, S., Flood, S., Goeken, R., Grover, J., Meyer, E., Pacas, J., & Sobek, M. (2018). *IPUMS USA (Version 8.0) [dataset]*. IPUMS: Minneapolis, MN. https://doi.org/10.18128/D010.V8.0
Schaefer, A., Mattingly, M. J., & Johnson, K. M. (2016, February). *Child poverty higher and more persistent in rural America (Brief)*. Durham, NH: Carsey School of Public Policy. Retrieved from https://carsey.unh.edu/publication/rural-child-poverty-higher
Sherman, J. (2009). *Those who work, those who don't: Poverty, morality, and family in rural America*. Minneapolis, MN: University of Minnesota Press.
Slack, T., & Jensen, L. (2002). Race, ethnicity and underemployment in nonmetropolitan America: A 30-year profile. *Rural Sociology, 67*(2), 208–233.
Smith, K. E. (2011). Changing roles: Women and work in rural America. In K. E. Smith & A. R. Tickamyer (Eds.), *Economic restructuring and family well-being in rural America* (pp. 60–81). University Park, PA: The Pennsylvania State University Press.
Smith, K. E., & Mattingly, M. J. (2012). Rural families in transition. In L. J. Kulcsar & K. J. Curtis (Eds.), *International handbooks of population: International handbook of rural demography* (Vol. 3, pp. 239–253). New York: Springer.
Smith, K. E., & Tickamyer, A. R. (2011). Introduction. In K. E. Smith & A. R. Tickamyer (Eds.), *Economic restructuring and family well-being in Rural America* (pp. 1–24). University Park, PA: The Pennsylvania State University Press.
Snyder, A. (2011). Patterns of family formation and dissolution in rural America and implications for well-being. In K. E. Smith & A. R. Tickamyer (Eds.), *Economic restructuring and family well-being in rural America* (pp. 124–135). University Park, PA: The Pennsylvania State University Press.
Toossi, M., & Morisi, T. L. (2017, July). *Women in the workforce before, during, and after the great recession* (Spotlight on Statistics). Washington, DC: Bureau of Labor

Statistics, U.S. Department of Labor. Retrieved from https://www.bls.gov/spotlight/2017/women-in-the-workforce-before-during-and-after-the-great-recession/pdf/women-in-the-workforce-before-during-and-after-the-great-recession.pdf

U.S. Census Bureau (1995). *Urban and Rural Population: 1900–1990*. Retrieved from https://www.census.gov/population/censusdata/urpop0090.txt

U.S. Census Bureau (2016). *The majority of children live with two parents, Census Bureau Reports* (Release No. CB16-192). Retrieved from https://www.census.gov/newsroom/press-releases/2016/cb16-192.html

Ulrich-Schad, J. D., & Duncan, C. M. (2018). People and places left behind: Work, culture, and politics in the rural United States. *The Journal of Peasant Studies, 45*(1), 59–79.

Wimer, C., Fox, L., Garfinkel, I., Kaushal, N., Laird, J., Nam, J., … Waldfogel, J. (2017). *Historical Supplemental Poverty Measure (SPM) data*. Center on Poverty and Social Policy at Columbia University. Retrieved from https://www.povertycenter.columbia.edu/historical-spm-data-reg

Young, J. R. (2012, Fall). *Underemployment in urban and rural America, 2005–2012*. (Issue Brief No. 55). Durham, NH: Carsey School of Public Policy. https://scholars.unh.edu/cgi/viewcontent.cgi?article=1178&context=carsey

Young, J. R., & Mattingly, M. J. (2016, December). *Underemployment among Hispanics: The case of involuntary part-time work* (Monthly Labor Review). Washington, DC: Bureau of Labor Statistics, U.S. Department of Labor. Retrieved from https://www.bls.gov/opub/mlr/2016/article/underemployment-among-hispanics.htm

Employment and Wages in the Places Left Behind

Mark D. Partridge, Rodrigo Pérez-Silva, and Sydney Schreiner

Declining U.S. labor force participation and a corresponding decrease in the employment-to-population ratio in recent decades have been trends widely debated in policy circles. While some of the existing literature points to structural changes in the labor market composition, such as an aging population as a primary driver (Aaronson et al., 2014), others argue that increasing take-ups of disability payments (and other welfare assistance) could explain a nontrivial part of reduced labor force participation (Blau & Goodstein, 2010). Notably, most existing studies document trends in labor market indicators at the national level, which are largely driven by changes in metropolitan areas where close to 86% of the U.S. population resides.[1]

In this chapter, we analyze recent trends in the U.S. employment-to-population ratio and real wages. However, unlike the past literature, we focus our discussion on nonmetropolitan areas and other places left behind (see Goetz, Partridge, & Stephens, 2018; Partridge & Olfert, 2011). We explore heterogeneity across places and among workers by documenting differences across education groups, gender, and industries. While national-level insights are important for understanding how the broader economy functioned in the wake of the Great Recession, there is significant variation in economic growth across space (Carlino & Mills, 1996; Rey & Montouri, 1999) and as a result, in how regions recover from economic downturns (Partridge & Tsvetkova, 2018). Understanding these differences is essential for crafting policy solutions to aid struggling residents in places left behind.

[1]According to U.S. Census 2017 population estimates. Using older metropolitan definitions would produce a higher rural/nonmetropolitan share.

M. D. Partridge · S. Schreiner (✉)
The Ohio State University, Columbus, OH, USA
e-mail: schreiner.77@osu.edu

R. Pérez-Silva
Centre for Economics and Social Policy, Universidad Mayor, Santiago, Chile

J. E. Glick et al. (eds.), *Rural Families and Communities in the United States*,
National Symposium on Family Issues 10, https://doi.org/10.1007/978-3-030-37689-5_3

Recent National Trends in Urban and Rural America

Nonmetro areas in particular, have been slow to recover due to their industrial composition and related technological changes. Historically, nonmetro regions are more likely to be dominated by agriculture or other resource-based industries, and labor-saving technological change has long led to fewer people being employed (Goetz et al., 2018; Partridge & Olfert, 2011). Similarly, employment in manufacturing, a relative rural economic success dating back at least 50 years, declined 32.5% since nonmetro manufacturing employment levels peaked in 1995, falling primarily due to productivity growth as well as global competition (Goetz et al., 2018).[2] In contrast, metropolitan manufacturing employment peaked in 1979 and has fallen by 41.1%. Of course, in both the metropolitan and the nonmetropolitan U.S., their respective manufacturing employment shares have steadily declined over most of this period. Using Federal Reserve Bank of St. Louis data (FRED), U.S. national *nonfarm wage & salary* manufacturing employment was at a cyclical high of 32.4% in July 1953 (just below the immediate World War II all-time high), and has been falling ever since. It seems likely the metropolitan manufacturing share has been steadily falling ever since 1953 as well, though there has been a slight rebound in nonmetro manufacturing share over the 2010–2016 period. As a result, technological change has disproportionately affected the mainstay industries in nonmetro economies.

The employment share of farming, the historic engine of rural American economies, in nonmetro areas declined from 15% in 1969 to just 5.7% in 2016 according to BEA data. Indeed, in terms of other extractive industries, forestry accounted only for about 1.4% and mining accounted for about 2% of nonmetro total employment. Similarly, 2016 nonmetro employment in manufacturing was nearly double nonmetro total farm employment. Even in 1969, total employment in manufacturing in rural areas was 38% higher than total farm employment. This trend illustrates that while farming was once the engine of a typical rural community's economy, that has long not been the case in the rural U.S.

Because nonmetro economies rely heavily on export-based industries like mining, manufacturing, and large-scale agriculture, the resulting labor market segmentation, enduring unemployment in nonmetro regions (Weiler, 2001), slower job growth due to technological change, and the positive rural trade surplus by definition mean that capital has been flowing out of the areas. In fact, by definition from national income accounting, the net goods and service balance equals the negative of the capital account balance. Metro areas with negative trade balances (or positive capital inflows) are the fastest growing and most dynamic economic growth areas (Kilkenny & Partridge, 2009; Krugman, 2018). Net capital flowing out of rural America suggests that new investments in their growth industries will lag. Finally, increasing global trade with low-wage countries has eliminated the wage and land cost advantages that manufacturers in nonmetro economies have historically enjoyed (Goetz et al., 2018).

---

[2] Source is U.S. Bureau of Economic Analysis (BEA) data.

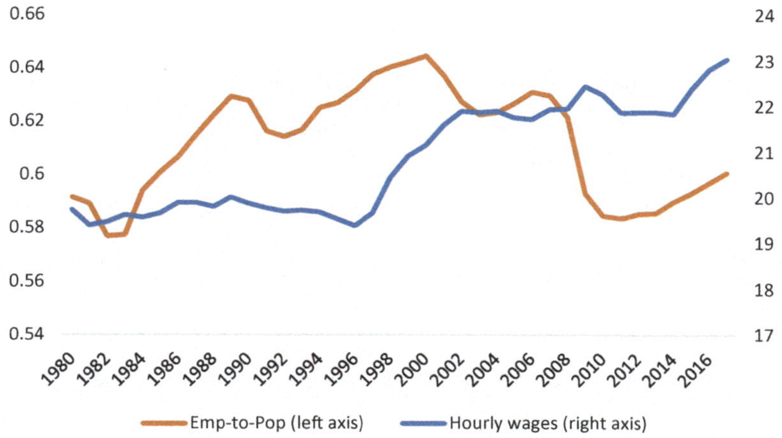

Fig. 1 U.S. employment-to-population ratio and real hourly wages, 1980–2017. Source: Authors' calculations based on Current Population Survey (CPS) data

As shown in Fig. 1, the U.S. employment-to-population ratio has been decreasing rapidly since the beginning of the recession in 2007, falling from 63% in 2005–2007 to a low of 58.4% in 2010–2011. It has not yet fully recovered with just 60% of the population being employed in 2017. Moreover, the employment-to-population ratio of 2017 is around 5 percentage points below the levels of 1999–2000. Real wages, on the other hand, remained mostly constant between 2008 and 2014 at around $22 per hour[3] and began to grow again in 2015, reaching a maximum of $23.05 in 2017. It is important to recognize that these national averages predominately reflect reality in metro areas. While many trends are similar for nonmetro areas, there is meaningful heterogeneity that must be explored in order to fully understand the extent to which the U.S. economy, and especially rural U.S., has recovered from the economic downturn beginning in 2008.

As an example, Fig. 2 shows the trends in the employment-to-population ratios and real wages for metro (solid lines) and nonmetro areas (dashed lines). First, note the differences in levels in terms of both ratios and wages between metro areas and nonmetro areas. Employment-to-population ratios and wages are on average 2% and 20% lower, respectively, in nonmetro areas than in metro areas over the 27-year period analyzed. Second, while the difference in wages between metro and nonmetro areas appears constant over time, there is a clear change in the trend in the employment-to-population ratio in nonmetro areas after the Great Recession. The employment-to-population ratio fell more in nonmetro areas during the Great Recession, and in contrast with the national average, has recovered significantly slower.

[3] In 2017 dollars.

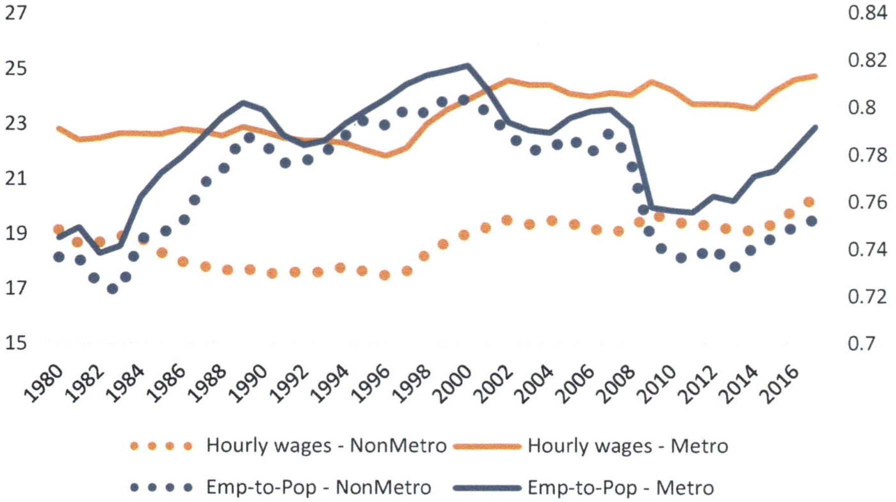

Fig. 2 Employment-to-population ratio and real hourly wages ($ of 2017). Metro versus non-metro, 1980–2017. Source: Authors' calculations based on Current Population Survey (CPS) data

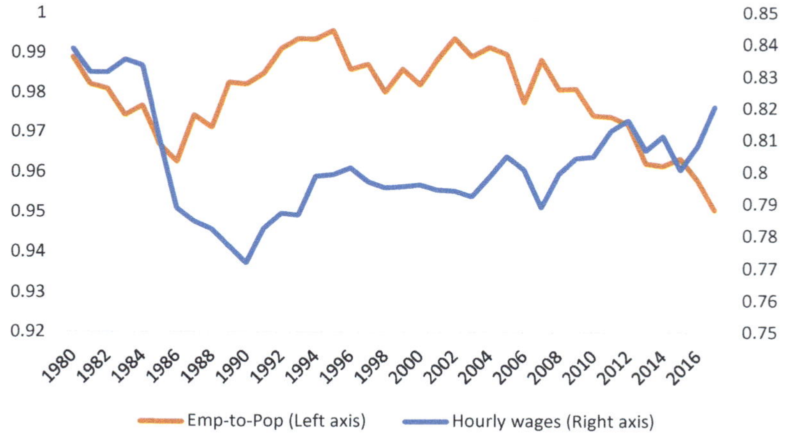

Fig. 3 Differences in the employment-to-population ratio and wages between nonmetro and metro areas, 1980–2017. Source: Authors' calculations based on Current Population Survey (CPS) data

Figure 2 shows how these metro/nonmetro wages and employment/population ratios evolve over time. The evolution of these changes can be easily observed in Fig. 3, which shows, for both variables of interest, the ratio between nonmetro and metro areas.[4] Over the period of study, both ratios are less than one (with both

[4]This is $Wages_{\text{NonM}}/Wages_{\text{Metro}}$ and $\left(\frac{Emp}{Pop}\right)_{NonM} / \left(\frac{Emp}{Pop}\right)_{Metro}$.

employment-to-population ratios and wages being higher in metro areas on average), though there are notable changes over time.

While the ratios of the nonmetro/metro employment-to-population rates fluctuated between 0.98 and 1 until the end of the Great Recession, it declined sharply after 2010, breaking the historical trend. This change indicates that the relative nonmetro employment-to-population ratio declined sharply compared to metro areas. In contrast, hourly wages in nonmetro areas appear to be slowly converging to those in metro areas, following a trend that has been mostly constant since 1990, probably reflecting a decline in relative rural labor supply due to out-migration. Overall, the difference in wages and employment-to-population ratios between metro and nonmetro areas have increased more than 2% and 4%, respectively, over the study period. To put these differences in perspective, if the employment-to-population ratio in metro and nonmetro areas were equal, there would be about 770,000 more jobs in nonmetro areas or 3.9% more rural jobs.

The economics literature points to several phenomena as possibly driving changes in nonmetro labor markets. The first is a reduction in labor supply driven by decreased willingness of people to work as a result of expanded unemployment insurance benefits implemented in the immediate wake of the Great Recession (Elsby, Hobijn, & Sahin, 2010; Rothstein, 2011). Second, increases in immigrant flows to lagging areas which, in the absence of an increase in productivity and of an equivalent out-migration of natives, increases labor supply, reducing the participation of natives and their employment-to-population ratio, and reduces wages (Ali, Partridge, & Rickman, 2011; Borjas, 2003, 2007; Orrenius & Zavodny, 2007). An opposing argument though, is that immigrants increase productivity in the areas in which they settle by increasing the demand for native workers due to the complementary nature of immigrant labor and native labor (Ottaviano & Peri, 2012).

Lower demand for labor among nonmetro employers, due to technological change, could also explain recent changes in nonmetro economies. Technological change has led to increased mechanization, which has the potential to displace low- and medium-skilled workers in routine-task jobs. In certain industries, such as health care and retail, mechanization will lead to larger operations. The result is that *mom-and-pop* shops that employ local workers are being replaced by big-box stores, which employ fewer workers on average (per unit of sales). As a result of these changes, employers on balance reduce employment and the wages of workers who remain employed decreases.

Skill-based technological change (Autor, Katz, & Kearney, 2008), outsourcing to foreign markets (Dube & Kaplan, 2010), and greater female labor force participation (Katz & Murphy, 1992) could all potentially contribute to an uneven recovery in nonmetro regions. Consequently, demand for local labor in lagging regions will be lower due to employers using more mechanized technologies and offshoring activities using more workers in foreign markets. At the same time, the supply of labor could rise as a result of increased labor force participation by women who were not previously participants.

Rural and Urban America's Economy

Before delving into relative economic conditions, we first have to define rural and urban for our purposes. Note that we will use the terms *rural* and *nonmetropolitan* interchangeably, as well as *urban* and *metropolitan*. The definition of metropolitan areas captures the notion of functional urban areas or labor markets. U.S. metropolitan areas are defined as counties that include a city of at least 50,000 and any other county with at least 25% commuting linkages with the metropolitan core. Thus, metro areas are defined as labor markets and even low-density outer areas/counties of a metropolitan area have urban labor market linkages. The landscape may look agricultural but the people are economically integrated with the urban area. Culturally though, they may remain quite rural. Of course, one could quibble, as we do, with the exact thresholds. For example, Canada uses a minimum principle-city threshold of 100,000 and commuting thresholds of 50% in determining their metro areas. We agree that a 100,000 threshold makes more sense to reflect contemporaneous agglomeration patterns and the U.S. 25% commuting thresholds should be increased say 30% to 35%.

Recent Rural/Urban Conditions

Rural America is stereotypically described as uniformly economically stagnate. It is also generally described as primarily agricultural and dominated by industries focused on resource extraction. However, the notion that rural areas are in perpetual decline is misleading because it depends on when you define rural for your assessment. Using 1950 metropolitan definitions, rural areas have grown significantly faster than urban—suggesting that nonmetro development is a success if one looks back 70 years (Goetz et al., 2018). However, over time most of the fastest-growing rural counties have either crossed the threshold to become their own metro area or were added to existing metro areas (Goetz et al., 2018). Thus, nonmetro performance declined over time as the fastest-growing rural counties were reclassified as metropolitan. What's left are the slower growing counties that are typically more remote from urban centers, making economic development even more challenging.

Access to urban labor markets is a critical component of rural economic development. Access to larger urban areas is just as important in describing rural growth as natural amenities are in describing population dynamics in the post 1950 period (Partridge, Rickman, Ali, & Olfert, 2008, 2010) Indeed, the advantage of urban access is primarily on the firm productivity side, and it is growing over time, with household changes being more neutral in their location preferences (Partridge, Rickman, et al., 2010). The growing importance of urban areas to rural areas is seen using Bureau of Economic Analysis (BEA) data examining the commuting income adjustment with metropolitan areas (i.e., how much income rural Americans earned by commuting to urban areas minus how much income urban Americans earned by commuting to rural areas). In 1969, rural America (using 2017 metropolitan area definitions) had a net commuting balance that equaled 4.3% of wage and salary earnings, but by 2016, this figured had doubled to 8.1%. Remember, this is **net**-commuting income, illustrating that commuting is an important source of rural income. Commuting to urban-led growth is an important component of rural economic development toolkits.

To give a feel for the potential importance of nonmetro commuting, in 2016, 73% of San Jacinto County, TX's (near Houston) wage and salary earnings came from net-commuting with metro areas. Corresponding totals for Camden County, NC (on the Atlantic coast) and Issaquena County, MS (in the Mississippi valley near Vicksburg) were respectively 72% and 69%. Illustrating the potential of this growth, Issaquena County's share of wage and salary earnings accounted for by net-commuting with metropolitan areas totaled only 10% in 1969.

More generally, at the 90th percentile, fully 36% of rural county wage and salary income is from net-metropolitan commuting income, while the corresponding shares at the 75th and 50th percentiles respectively equal 22.7% and 8.8%. However, over 28% of nonmetro counties had a *negative* net-commuting balance with metro areas, suggesting that while rural areas are usually on balance a source of labor for urban areas, the reverse can also be true. On the whole, interlinking with urban economies is a key part of rural economies, and for many, their survival.

The analysis of commuting income vastly understates the importance of rural commuting. Between 1973 and 2013, 520 counties were reclassified to metropolitan, many of which had very high shares of net-commuting income before being reclassified. For example, decennial census data shows that in 1970 (using 1970 metro definitions) approximately 21.2% of nonmetropolitan workers commuted outside their county of residence, while in 2016, approximately 23.9% of employed workers commuted outside their county (using American Community Survey, with 2016 definitions). Such high commuting rates illustrate that successful rural development for a county is about successful *regional* development with neighboring communities.

Figure 4, panels a and b respectively show post Great Recession 2010–2016 job growth for urban and rural areas. The classification splits urban into five equal-sized job growth categories for metropolitan areas. It uses the same numerical categories for rural areas so that the maps can be directly compared in terms of how rural areas are faring relative to urban areas. Metro areas have fared better with average job growth of 13.1%, while job growth is only 4.2% in nonmetro areas. Figure 4 shows that metro job growth is more widespread than rural job growth, with nonmetro job growth in the eastern U.S. particularly lagging. There are several other clusters of weak rural job performance in Texas, Kansas, and the Dakotas, for example.

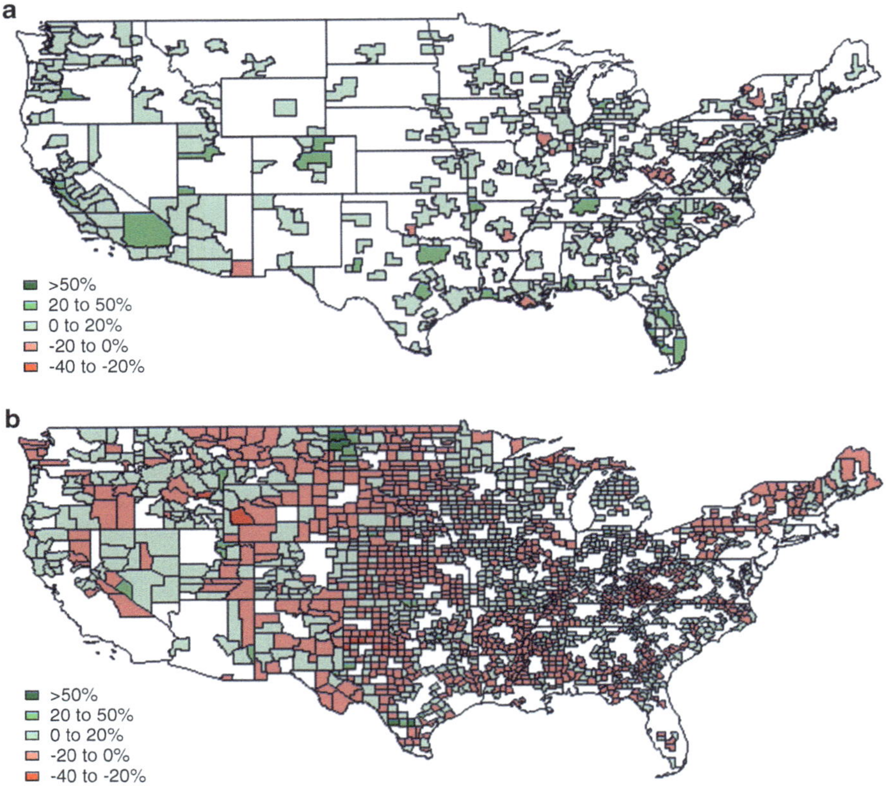

Fig. 4 (**a**) Job growth in U.S. counties, 2010–2016: Metro areas. (**b**) Job growth in U.S. counties, 2010–2016: Nonmetro areas

It is also clear that not all of rural America is an economic basket case. First, oil and gas drilling regions such as the Bakken in northwestern North Dakota and traditional oil patches in Texas, Oklahoma, and New Mexico have grown rapidly. It is also clear, though, that not all rural drilling regions have fared well as shown by the Marcellus in Pennsylvania. Generally, the most widespread rural prosperity is in high-amenity Rocky Mountain areas that have been faring well for decades. Yet, there can be surprises such as rural Ohio outperforming metropolitan Ohio in terms of job growth in 2010–2018 (using Bureau of Labor Statistics Current Employment Statistics data) and continued growth in rural areas in other Midwestern states like Michigan, Wisconsin, and Minnesota.

One change, discussed further below, is that counties adjacent to metro areas are not necessarily faring well even though they had strong growth in the past. One reason is that as metropolitan areas expanded, previously nonmetro adjacent counties were reclassified as metro. Thus, many of the prosperous metro-adjacent rural counties are *now* known as metropolitan.

Is It True that Places Are Being Left Behind?

The general U.S. story has been one of economic convergence in which the gap between the lowest income places and the highest income places declined. Economists argued this was the natural movement of capital to the capital-poor locations. Take the cases of Mississippi versus New York and Tennessee versus Massachusetts. In 1929 (using BEA data), the poorest state, Mississippi, had per-capita personal income equaling 24% of the richest state, New York, and 40% of the national average. Tennessee, one of the poorest states, had per capita income that totaled 41% of Massachusetts, one of the richest states, and 54% of the national average.

By 1979, Mississippi's per capita personal income was 66% of New York and 71% of the national average. The respective figures for Tennessee were 80% of Massachusetts and 83% of the national average. However, since about 1979, convergence has slowed. By 2017, Mississippi's per capita income retreated to 57% of New York's and 71% of the national average. Tennessee's per capita income decreased to 67% of Massachusetts's, though its per capita income had modestly risen to 88% of the national average. The general point is that lagging regions are not catching up nearly to the extent as in the past, further supporting the argument that many places are increasingly being left behind.

Furthermore, population-weighted standard deviation of county per capita income has increased by about 60% since the mid-1970s, with even more stark increases when removing government transfer payments, leaving market income (Partridge & Tsvetkova, 2018). Similarly, while the standard deviation of county employment growth decreased over the 1969–2010 period, since the Great Recession the standard deviation of job growth has also increased, with the gap between economic winners and losers growing wider.

This divergence pattern is quite apparent when examining Fig. 5a, b. Figure 5a shows 1990–2017 population growth and Fig. 5b shows population growth over the postrecession 2010–2017 period. When considering the longer period, population growth was negative only in the low-density Great Plains, Mississippi Valley, parts of the Black Belt, Central Appalachian, and Western New York. The vast majority of the country experienced population growth with much of the Sun Belt and Western U.S. being leaders. Yet, since the Great Recession, the portion of the nation that lost population has expanded—especially in the eastern 60% of the country (despite a commodity boom in agriculture and mining/oil/gas). For example, between 1990 and 2017, the percentage of metropolitan and nonmetropolitan counties that experienced positive growth was 87.8% and 58.4%, respectively, while the number that experienced more than twice the national growth rate was respectively, 22.9% and 3.8% (Table 1).

Overall, the metro and nonmetro population growth was 34.3% and 11.2%, respectively, for the 1990–2017 period. Yet, in the postrecession period 2010–2017, the urban advantage grew even larger. Specifically, the number of metropolitan counties that experienced positive growth was 69.8% versus just 32.6% for

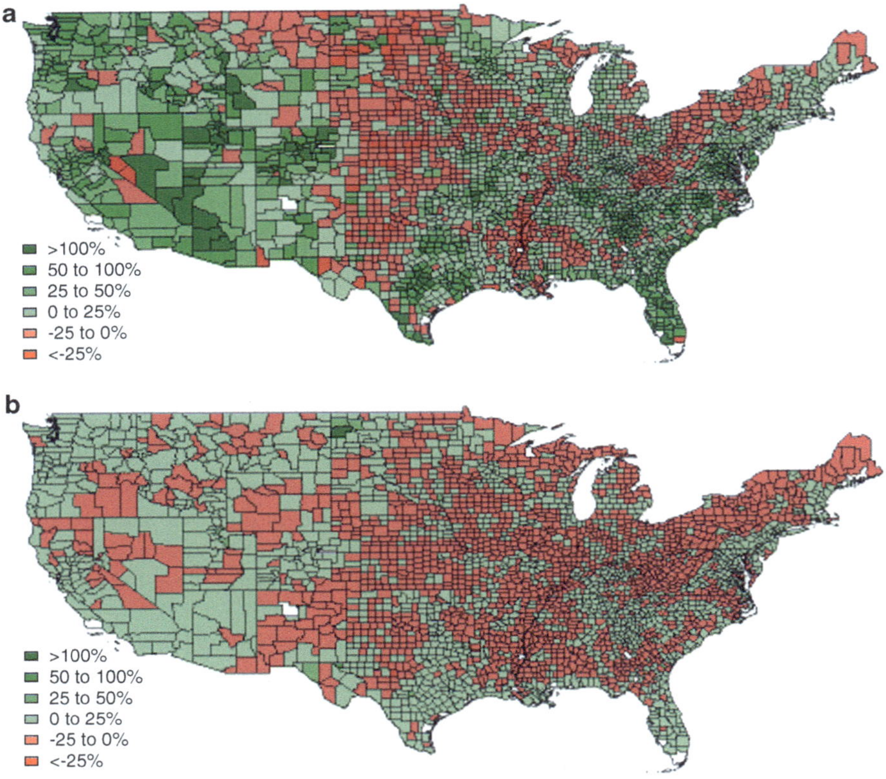

Fig. 5 (**a**) Population growth in U.S. counties: 1990–2017. (**b**) Population growth in U.S. counties: 2010–2017

nonmetropolitan counties. Whereas 15.7% of urban counties experienced more than twice the national growth rate, only 1.5% of rural counties did so. That is, there has been an increasing concentration of places being left behind, with fewer places prospering. These changes can be seen in Table 1.

What Types of Places Are Left Behind?

A stereotype is that the largest coastal cities are faring well while smaller cities and rural areas are faring poorly. To assess the recent past, we must again consider that the fastest-growing places are typically reclassified to metropolitan status. That is, if we use the recent contemporaneous categories for analysis, we will miss that many of the fastest-growing places were recategorized, producing a misleading assessment that favors the larger category groupings.

Table 1 Population and population growth 1990–2017, 2010–2017

	Nonmetro				
Population level year	Nonadjacent	Adjacent	Total	Metro	U.S. Total
1990	18,563,548	22,820,635	41,384,183	208,238,817	249,623,000
2010	20,071,333	26,173,406	46,244,739	263,093,682	309,338,421
2017	19,909,962	26,111,196	46,021,158	279,698,020	325,719,178
National growth					
1990–2017	7.25%	14.42%	11.20%	34.32%	30.48%
2010–2017	−0.80%	−0.24%	−0.48%	6.31%	5.30%
Percentage (%)					
Counties that gained population 1990–2017	53.6%	74.2%	62.6%	88.0%	69.3%
Counties that gained population 2X national average 1990–2017	4.2%	7.5%	5.7%	25.2%	10.9%
Counties that gained population 2010–2017	34.4%	38.5%	36.2%	74.8%	46.5%
Counties that gained population 2X national average 2010–2017	1.8%	3.6%	2.6%	18.5%	6.8%

Figure 6 shows how metropolitan areas fared based on population size for 1990–2017. For rural areas, the division is based on adjacency/nonadjacent to metropolitan areas. As noted above, being closer to urban areas gives rural areas access to markets and jobs. We use one million as the dividing line for adjacent for "small" and "large." Larger cities have agglomeration economy advantages that lead to higher productivity, but this is eventually offset by congestion effects, such as rising transportation costs in crowded cities.

The difference between panels a and b of Fig. 6 is that Panel a uses 1990 population sizes for total metropolitan population and for rural counties, while using 1993 metro definitions to define the metro areas and determine whether rural counties are adjacent to metro areas. Panel b uses 2017 population categories and 2013 metro area definitions to provide a backward look at recent patterns. In other words, it is the typical rearview mirror approach that the media uses to make sweeping claims that larger coastal cities are doing well and most rural areas are dying.

Figure 6a shows that the fastest-growing category is larger-medium-sized metro areas of one to three million in the 1990 population. However, the second-fastest-growing category is rural counties adjacent to metro areas larger than one million people. The largest urban areas over three million population (in 1990) did not grow faster than smaller-medium-sized cities of 250,000 to one-million. The largest urban areas only grew faster than metro areas of 50,000–100,000 (1990 population), areas of 100,000–250,000 (1990 population), nonadjacent rural areas, and rural areas adjacent to metro areas with a 1990 population of less than one million.

The weakest performers in order of fastest- to-slowest growing are the smallest metro class of 50,000–100,000, nonmetro adjacent to smaller metropolitan areas, and rural areas that are not adjacent to metropolitan areas. However, even nonmetro counties adjacent to smaller metro areas grew an average of 17% over the 27-year period.

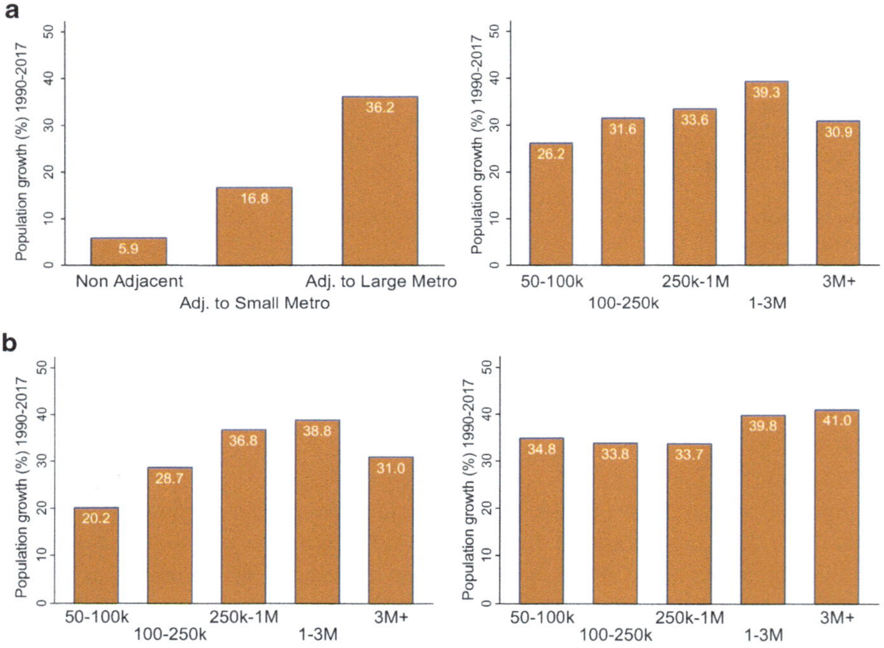

Fig. 6 (**a**) Population growth (%) 1990–2017 by city size. Nonmetro counties (left) and metro counties (right) classified using 1990 population, 1993 USDA RUCC and UIC codes, and 1993 U.S. Census Bureau MSA definitions. Notes: RUCC stands for Rural Urban Continuum Codes for USDA Economic Research Service. UIC stands for Urban Influence Codes. For 1993, "Non-Adjacent" are counties defined as RUCC = 5, 7, or 9 in 1993 regardless of population. Counties classified as UIC = 8 are also included in this category, regardless of population if they did not belong to an MSA. "Adjacent to Small Metro" are counties classified as UIC = 5 in 1993. Counties classified as UIC = 6 are also in this category, regardless of population if they are not in an MSA. "Adj. to Large Metro" are counties defined as UIC = 3, or 4 in 1993. For 2013, "Non-Adjacent" are counties defined as RUCC = 5, 7, or 9 regardless of population. "Adjacent to Small Metro" are counties classified as RUCC = 4, 6, or 8 in 2013. Counties classified as UIC = 2 but with population less than 50,000 are also included in this category. "Adj. to Large Metro" are counties defined as UIC = 3, or 4 in 2013. Other counties classified as UIC = 1 but with population less than 50,000 are included here as well. (**b**) Population growth by area size. Metro counties classified according to 1990 population (left), and to 2017 population (right). Notes: Metro counties are classified according to their 1990/2017 population if they were previously classified as nonmetro

Figure 6b shows what happens if we choose the rearview mirror approach of using contemporaneous definitions and population categories after counties are reclassified and population growth pushed groupings above the various thresholds over time. Now after reclassification, the fastest-growing urban areas are the largest two and smallest categories, with those in the middle now growing slower. All rural areas now significantly lag behind their urban counterparts, with each nonmetropolitan category having lower growth than in Fig. 6a. Thus, looking backward, one might draw the mistaken conclusion that growth has significantly favored urban areas, especially the largest, with all rural areas lagging considerably behind.

Industry Mix in Urban and Rural America

Figure 7 shows the relative one-digit industry employment shares in urban and rural places—while the top of each bar shows the relative different shares for nonmetropolitan versus metropolitan for each industry.[5] It is not surprising that rural America has much higher shares of farming, forestry, and mining, while it may be surprising that rural manufacturing is 71% more intensive than in urban areas. Thus, rural America is much more dependent on export industries, which presents a host of problems that were described before (i.e., capital outflows, labor-saving productivity growth). That is, modern-day mercantilist approaches are problematic whether conducted at the local or national levels. If not, the rural farm-based economies in the Great Plains would be exceptionally prosperous given their massive shares of value added they export.

Figures 8, 9, and 10 show nonmetropolitan and metropolitan total employment shares for farming (including forestry), mining, and manufacturing between 1969 and 2016. In both rural and urban areas, farming has become much less important with a sharp decline in rural areas. Mining employment shares are more variable depending on the state of the worldwide commodity cycle—though the total employment share is quite modest over the entire period.

Rural manufacturing is a success story in that manufacturing was primarily an urban phenomenon at the beginning of the period with the 1969 manufacturing total employment share being 23.0% in the metro U.S. and just 20.3% in nonmetro areas. Rural areas surpassed urban ones in terms of relative manufacturing intensity in 1976. The relative manufacturing intensity gap in rural America continued to grow before stabilizing after 1989 at 4–5 percentage points higher share even as manufacturing shares generally declined. The 2016 manufacturing total employment shares were 10.7% in nonmetro areas and 6.2% in metro areas. Indeed, Fig. 11 shows the relative share of manufacturing employment in rural areas over the period. It is clear that the trend is positive with 17.3% of manufacturing being in rural America in 1969 and steadily increasing to 24% in 2016. In fact, since 2010, rural manufacturing growth exceeded

[5] For example, if the rural manufacturing employment share is 10.7% and the metropolitan manufacturing share is 6.2%, then 100∗10.7/6.2 equals a 171.3% higher nonmetro farm share.

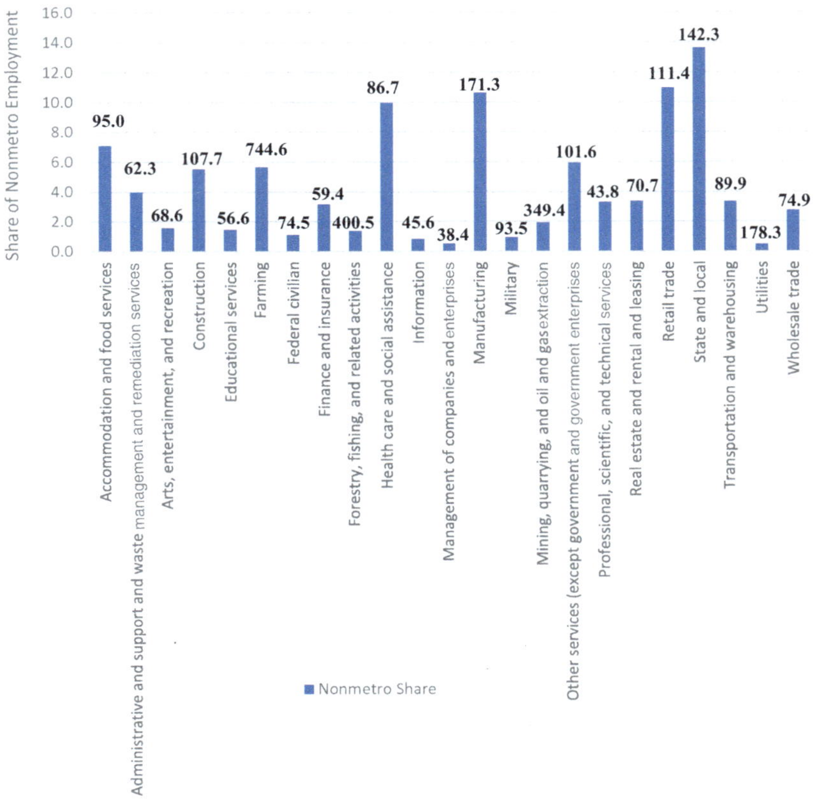

Fig. 7 Relative employment by industry, 2016. Source: BEA. The relative shares are the nonmetropolitan employment share divided by the metropolitan share

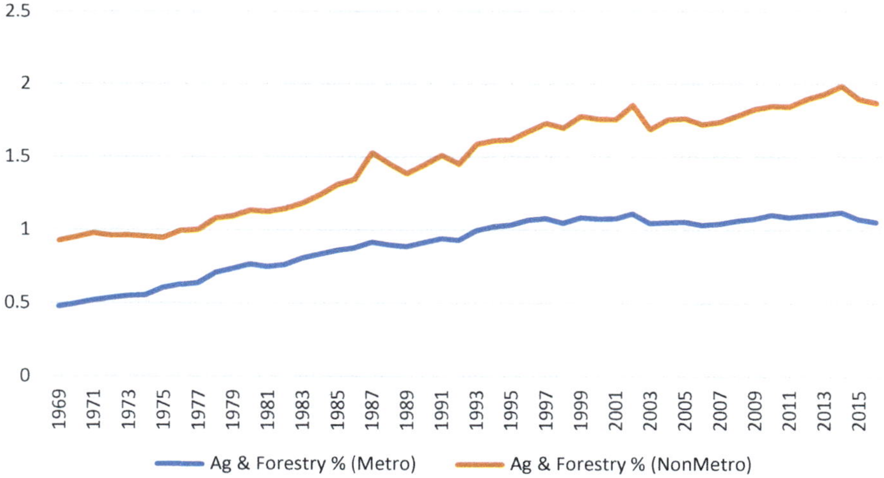

Fig. 8 Share of employment in agriculture and forestry, 1969–2016. Source: BEA

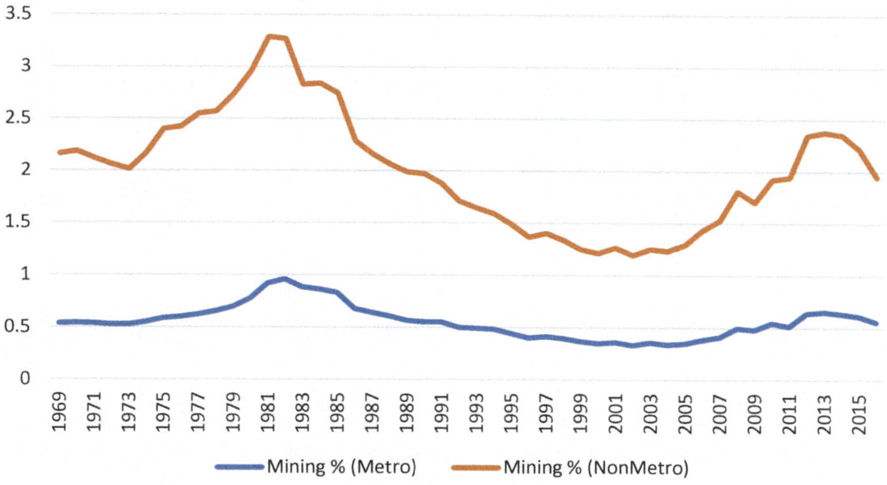

Fig. 9 Share of employment in mining, 1969–2016. Source: BEA

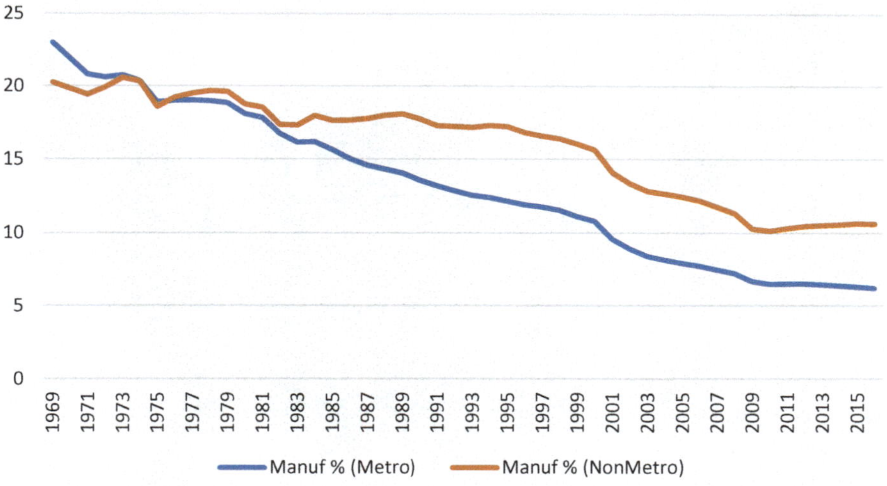

Fig. 10 Share of employment in manufacturing, 1969–2016. Source: BEA

total rural job growth as a whole, which is rather remarkable given the decline of manufacturing's relative national importance since the 1950s.

Figure 12 shows the 2016 manufacturing employment shares by county. Basically, rural manufacturing is a mainstay of local economies in the upper Midwest, middle-south, and in the southeast centered in the Carolinas. However, a weakness is that any rural U.S. manufacturing edge is primarily based on cost advantages from lower wages, lower land costs, and in the past, less unionization. Yet, that makes rural U.S. manufacturing vulnerable to exchange rate fluctuations as well as to competition from low-wage countries with far lower labor costs.

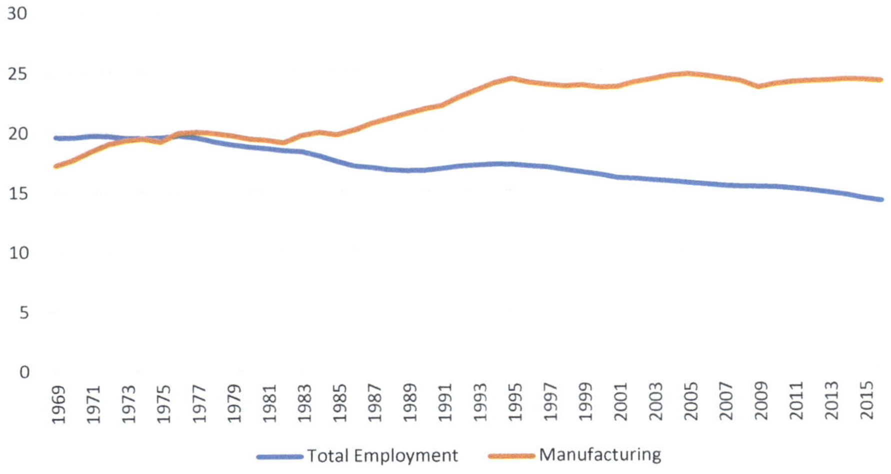

Fig. 11 Nonmetro share of total and manufacturing employment. Source: BEA

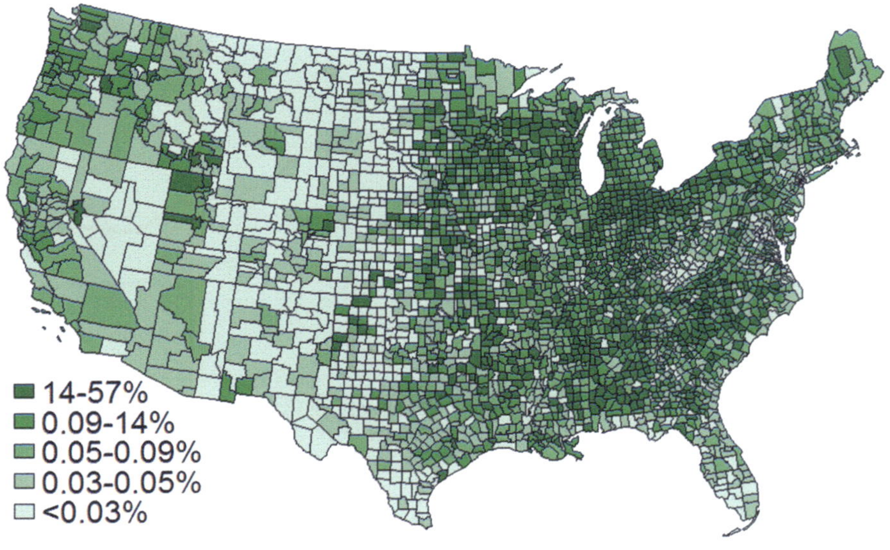

Fig. 12 Share of employment in manufacturing by county, 2016. Source: BEA. Note: Share in counties with no data was imputed using the average difference between the share of manufacturing in the county and the national level in the period 2013–2015. If no information was available during that period, shares were imputed using county data from 1980 to 2015

While rural America depends on export-oriented industries, it is considerably less dependent on key knowledge-intensive industries that benefit urban areas. For example, finance; real estate; information; professional, scientific and technical services; management; administrative and support services; waste management and remediation services; and educational services are considerably more intensive in urban areas and these sectors tend to have above-average job growth. By contrast, the nonmetro U.S. is about 30% more intensive in government employment—especially state and local government. Also showing rural dependence on government, transfer payments as a share of personal income rose from 10.5% in 1969 to fully 25.9% in 2016 versus a corresponding rise of just 7.5% to only 16.3% in urban areas.

Another source of concern is rural America's lack of dynamism as reflected by slow self-employment growth. This is problematic because small business development is linked to faster growth for a host of reasons such as the propensity to buy more inputs locally and for profits to remain local. Also, local employment multipliers are higher for small business development than equal-sized increases in wage and salary employment growth (Bartik, 1993; Goetz, Partridge, Rickman, & Majumdar, 2011; Stephens & Partridge, 2011; Tsvetkova & Partridge, 2018). In general, rural economies have higher shares of *nonfarm* self-employment due to technological reasons. As an example, a plumbing service may have two employees in a small village but hundreds in a large city; one is a pass-through self-employment partnership versus a corporation in urban settings.

The lack of relative growth of *nonfarm* self-employment is problematic for rural America. For example, in 1969, the self-employment share of rural nonfarm employment totaled 24.3%, but it rose only to 26.4% by 2016. By contrast, corresponding urban self-employment shares rose from 11.3% to 22.0%, suggesting a much stronger degree of dynamism in urban areas.

How Much Does Rural America's Industry Composition Explain Lower Growth?

Rural U.S. areas have lagged urban areas in job growth for decades, since at least before the Civil War. Between 2010 and 2016, nonmetro job growth equaled 4.2%, while metropolitan job growth totaled 13.1%. There are two ways that rural areas lag urban ones in terms of industrial performance. One is that rural industry composition is slow growing, which can be shown by the industry mix term from shift-share analysis (or sometimes called the Bartik instrument):

$$\mathrm{SSIM}_{\mathrm{it}} = \sum_{j=1}^{n} \left[\mathrm{Sh}_{ijt-1} \cdot \frac{E_{jt} - E_{jt-1}}{E_{jt-1}} \right] \quad (1)$$

where $\mathrm{SSIM}_{\mathrm{it}}$ is the shift-share industry mix term in time t in area i. Sh_{ijt-1} is the share of employment in industry j at time $t - 1$ in area i, and E_{jt} is the national employment in industry j at time t. In our analysis, $t = 2016$, $t - 1 =$ is 2010, and $i =$ rural, urban. The outcome indicates how fast rural (urban) employment would have grown if all of its industries had grown at the national average. (i.e., Does the rural [urban] U.S. have a fast or slow-growing industry mix?)

The results suggest that over 2010–2016, urban areas had an average 6.8% advantage over rural due to having a faster growing industry composition (note this advantage was 15% between 2001–2016). In terms of policy, this does not mean that rural areas should entice fast-growing industries with tax breaks and subsidies. Picking winners is notoriously difficult. Rather, it would be better to create an environment to attract the next generation of winners with a high-skilled workforce and an entrepreneurial climate—that is, let the future winners choose you rather than the reverse.

The second way rural areas lag urban areas in terms of industrial performance is that rural growth in each industry generally lags the corresponding growth in urban areas. To assess how important this factor is, we use the following:

$$\mathrm{MSSIM}_{\mathrm{it}} = \sum_{j=1}^{n} \mathrm{Sh}_{ijt-1} \cdot \left[\frac{\mathrm{EM}_{jt} - \mathrm{EM}_{jt-1}}{\mathrm{EM}_{jt-1}} - \frac{\mathrm{ENM}_{jt} - \mathrm{ENM}_{jt-1}}{\mathrm{ENM}_{jt-1}} \right] \quad (2)$$

In Eq. (2), $\mathrm{MSSIM}_{\mathrm{it}}$ stands for the modified version of SSIM presented in Eq. (1). Different from the previous specification, here EM_{jt} is the national employment in metro areas in industry j at time t, and ENM_{jt} is the national employment in nonmetro areas in industry j at time t. The formula derives how much faster rural total employment growth would be if each rural industry grew at their urban growth rate—or how much rural areas potentially lag because their industries are growing slower than in urban areas. The results show that rural areas lag urban ones by 6.2%. Overall, of the 8.9% metropolitan/nonmetropolitan job–growth gap between 2010 and 2016, approximately 6.8% can be explained by rural areas having a slower growing industry composition (i.e., slowly growing industries tend to be located in rural areas) and 6.2% is due to having rural industries that grow slower than their metropolitan counterparts (i.e., for any given industry, growth is slower in rural than in metro areas; with a 4.1% residual that favors rural areas). Figure 13 depicts these changes across metropolitan areas for 2010–2016, and Fig. 14 shows the distribution of the shift share for the industry mix in nonmetro *counties*. Notice that both figures present the results from Eq. (1).

Labor Market Framework

We turn our attention to what were the underlying supply and demand factors that drove these changes to help us understand the appropriate policy conclusions. The theoretical underpinnings for the analysis to follow come from a basic supply and demand framework that explains how shifts in labor demand and supply cause changes in wage rates and employment. The labor supply curve is upward sloping because workers will supply more labor as wage rates rise. The labor demand curve

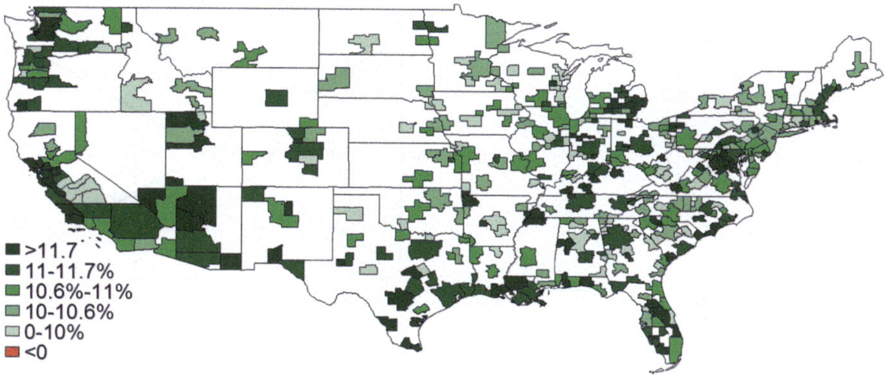

Fig. 13 Shift share of industry mix, Metro areas 2010–2016 classified by quintiles of growth

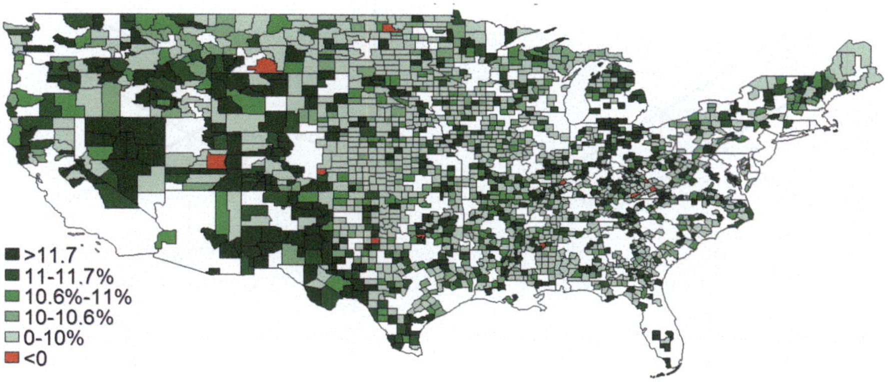

Fig. 14 Shift share of industry mix, Nonmetro areas 2010–2016 classified by quintiles of growth

slopes downward because as real wages increase, labor becomes more expensive for firms, and they substitute other factors such as capital as a result. Factors that affect worker willingness to work shift the labor supply (e.g., the generosity of welfare benefits or new migrants moving into an area). Factors that affect a firm's willingness to hire workers shift labor demand (e.g., shifts in firm product demand, productivity, and costs of other inputs). Figure 15 depicts equilibrium in a perfectly competitive labor market, where equilibrium wages are equal to W∗ and equilibrium employment is equal to Q∗.

Turning to specific examples, a leftward shift in the labor demand curve (reduced labor demand) as a result of decreased firm productivity, increased outsourcing, or skill-based technological change that reduces employment opportunities for middle-skill workers will decrease nominal wages, all else equal. In the new equilibrium, Fig. 16a shows that total employment will decrease through lower labor force participation rates and out-migration from the area. A reduction in labor demand,

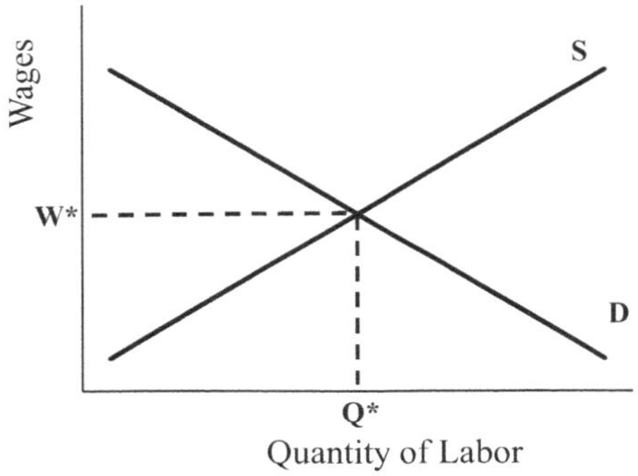

Fig. 15 Equilibrium in a perfectly competitive labor market

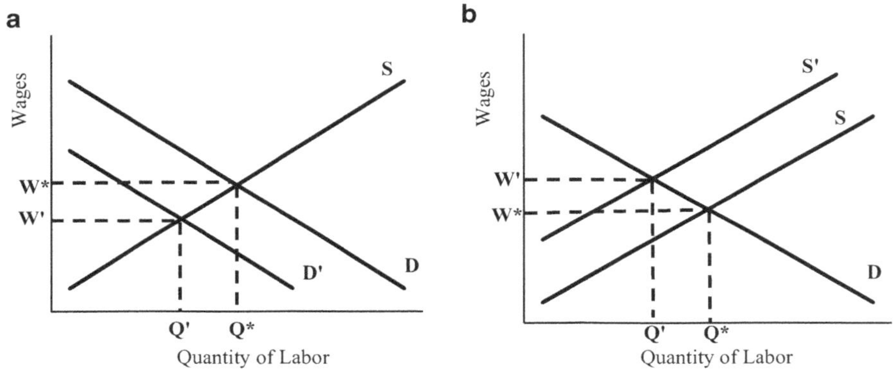

Fig. 16 (**a**) Reduction in labor demand. (**b**) Reduction in labor supply

therefore, could explain both lower employment-to-population ratios and lower wages in struggling regions.

Lower employment-to-population ratios, however, could be explained by a leftward shift of the labor supply curve (lower labor supply). If workers exit the labor force due to, for instance, a desire to substitute unemployment insurance benefits for earnings or a general unwillingness to work when they have high daycare costs, the labor supply curve will shift left, resulting in higher wages for the remaining workers but lower total employment (Fig. 16b).

Notice that in both cases, the effect is a reduction in total employment, or more specifically, lower employment/population rate. Yet, in the first case wages decline and in the second case wages increase from $W*$ to W'.

A reduction in wages could also be the result of a rightward shift in labor supply (greater labor supply; Fig. 17). Among other reasons, this can be caused by increased labor force participation due to women joining the workforce or by greater in-migration or foreign immigration to the local area, all else equal. However, the latter will generally reduce the employment-to-population ratio, in particular for the

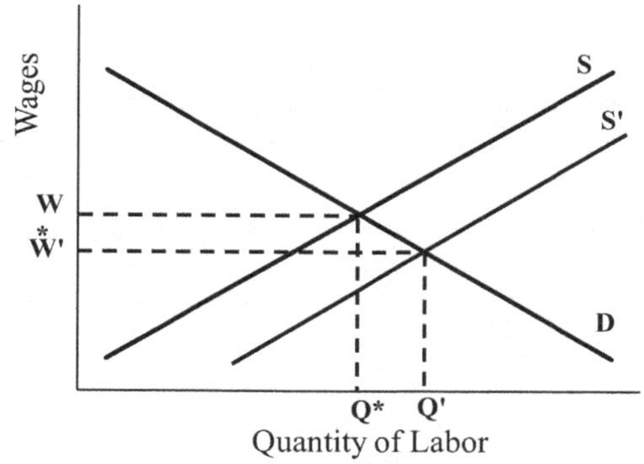

Fig. 17 Consequences of an increase in labor supply

workforce that was originally in the locale. The former would increase the employment-to-population ratio unless under the unlikely scenario that men equally drop out of the workforce as new women enter it. Note that these situations assume that the demand curve is fixed despite labor supply changes. Further adjustments will occur if the labor demand also shifts. Suppose that the influx of new workers (migrants or women) produces an increase in productivity, as it is the case when looking at highly educated immigrants (e.g., Hunt & Gauthier-Loiselle, 2010; Perez-Silva, Partridge, & Foster, 2018). If so, wages should rise, and the final equilibrium in terms of wages and quantity of labor will be a function of the magnitude of these changes.

Thus, examining whether wages increase or decrease in conjunction with the actual decline in labor force participation allows us to understand whether labor demand or supply is the primary cause for the observed changes. Once that is identified, we can determine the most likely (primary) cause of an area's economic conditions in lagging regions. In the following sections, we describe recent changes in employment-to-population ratios and wages with a focus in rural areas in identifying the key causal factors behind why the region lags.

Data and Methods

To examine supply and demand shifts, we use monthly data on wages and labor force participation from the Current Population Survey (CPS), obtained from the CEPR (Center for Economic Policy Research) Uniform Data Extracts between 1980 and 2017. We include data for all U.S. counties that can be accurately identified as metro or nonmetro. We construct our hourly wage measure by taking annual wages constructed by the CEPR and dividing it by the typical workweek hours. When the number of typical workweek hours is missing and the reported wage is zero, we treat the wage as missing. When hours worked in a typical week is missing, we use the number of hours worked last week in the primary job to construct our hourly wage measure. When none of the aforementioned variables are available, we use the number of weekly hours worked in all jobs. We use the Consumer Price Index for all Urban Consumers from the Bureau of Labor Statistics (BLS) to convert from nominal to real wages and express all wages in 2017 dollars.

To mitigate potential biases introduced by schooling, an aging population, or retirement, we consider only workers between 25 and 54 years old in the *active* labor force. Therefore, our employment-to-population rate refers to the number of employed workers relative to the sum of employed workers, unemployed workers, and people not in the labor force that are 25–54 years old only, unless otherwise noted. This is an important distinction because our participation rates are higher than those that consider the entire labor force (e.g., Aaronson et al., 2014). Other sources of information include employment data from the BEA and population data from the Decennial Census for 1970, 1990, and 2000, as well as the 2017 American Community Survey (ACS).

Heterogeneity Between Workers: Educational Groups, Industry, and Gender

We have established that important differences exist across local labor markets when analyzing trends in the employment-to-population ratio and wages. We have also shown how nonmetro areas are faring worse than metro areas. Thus, an examination of the differences between them is needed to focus on the areas left behind. However, worker outcomes are a function not only of local labor market-specific characteristics but also of worker-specific characteristics like education, occupation, and gender. Not all industries respond equally to shocks and recover similarly after recessions. As a result, we not only examine differences in labor market outcomes across local labor markets, but we also examine differences in outcomes within local labor markets for groups with different characteristics. In this section, we analyze changes in the employment-to-population rate and wages by educational groups, industry of employment, and gender. In the following section, we repeat the analysis focusing specifically on nonmetro areas to illustrate heterogeneity across areas left behind.

Differences Across Educational Groups

On average across all U.S. counties, real hourly wages have increased slightly since 2014 after more than ten years of stagnation, and the employment-to-population ratio started to slowly recover after a significant decrease that began around 2000. While current wage levels are about \$1 above real wage levels in 2002–2014, the employment-to-population ratio remains below its 1990s level. As expected, these trends hide an important heterogeneity in outcomes across educational groups. While real wages have increased for workers with a college degree and especially for those with an advanced degree, they have decreased for high school dropouts, high school graduates, and individuals with some college. Table 2 shows that real wages have declined for high school dropouts, high school graduates, and workers with some college by 19.1%, 8.1%, and 10.2%, respectively, between 1980 and 2017. In contrast, wages of those with bachelor's and advanced degrees increased by 11.9% and 17.4%, respectively. Similarly, the employment-to-population ratio fell from 62% to 61.2% for high school dropouts and remained constant for high school graduates. Employment-to-population ratios increased for workers with some college and college graduates on average, but surprisingly fell for those with advanced degrees. Figures 18, 19, 20, and 21 depict these changes over the study period.

In contrast with the national average, both the wages and the employment-to-population ratio of high school dropouts have declined. However, employment-to-population ratios have recovered slightly since 2010, and wages recovered slightly after 2014 (Fig. 18). Employment-to-population rate of those with a high school education is as low as in 1980 and is significantly below the levels of 1989–2008 as shown in Fig. 19. Real wages, on the other hand, declined sharply from 2009 to 2014. They have since recovered partially, although they remain significantly lower than they were between 2003 and 2009. In 2017, they are just above $18 per hour on average.

As mentioned, college-educated workers faced more favorable labor market outcomes than their less-educated counterparts. Their wages remained mostly unchanged in real terms between 1980 and 1996 and then increased until peaking at $31.1 per hour in 2002 (Fig. 20). Following a decline in real terms toward the end of the recession, wages for college-educated workers have increased steadily since 2014 to reach 2010 levels, but still below pre-recession levels. The employment-to-population ratio for college-educated workers, on the other hand, has been decreasing since 1990 to a low of 83% in 2010, the year in which it started a slow recovery, reaching 85% in 2017, but well below the levels before 2000.

Table 2 Change in wages and employment-to-population ratio by education, 1980–2017

	Hourly wages (2017$)			Emp-to-pop ratio		
	1980	2017	% Change	1980	2017	PP Change
Less than high school	17.20	13.92	−19.1%	62.0%	61.2%	−0.76
High school	19.64	18.05	−8.1%	72.7%	72.8%	0.09
Some college	22.40	20.12	−10.2%	78.6%	79.1%	0.49
College degree	27.03	30.25	11.9%	83.7%	84.9%	1.17
Advanced degree	30.78	36.14	17.4%	90.2%	88.8%	−1.38
All workers	21.85	24.26	11.0%	74.4%	78.4%	4.01

Note: Considers workers aged 25–54 years
Source: Authors' calculations based on the CPS extracts from CEPR

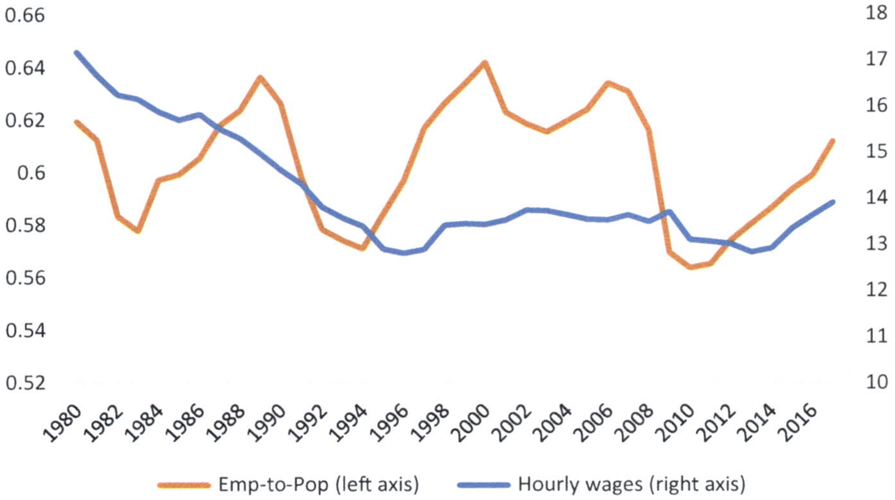

Fig. 18 Employment-to-population ratio and real hourly wages. Less than high school workers, 1980–2017. Source: Authors' calculations based on Current Population Survey (CPS) data

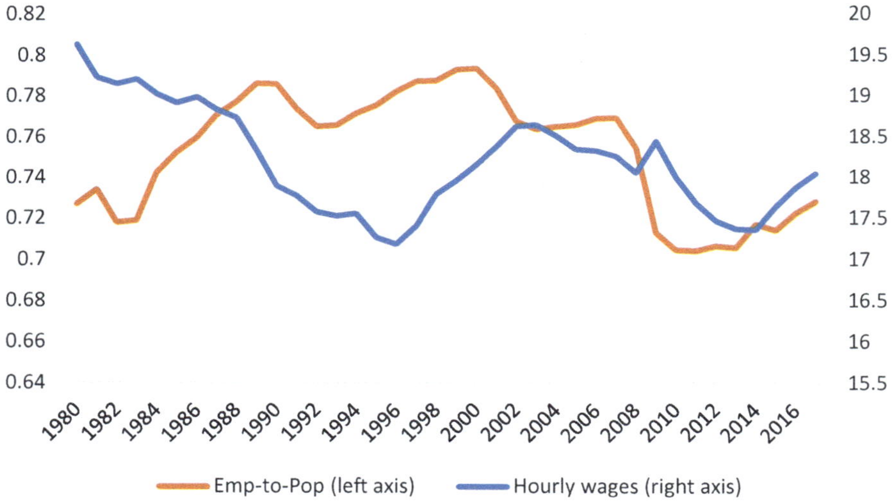

Fig. 19 1980–2017 Employment-to-population ratio and real hourly wages. High school graduates. Source: Authors' calculations based on Current Population Survey (CPS) data

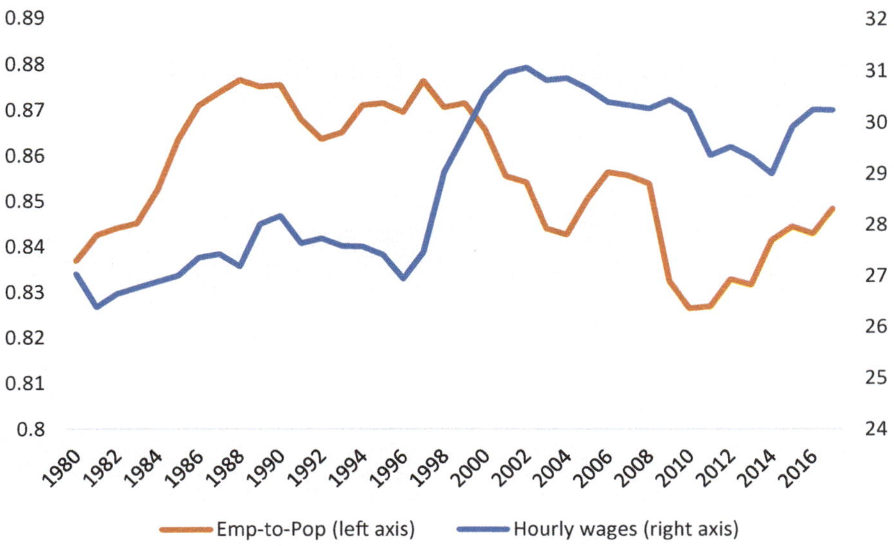

Fig. 20 1980–2017 Employment-to-population ratio and real hourly wages. College graduates. Source: Authors' calculations based on Current Population Survey (CPS) data

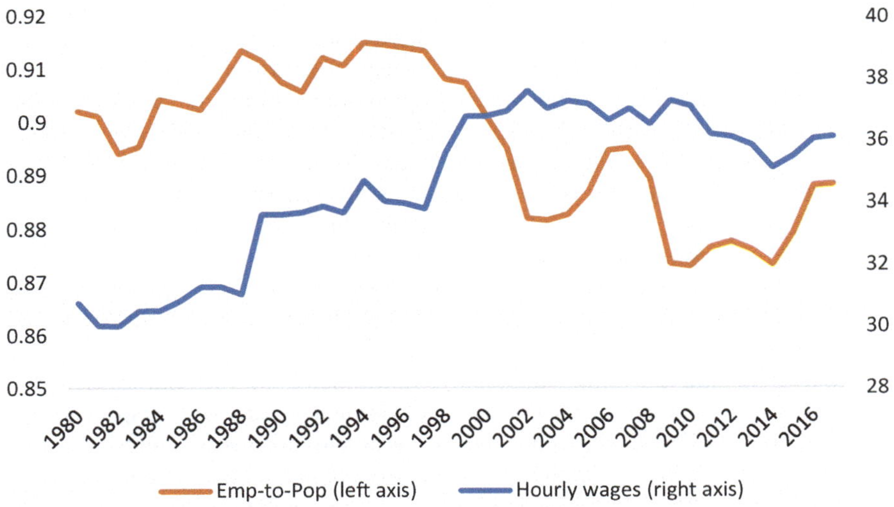

Fig. 21 1980–2017 Employment-to-population ratio and real hourly wages. Advanced degree graduates. Source: Authors' calculations based on Current Population Survey (CPS) data

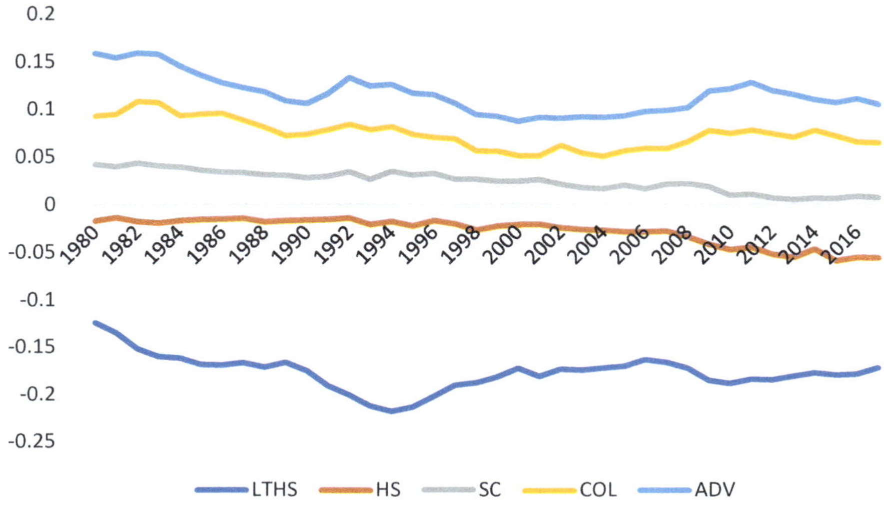

Fig. 22 Demeaned employment-to-population ratios by educational groups, 1980–2017. Source: Authors' calculations based on Current Population Survey (CPS) data

Finally, wages of workers with advanced degrees have increased nearly constantly since the beginning of the period (Fig. 21). As in the case of college-educated workers, wages for workers with advanced degrees peaked in 2002, 2005, and then again in 2009, when the hourly salary reached $37, one dollar above 2017 levels. The employment-to-population ratio for workers with advanced degrees, on the other hand, has decreased since 1997, recovering slightly since 2014. It is important to note that despite the changes in the labor force participation rate, the employment rates are remarkably high, remaining around 90% for the entire period. Also note that these data describe individuals between 25 and 54 years old, so population aging, suggested as a cause for the decrease in the employment-to-population ratio in previous studies, cannot explain the overall decrease observed here, though labor supply reductions are the likely culprit.

Figures 22 and 23 show the relative movements of the employment-to-population ratio and wages for different educational groups with respect to the national average. The downward trend in the employment-to-population rate is evident in Fig. 22, but the figure also clearly documents the differences in outcomes between educational groups. Employment-to-population rates for workers with some college, college graduates, and workers with advanced degrees are higher than average, while employment-to-population ratios for high school dropouts and high school graduates are below average. Note that for workers with some college experience, the differences with respect to the national average tend to diminish over the last three years of the period.

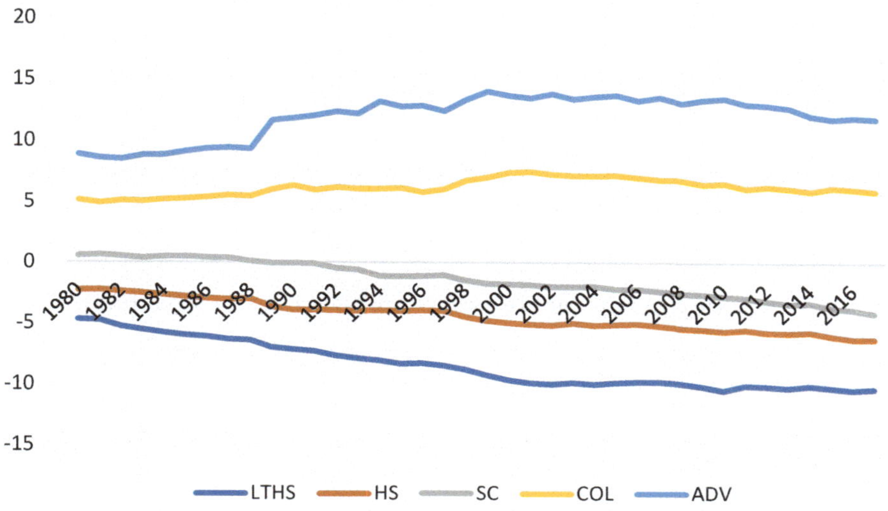

Fig. 23 Demeaned wages by educational groups, 1980–2017. Source: Authors' calculations based on Current Population Survey (CPS) data

As shown in Fig. 23, there is a sharp decline in relative wages for high school dropouts, high school graduates, and workers with some college experience across all years, and a slight increase in relative wages for college-educated workers. As a consequence, most of the positive wage variation in aggregate trends is driven by wage increases for workers with advanced degrees.

Differences Across Industries of Employment

Not only the trends in wages and employment are likely to differ across education groups. The aggregate trends could also hide an important heterogeneity across occupations, as industries respond differently to economic shocks. Here we analyze these heterogeneous effects across industries between 2003 and 2017, as shown in Fig. 24, benchmarked to 2003 = 100.

Real wages in Manufacturing and Construction were relatively stagnant over the period, growing between 0.5% and 2.8% after several years of negative growth. In contrast, workers in Professional and Business Services, Financial Services, and Information experienced the largest wage increases, with real wages rising around 5 to 6.4% between 2003 and 2017. Mining workers experienced a notable increase in wages during the middle of the period, but real wages decreased after 2016, converging to wage levels in other industries (Fig. 24).

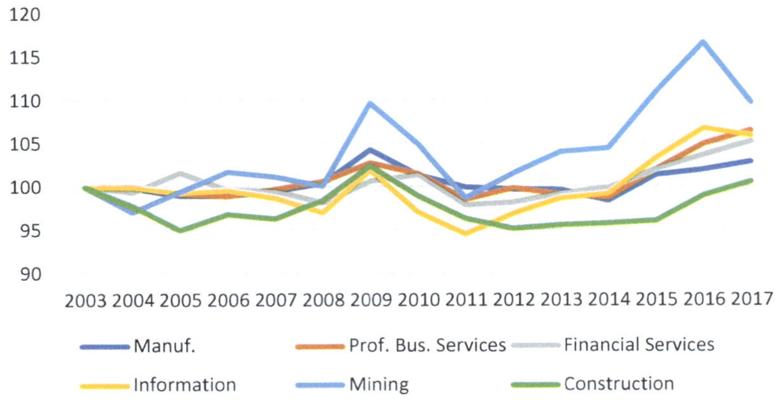

Fig. 24 Wages by industries (2003 = 100), 2003–2017. Source: Authors' calculations based on Current Population Survey (CPS) data

Differences Across Genders

As mentioned above, recent increases in female labor force participation are one plausible explanation for the reduction in the overall employment-to-population rate. If relatively more women become employed, labor supply will increase (shift the curve rightward), reducing wages (especially if these new workers are low-skilled). However, note that an increase in female labor supply does not explain a reduction in the employment-to-population ratio without a corresponding contraction in labor demand because an increase in labor supply alone yields higher employment than would be observed otherwise. Figures 25 and 26 show changes in the employment-to-population ratios and wages of male and female workers, respectively.

The male employment-to-population rate has fallen from close to 90% in 1980 to 85% in 2017, masking an 88–80% decline during the Great Recession. Since 2010, there has been a steady recovery in the male participation rate that is consistent with small increases in wages, especially in the last three years. Despite a downward trend starting in 2008, average male wage levels have remained well above the levels of the 1980s and 1990s, reaching $26 per hour in 2017.

These labor market indicators look completely different for females, as shown in Fig. 26. Hourly wages have increased significantly since 1980 from less than $17 in 1980 to $22.40 in 2017. Similarly, the employment-to-population rate increased from 60% in 1980 to 72% in 2017, with a peak of about 75% in 2000. Notice that despite these significant increases in participation and wages for women, there is still a significant gap in these levels relative to men.

These results suggest that the national trends in employment-to-population ratio and wages hide important worker-specific heterogeneity, in addition to heterogeneity across local labor markets. Nonmetro workers, workers employed in industries

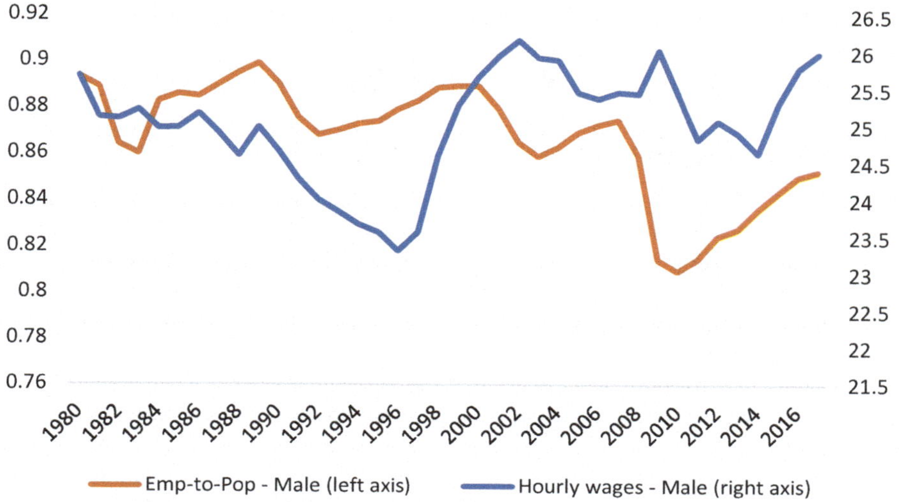

Fig. 25 Employment-to-population ratio and real hourly wages. Males, 1980–2017. Source: Authors' calculations based on Current Population Survey (CPS) data

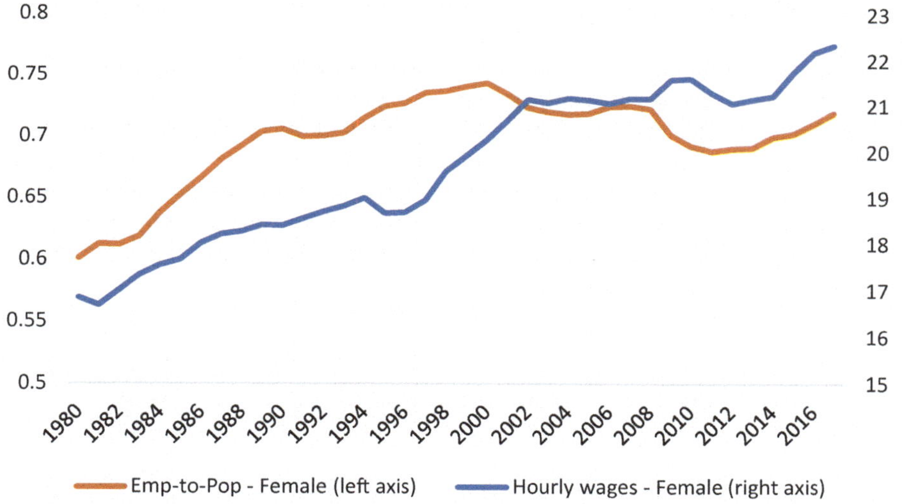

Fig. 26 Employment-to-population ratio and real hourly wages. Females, 1980–2017. Source: Authors' calculations based on Current Population Survey (CPS) data

with a higher concentration of low-skilled workers, and workers with less education appear to have been more affected by the recession starting in 2008 and have not yet fully recovered. In particular, wages of affected workers have mostly decreased or have just recovered to the levels observed more than 30 years ago, while their labor market participation has not returned to pre-recession levels. Finally, women have experienced wage increases and have increased their labor market participation, as is evident from more favorable trends relative to men, but their employment-to-population ratio and wage levels are still far below those for men.

The Places Left Behind

Differences between metro and nonmetro areas in terms of wages and labor force participation, measured by the employment-to-population ratio, are constant over time. There is a clear gap in favor of urban areas in the pre-recession period. Still, the employment-to-population ratio of rural areas has separated from the metro and national trajectory since the recession. While the employment-to-population ratio was around 76% for both areas in 2009, it has since increased to more than 79% in metro areas but remained at around 76% in nonmetro areas, after falling to as low as 73% in 2013.

Wages, on the other hand, have started to recover slightly in nonmetro areas, but they still lag far below metro wages. This poor performance is partly due to the composition of the labor market with a higher percentage of less-educated workers in rural areas. It is also due to nonmetro industry composition, with relatively high levels of employment in manufacturing, mining, and agriculture. As we have shown, whereas mining has grown recently mainly due to the shale gas "boom" (Brown, 2014; Munasib & Rickman, 2015; Rickman, Wang, & Winters, 2017), manufacturing employment has declined since 2000. Similarly, wages have only increased in real terms for workers with a college degree or advanced degree, leaving the rest at a disadvantage. This triple interaction between lack of opportunities in rural areas, a relatively low rural educational attainment, and a relatively large presence of declining industries, such as manufacturing, create conditions that produce adverse outcomes in rural America. As above, we will next explore outcomes for workers in nonmetro areas by level of educational attainment and industry in order to better understand outcomes for different types of workers.

Differences Across Educational Groups in Nonmetro Areas

Similar to the trends observed for the U.S. as a whole, wages in nonmetro areas have declined for less-educated workers and have increased for college-educated workers (9.9%) and workers with advanced degrees (19.8%). In particular, wages of workers with less than high school fell almost 13% in real terms between 1980 and 2017, while high school graduates experienced a 5.3% decrease in real wages. Workers with some college have also been penalized, even more so than high school graduates, with a total reduction in real hourly wages of 7.2% between 1980 and 2017. Similarly, the employment-to-population ratio declined from 62.8% in 1980 to 54.7% in 2017 for high school dropouts and from 73.9% to 70.4% for workers with a high school education (Table 3).

Table 3 Total change in wages and employment-to-population ratio by education, nonmetro areas, 1980–2017

	Hourly wages (2017$)			Emp-to-pop ratio		
	1980	2017	% Change	1980	2017	PP Change
Less than high school	15.88	13.83	−12.9%	62.8%	54.7%	−8.06
High school	18.14	17.18	−5.3%	73.9%	70.4%	−3.48
Some college	20.36	18.89	−7.2%	78.1%	78.6%	0.51
College	23.55	25.87	9.9%	84.7%	86.7%	1.95
Advanced degree	26.57	31.82	19.8%	91.7%	91.2%	−0.47
All workers	19.16	20.30	5.9%	73.7%	75.3%	1.59

Note: Considers workers aged 25–54 years
Source: Authors' calculations based on the CPS extracts from CEPR

Smaller participation rate changes (less than 1 percentage point) are observed for workers with some college (0.51 percentage points between 1980 and 2017) and for those with advanced degrees (a reduction of 0.47 percentage points). Workers with a college degree had the highest increase in the employment-to-participation rate with a total change of 1.95 percentage points.

The trajectory of these changes is shown in Figs. 27, 28, 29, and 30 for high school dropouts, high school graduates, college graduates, and advanced degree recipients, respectively. In the case of high school dropouts, the employment-to-population ratio persistently declines over the period, despite some brief recoveries. During the Great Recession, this ratio fell from 57% in 2006 to 50.7% in 2009 and remained near 50% until 2015. The ratio recovered between 2015 and 2017 but is still below the pre-recession levels at 54.7% in 2017.

Wages fell at the beginning of the period, from a high of $16.20 in 1980 (in 2017$) to a low of $12.50 per hour in 1995 (Fig. 27). Wages began to slightly recover in 1997 but did not recover completely, stabilizing between $13 and $14. In 2017, real hourly wages reached $14 per hour, still more than $2 below the beginning of the study period.

An even more dramatic picture is presented for high school graduates. While they have not experienced a constant decrease in the employment-to-population ratio, they also have not yet recovered from the recession. Moreover, the ratio continued to trend downward several years after the recession. As for high school dropouts, the 2017 employment-to-population ratio of high school graduates is at its lowest level (70%) after a sharp decline that started at around 2007.

Wages of high school graduates have also declined significantly in the first decade of analysis, but they tend to recover, growing until 2002 (Fig. 28). Despite minor movements in the trajectory, wage levels have remained similar to those in 2002 until the end of the series, reaching $17.20 in 2017. Yet, this wage rate is still below its 1980 level.

As shown in Table 3, both wages and the employment-to-population ratio have increased for college graduates in nonmetro areas, but important differences in outcomes exist between the two measures. Wages have increased since 1997, reaching

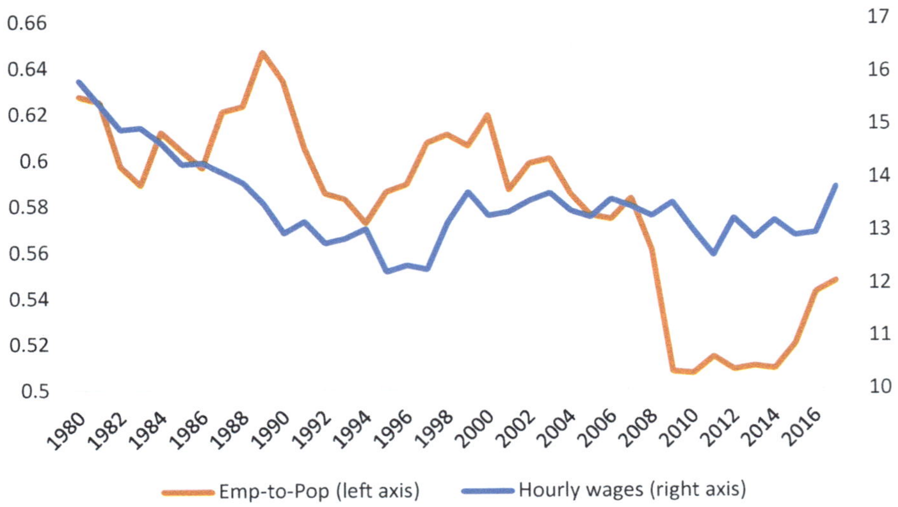

Fig. 27 Employment-to-population ratio and real hourly wages. High school dropouts in nonmetro areas, 1980–2017. Source: Authors' calculations based on Current Population Survey (CPS) data

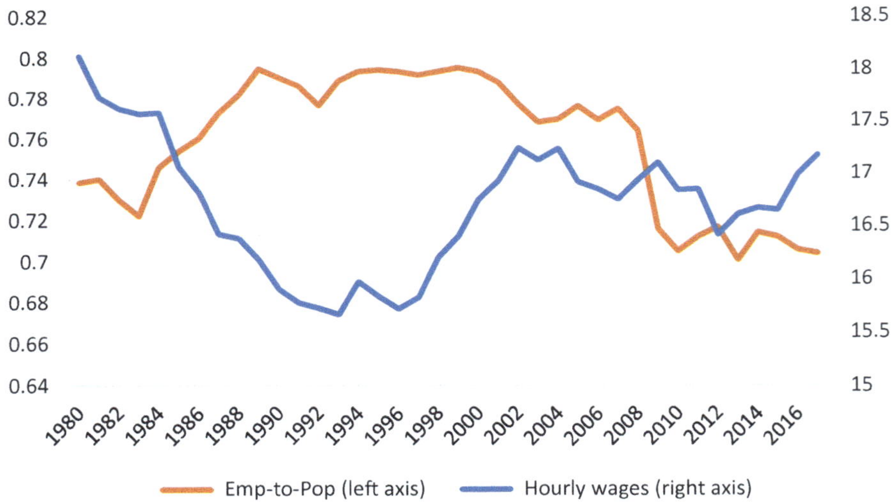

Fig. 28 Employment-to-population ratio and real hourly wages. High school workers in nonmetro areas, 1980–2017. Source: Authors' calculations based on Current Population Survey (CPS) data

$26 per hour in 2017. The employment-to-population ratio, on the other hand, is higher than it was in 1980 but still below pre-recession levels. More importantly, as with high school graduates, the employment-to-population ratio trends downward since 2016, as shown in Fig. 29. In 2017, the employment-to-population ratio of rural college-educated workers is below 87%.

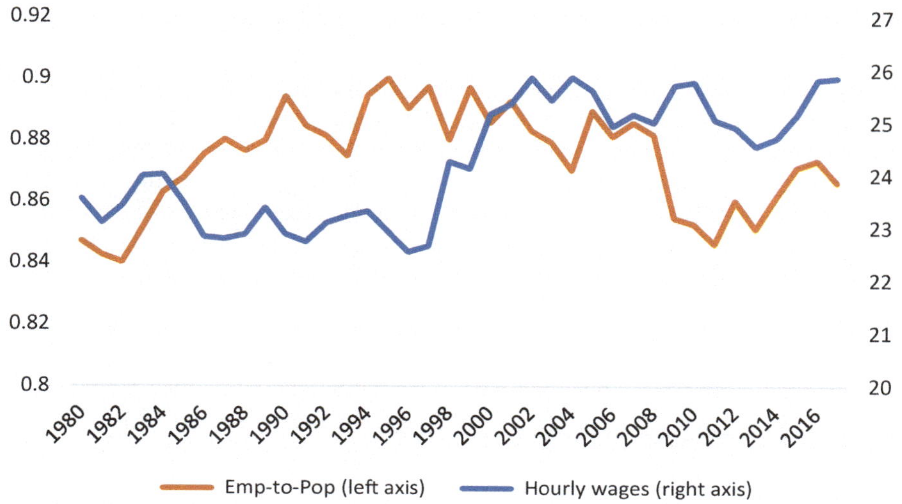

Fig. 29 Employment-to-population ratio and real hourly wages. College workers in nonmetro areas, 1980–2017. Source: Authors' calculations based on Current Population Survey (CPS) data

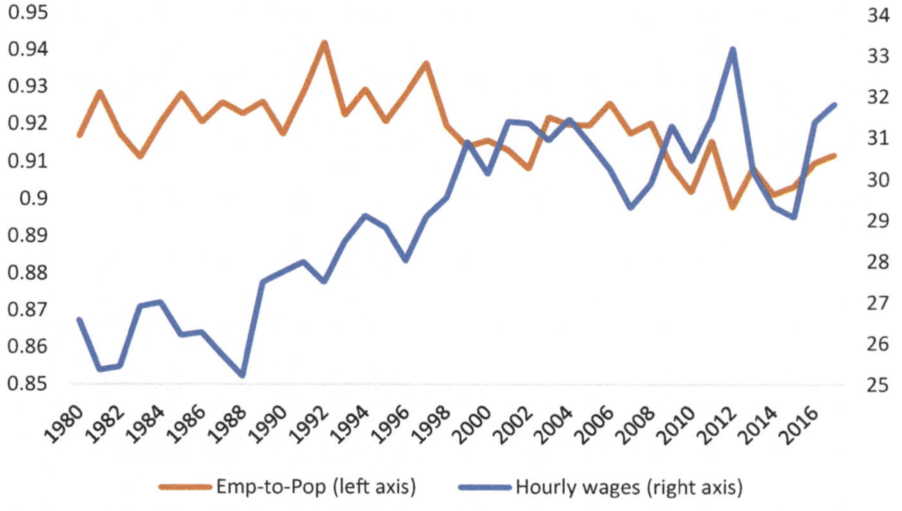

Fig. 30 Employment-to-population ratio and real hourly wages. Advanced degree workers in non-metro areas, 1980–2017. Source: Authors' calculations based on Current Population Survey (CPS) data

Wages of workers with advanced degrees almost constantly increased between 1980 and 2017, rising from \$26.6 to \$31.80 per hour, despite a relative stagnation between 2000 and 2010 (Fig. 30). The employment-to-population ratio of workers with advanced degrees has slowly and steadily declined throughout the period, but remains at high levels with more than 91% of the working age population employed.

Differences Across Nonmetro Industries of Employment

When looking at differences across industries in nonmetro areas (Fig. 31), wages have increased more for workers in Financial Services, Information, Mining, and Construction in recent years. Mining's growth has been above the U.S. average, but has declined in the last 3 years due to the 2014–2016 energy bust. Finally, nonmetro Manufacturing exhibits the lowest wage growth among these industries—consistent with fierce global competition keeping a lid on wages. Unlike metro areas, no nonmetro industry seems to dominate the others with all industries growing at a relatively slow pace.

Gender Differences in Nonmetro Areas

It is important to note that the same national trends by gender are present in rural areas. Female workers face lower wages and lower employment-to-population ratios than men but are significantly increasing their labor force participation and enjoying increases in real hourly wages. Female workers in nonmetro areas earned close to $19 per hour in 2017, with conditions improving after the recession (Fig. 32). The female employment-to-population ratio, on the other hand, dropped significantly since 2008 to less than 68% in 2013 and continues to be less than 70% in 2017.

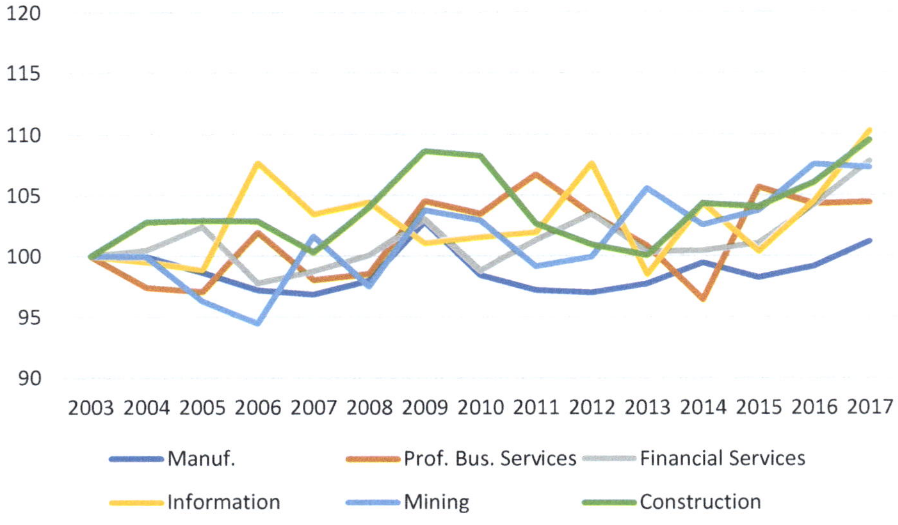

Fig. 31 Wages by industries (2003 = 100), nonmetro areas 2003–2017. Source: Authors' calculations based on Current Population Survey (CPS) data

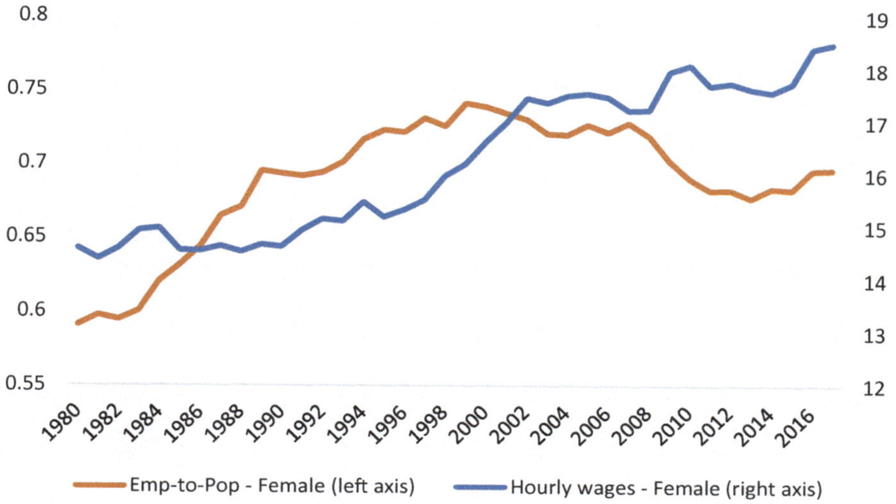

Fig. 32 1980–2017 female nonmetro employment-to-population rate and real hourly wages. Source: Authors' calculations based on Current Population Survey (CPS) data

Matching the Theory with the Evidence: Post-Recession Analysis

The results presented here suggest that overall wages have remained mostly stable while the employment-to-population ratio declined slightly over the last 4 decades. Nonetheless, these trends hide clear heterogeneity across workers, areas, gender, and industry. The national data finally signals a slow recovery in both wages and employment-to-population ratio after the Great Recession. Recovery in those two areas is consistent with an increase in labor demand, most likely accompanied by a similar increase in labor supply in order to keep wages nearly constant in real terms.

For rural areas, wages seem to have started to recover, but the employment-to-population rate has not recovered, which could relate to a slight decline in labor supply. This potential reduction in rural labor supply appears to relate to the out-migration from rural to metro areas as shown in Fig. 33. Only between 1992 and 1998 did rural areas exhibit positive net migration. Net migration has been negative in nonmetro areas at least since 1999 (also see Cromartie, 2017). Yet, there has been a dramatic improvement since 2014, to almost a zero net balance in 2017.

Despite these results, the changes mostly reflect trends for highly educated workers, especially those with advanced degrees. Less-educated rural workers have experienced a marked reduction in both wages and employment-to-population rate, mostly consistent with reductions in productivity and a reduction in labor demand.

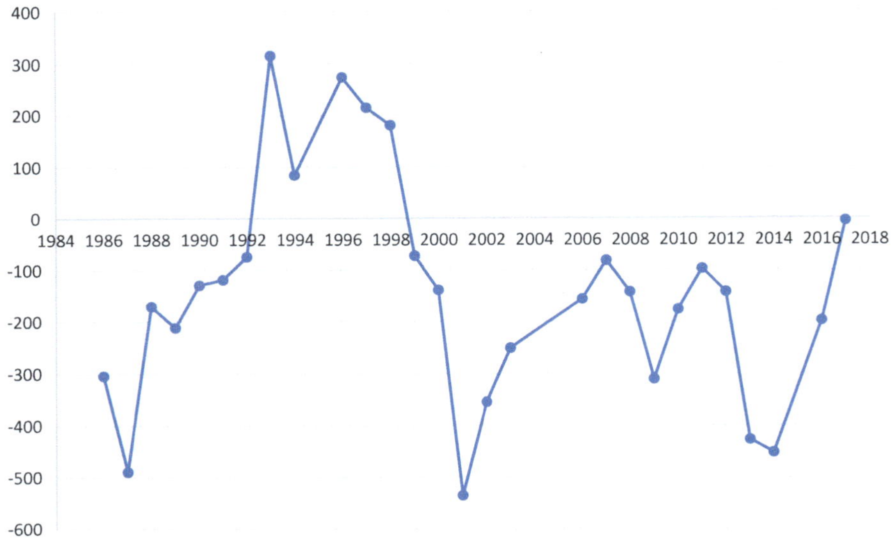

Fig. 33 Net domestic migration of nonmetro to metro areas, 1986–2016 (1000 s). Source: U.S. Census Bureau, Current Population Survey

The latter two reductions, in turn, are highly consistent with wage declines in industries such as manufacturing and mining (with the notable exceptions of boom towns (Tsvetkova & Partridge, 2018)), at least in the last couple of years.

Overall, our results suggest that the decline in participation rates in rural areas can be explained by a relative reduction in productivity, rather than intentions of workers to depend on public welfare benefits, consistent with the findings of Partridge et al. (2010). Similarly, because we exclude workers aged 55 years and older, we can eliminate concerns that an aging population is the main cause for the findings.

Conclusion

This chapter documents heterogeneity in labor market outcomes both across and within U.S. local labor markets for workers with differing levels of educational attainment, for workers employed in different industries, and for men and women. We underscore the need to examine specific areas and subpopulations more closely in order to more accurately understand the extent to which the U.S. has recovered from the Great Recession, as national-level trends often mask important variations in local labor markets.

We show that, in general, nonmetro areas have not recovered as quickly as metro areas, and nonmetro less-educated workers employed in manufacturing appear to fare the worst in terms of wages. Our analysis identifies pockets within the national economy that are struggling relative to others in the wake of the most recent economic downturn, and as a result, identifies where policymakers should focus their efforts in order to improve labor market outcomes for workers in places that have been left behind. Future research should focus on examining the effects of local policies targeted at improving labor market outcomes for less-educated workers in nonmetro areas, particularly those employed in manufacturing. In addition, research should seek to understand how national policies can support lagging regions in their effort to catch up to areas that have successfully recovered.

References

Aaronson, S., Cajner, T., Fallick, B., Galbis-Reig, F., Smith, C., & Wascher, W. (2014, September). *Labor force participation: Recent developments and future prospects* (Finance and Economics Discussion Series Working Paper). Washington, DC: Federal Reserve Board. Retrieved from https://www.federalreserve.gov/pubs/feds/2014/201464/201464pap.pdf.

Ali, K., Partridge, M. D., & Rickman, D. S. (2011). International immigration and domestic out-migrants: Are domestic migrants moving to new jobs or away from immigrants? *The Annals of Regional Science, 49*(2), 397–415. https://doi.org/10.1007/s00168-011-0456-2

Autor, D. H., Katz, L. F., & Kearney, M. S. (2008). Trends in U.S. wage inequality: Revising the revisionists. *Review of Economics and Statistics, 90*(2), 300–323. https://doi.org/10.1162/rest.90.2.300

Bartik, T. J. (1993). Who benefits from local job growth: Migrants or the original residents? *Regional Studies, 27*(4), 297–311. https://doi.org/10.1080/00343409312331347575

Blau, D. M., & Goodstein, R. M. (2010). Can social security explain trends in labor force participation of older men in the United States? *The Journal of Human Resources, 45*(2), 328–363. Retrieved from https://www.jstor.org/stable/25703459

Borjas, G. J. (2003).*The labor demand curve is downward sloping: Reexamining the impact of immigration on the labor market* (Working Paper No. 9755). Cambridge, MA: National Bureau of Economic Research. Retrieved from http://www.nber.org/papers/w9755.

Borjas, G. J. (Ed.). (2007). *Mexican immigration to the United States*. Chicago: University of Chicago Press.

Brown, J. P. (2014). Production of natural gas from shale in local economies: A resource curse or blessing? *Economic Review, 99*(1), 119–147.

Carlino, G., & Mills, L. (1996). Convergence and the U.S. states: A time-series analysis. *Journal of Regional Science, 36*(4), 597–616. https://doi.org/10.1111/j.1467-9787.1996.tb01120.x

Cromartie, J. (2017). *Rural America at a glance*. (Economic Information Bulletin 182). Washington, DC: United States Department of Agriculture, Economic Research Service. Retrieved from https://www.ers.usda.gov/webdocs/publications/85740/eib-182.pdf?v=0.

Dube, A., & Kaplan, E. (2010). Does outsourcing reduce wages in the low-wage service occupations? Evidence from janitors and guards. *ILR Review, 63*(2), 287–306. https://doi.org/10.1177/001979391006300206

Elsby, M. W., Hobijn, B., & Sahin, A. (2010). *The labor market in the great recession* (Working Paper No 15979). Cambridge, MA: National Bureau of Economic Research. Retrieved from http://www.nber.org/papers/w15979.

Goetz, S. J., Partridge, M. D., Rickman, D. S., & Majumdar, S. (2011). Sharing the gains of local economic growth: Race-to-the-top versus race-to-the-bottom economic development. *Environment and Planning C: Politics and Space, 29*(3), 428–456. https://doi.org/10.1068/c1077r

Goetz, S. J., Partridge, M. D., & Stephens, H. M. (2018). The economic status of rural America in the President Trump era and beyond. *Applied Economic Perspectives and Policy, 40*(1), 97–118. https://doi.org/10.1093/aepp/ppx061

Hunt, J., & Gauthier-Loiselle, M. (2010). How much does immigration boost innovation? *American Economic Journal: Macroeconomics, 2*(2), 31–56. https://doi.org/10.1257/mac.2.2.31

Katz, L. F., & Murphy, K. M. (1992). Changes in relative wages, 1963–1987: Supply and demand factors. *The Quarterly Journal of Economics, 107*(1), 35–78. https://www.jstor.org/stable/2118323

Kilkenny, M., & Partridge, M. D. (2009). Export sectors and rural development. *American Journal of Agricultural Economics, 91*(4), 910–929. https://doi.org/10.1111/j.1467-8276.2009.01320.x

Krugman, P. (2018, March 24). Trade and the cities (Wonkish). *The New York Times*. Retrieved from https://www.nytimes.com/2018/03/24/opinion/trade-and-the-cities-wonkish.html

Munasib, A., & Rickman, D. S. (2015). Regional economic impacts of the shale gas and tight oil boom: A synthetic control analysis. *Regional Science and Urban Economics, 50*(1), 1–17.

Orrenius, P. M., & Zavodny, M. (2007). Does immigration affect wages? A look at occupation-level evidence. *Labour Economics, 14*(5), 757–773. https://doi.org/10.1016/j.labeco.2006.09.006

Ottaviano, G. I. P., & Peri, G. (2012). Rethinking the effect of immigration on wages. *Journal of the European Economic Association, 10*(1), 152–197. https://doi.org/10.1111/j.1542-4774.2011.01052.x

Partridge, M. D., Ali, K., & Olfert, M. R. (2010). Rural-to-urban commuting: Three degrees of Integration. *Growth and Change, 41*(2), 303–335. https://doi.org/10.1111/j.1468-2257.2010.00528.x

Partridge, M. D., & Olfert, M. R. (2011). The winners' choice: Sustainable economic strategies for successful 21st-century regions. *Applied Economic Perspectives and Policy, 33*(2), 143–178. https://doi.org/10.1093/aepp/ppr006

Partridge, M. D., Rickman, D. S., Ali, K., & Olfert, M. R. (2008). Lost in space: Population growth in the American hinterlands and small cities. *Journal of Economic Geography, 8*(6), 727–757. https://doi.org/10.1093/jeg/lbn038

Partridge, M. D., Rickman, D. S., Ali, K., & Olfert, M. R. (2010). Recent spatial growth dynamics in wages and housing costs: Proximity to urban production externalities and consumer amenities. *Regional Science and Urban Economics, 40*(6), 440–452. https://doi.org/10.1016/j.regsciurbeco.2010.05.003

Partridge, M. D. & Tsvetkova, A. (2018). *Local ability to "rewire" and socioeconomic performance: Evidence from U.S. counties before and after the Great Recession*. (Unpublished manuscript).

Perez-Silva, R., Partridge, M. D., & Foster, W. E. (2018). Are foreign-born researchers more innovative? Self-selection and the production of knowledge among PhD recipients in the USA. *Journal of Geographical Systems*, 1–38. https://doi.org/10.1007/s10109-018-0281-6

Rey, S. J., & Montouri, B. D. (1999). US regional income convergence: A spatial econometric perspective. *Regional Studies, 33*(2), 143–156. web.pdx.edu/~crkl/SEAUG/papers/Rey_RS99.pdf.

Rickman, D. S., Wang, H., & Winters, J. V. (2017). Is shale development drilling holes in the human capital pipeline? *Energy Economics, 62*(1), 283–290.

Rothstein, J. (2011). *Unemployment insurance and job search in the Great Recession* (pp. 143–214). Washington, DC: Brookings Papers on Economic Activity. https://www.brookings.edu/wp-content/uploads/2011/09/2011b_bpea_rothstein.pdf

Stephens, H. M., & Partridge, M. D. (2011). Do entrepreneurs enhance economic growth in lagging regions? *Growth and Change, 42*(4), 431–465. https://doi.org/10.1111/j.1468-2257.2011.00563.x

Tsvetkova, A., & Partridge, M. D. (2018). Knowledge-based service economy and firm entry: An alternative to the Knowledge Spillover Theory of Entrepreneurship. *Small Business Economics*. https://www.researchgate.net/publication/329911566_Knowledge-based_service_economy_and_firm_entry_An_alternative_to_the_Knowledge_Spillover_Theory_of_Entrepreneurship
Weiler, S. (2001). Unemployment in regional labor markets: Using structural theories to understand local jobless rates in West Virginia. *Industrial and Labor Relations Review, 54*(3), 573–591. https://doi.org/10.2307/2695990

Part II
Economic and Health Challenges Facing Families in the Rural U.S.

Rural Job Loss to Offshoring and Automation

Srikant Devaraj, Emily J. Wornell, Dagney Faulk, and Michael Hicks

Social and political unease surrounding the wide differences in regional economic performance has troubled the U.S. for more than a generation. While geographic variation is not new, it appears more pronounced today than in the recent past. Over the past decade, several important studies have addressed the issue itself—implicating trade, automation, and the forces of urban agglomeration—while other studies have examined the corresponding impacts on individuals, families, and communities. In this study, we consider the geographic and socioeconomic concentration of job risk due to both offshoring and automation, and examine which poses a greater threat to U.S. jobs.

It has been argued that urbanization effects on labor markets ultimately culminate in a "new geography of jobs" in the U.S. (Moretti, 2012). Similarly, labor market polarization is argued to move workers from the middle into low skill or high skill occupations (Autor & Dorn, 2013). Offshoring of job tasks could well be part of a new industrial revolution (Blinder, 2006), and economic growth resulting from recent innovations such as artificial intelligence, are said to be part of "the new machine age" (Brynjolfsson & McAfee, 2014). Notably, these concerns are not new. As early as in 1817, the basic outline of both the benefits and costs of trade and technological unemployment was presented (Ricardo, 1817).

Our interest in these issues reflects a growing concern that the concentration of labor market shocks in particular geographies and for workers with lower levels of educational attainment have the potential to be far worse in the immediate future than in past decades. Indeed, in a 2016 study of the past three recessions (1991, 2001, and 2007–2009), the Economic Innovation Group (EIG) finds that half of all new business formation occurred in a small number of counties (125, 64, and 20, respectively), meaning that half of all establishment growth in the U.S. since the

S. Devaraj · E. J. Wornell (✉) · D. Faulk · M. Hicks
Ball State University, Muncie, IN, USA
e-mail: ejwornell@bsu.edu

J. E. Glick et al. (eds.), *Rural Families and Communities in the United States*,
National Symposium on Family Issues 10, https://doi.org/10.1007/978-3-030-37689-5_4

last recession occurred in just 0.64% of the more than 3100 U.S. counties (EIG, 2016).

The differences in geographic volatility are exemplified by a comparison of two counties, based on our analysis of the Bureau of Economic Analysis (BEA) Regional Economic Information Systems data (2017): Montgomery County, Maryland, and Elkhart County, Indiana. Montgomery County is in the Washington, D.C. metropolitan area and is heavily dependent on government employment. Elkhart, Indiana is predominately rural (although technically part of the Elkhart-Goshen Metropolitan Statistical Area), and relies heavily on manufacturing, with roughly 45% of wages directly tied to the production of goods. Over the past two recessions (2001 and 2007–2009), the unemployment rate in Montgomery County peaked at 3.8 and 6.0%, respectively. Comparatively, Elkhart County experienced an unemployment rate of 10.1 and 20.0% during the same business cycles. (Results presented in the next two paragraphs are the authors' calculations using the BEA Regional Economic Information Systems data, 2017.)

Our analysis of this data shows that it is not only regions experiencing this divergence, however. While real weekly wages for the average worker have increased only by 2% since the immediate aftermath of the 2001 recession, and less than 4% since 1979, even this slow growth is not shared equally. High-income workers have seen significant wage gains, while low-income workers are experiencing declines (BEA, 2017). Similarly, job opportunities are bifurcated by educational attainment. Since 1992, the U.S. has seen an increase of more than 35 million jobs for workers with some post-secondary education. Over the same time, however, there were two million fewer employed workers with only a high school diploma and five million fewer jobs for those without a high school degree (BEA, 2017). Accompanying this, was a decline in the labor force participation rate of high school graduates from 63% to 57% (BEA, 2017). Though some of these changes reflect a higher share of adults participating in post-secondary education, it is clear that while employment options for those with education beyond high school are growing, jobs for workers who have not been to college are declining.

One critical element of this trend for both regions and individual workers is declining employment in manufacturing. Historically viewed as a pathway to the middle class, jobs in manufacturing have been declining since the late 1970s and have seen roughly a 30% drop since the turn of the twenty-first century. The contrast between manufacturing production and employment, however, is stark. Since 2000, manufacturing production in the U.S. has risen more than 10% (in inflation-adjusted terms), while manufacturing employment has declined by almost 5.5 million jobs (BEA, 2017). Though automation and trade alone do not account for the regional disbursement of economic changes, the fortune of manufacturing has special resonance for several reasons. First, manufacturing tends to be highly geographically concentrated, with job losses focused by location and industry. Second, manufacturing jobs have been an important source of middle-class wages throughout the middle part of the twentieth century. The loss of these employment options interacts with the observed bifurcation of jobs (see Acemoglu & Autor, 2010), and geographic concentration interacts with additional factors, including a compelling portrait of agglomeration-related changes and the ensuing impact on population and employment change (see Moretti, 2012). Agglomeration forces—the clustering of firms and concentration of economic activity—occur in more densely populated places with thick labor markets (those with a high number of buyers and sellers, typified by much competition between businesses and lower costs of job searches for workers) and an abundance of highly educated workers. This trend offers a clear explanation for the observed population dynamics of the past two decades—all net U.S. population growth has occurred in large urban places. While prior research on such trends focuses primarily on urban places (Moretti, 2012), the impact in counties that are not part of large metropolitan areas is also clear. After all, migration-related population growth in urban places necessarily comes at the expense of rural communities (Cromartie, chapter "Demographic Components of Aging in the Nonmetropolitan U.S., 1980–2017"). The problems these trends generate are not confined to commercial economic activity. Prior research has provided causal explanations for inequality of opportunity at the commuter zone level, focusing on a broad suite of effects that limit intergenerational income mobility (Chetty, Hendren, and Katz (2016). What is clear from this work is that a bifurcation of economic experience is underway, across geography and education.

One need not accept the causative interpretations of any of these studies to acknowledge that the issues they explore are worthy of much fuller understanding and illumination. Thus, we highlight divergence in regional economic performance and the potential impact of this divergence on households and communities. The intent is to guide researchers and policy makers toward a better appreciation of the complexities of interregional economic differences, including how differences may be related to income inequality at the household level. To accomplish this, preliminary analysis of two important characteristics of regional economies are provided: the degree to which counties in the U.S. are exposed to automation-related job losses and the offshoring of employment.

What follows is a series of relatively straightforward data presentations and analyses of these issues. The proximal goal is to combine existing research in a comparable and intuitively useful way to guide future research on these matters. This is a work of synthesis, which argues that the divergence of labor market opportunities for people and places necessitate an urgent call to research and policy analysis. To begin, we offer a brief discussion of automation, trade, and regional economic vulnerability. This is followed by a presentation of the data and potential impacts on families and communities, and then concludes with local, state, and national policy considerations.

Automation, Trade, and Regional Economies

A number of studies have sought to identify the relative effect of automation and trade on manufacturing job losses in recent decades. Employment losses in the U.S. due to imports from 1999 to 2013 are estimated in the 2.0 million to 2.4 million range (Acemoglu, Autor, Dorn, Hanson, & Price, 2016). The direct manufacturing estimates resulting from this would appear to be in the 1.0 million to 1.3 million range. This would account for between 80 and 90% of total manufacturing job losses since the peak of manufacturing employment in the late 1970s. Other contemporary studies report similar findings. Roughly 88% of job losses in manufacturing from 2000 to 2010 were due to productivity changes, not import substitution (Hicks and Devaraj (2015). Statistical measurement of the value of intermediate goods is argued to be biased toward import substitutes (Houseman, Kurz, Lengermann, & Mandel, 2011). Thus, the official statistical data overstates worker productivity growth in the U.S. and understates import substitution. Exposure to Chinese trade in commuter zones is reported to be responsible for 26 to 55% of job losses associated with manufacturing employment decline in the 1999–2013 period (Autor, Dorn, & Hanson, 2016). (Commuter zones are broadly defined as connected urban centers and the surrounding non-metropolitan that share a market; or home-to-work travel areas in which workers live outside the immediate area of their workplace and commute to work.)

A very detailed account of job losses associated with extending Permanent Normal Trading Relations (PNTR) to China in 2001 has been reported (Pierce & Schott, 2016). Significant declines in manufacturing employment are linked to import substitution, with a contribution of roughly 1.3% of the percent of employment declines during the 2000–2007 period (combined job creation and destruction changes). This accounts for roughly half of the total manufacturing employment losses over this time period.

All of these studies conclude that both productivity gains and trade have played a role in the loss of manufacturing jobs over the past generation. Importantly, none of these studies argue that there are net losses to trade, simply that understanding the distribution of job losses offers a better understanding of the distribution of benefits and costs across occupations and geography.

The implications of these studies are useful in understanding and preparing for the future. Employment declines since the 1990s have been concentrated within a few industries, occupations, and levels of educational attainment. Indeed, these forces are also associated with political changes, which potentially impact trade and technology policy. According to the related analysis of voting patterns at the congressional district level, these job losses have led to a significant polarization of voting patterns (Autor, Dorn, Hanson, & Majlesi, 2016). Restating their conclusions simply: with broad job losses, red districts get redder, and blue districts get bluer. Any observer of the 2016 presidential election will appreciate this trend.

Still, the manufacturing job losses described here account for trade job losses of between one and 2% of all U.S. jobs, with total job losses in manufacturing alone accounting for less than 5% of current employment (Hicks & Devaraj, 2015). This manufacturing job loss occurred during a period of general employment growth, tight labor markets, and near full employment by 2017. Importantly, the apparently high levels of political tension and social discord resulting from these changes in the economy have occurred within the context of modest employment growth, not declines. However, there is ample evidence that automation will continue to replace specific human tasks and trade will continue to reflect regional comparative advantage resulting in a distribution of job losses that may continue to polarize both regions and households through very different economic outcomes. As such, evidence regarding which occupations may be most impacted offers important insight into regional economic conditions.

Data and Methodology

To better understand the scope, concentration, and impact of future economic conditions, we ask the following questions:

1. What is the risk of job loss due to automation and trade at the county level?
2. To what degree is job loss risk concentrated by geography and/or socioeconomic characteristics?

We approach these questions using data from two existing studies: Frey and Osborne, (2017) and Blinder (2009). The Frey and Osborne study (Frey & Osborne, 2017) estimated the probability of automation-related employment losses at the occupation level for the U.S. By examining the specific tasks through recent Bureau of Labor Statistics O∗NET job function data, they were able to assign a probability of automation to each occupation. The Frey and Osborne approach has been supplemented by other analyses which largely corroborates the range of automation effects they report (Bowles, 2014; Manyika et al., 2017), and has been replicated in other geographies (Frey, Osborne, & Holmes, 2016). A much smaller share of automatable jobs (under 10%) has been reported, focusing on heterogeneity within occupations as an explanation for the different estimates (Arntz, Gregory, & Zierahn, 2016). The estimates of automation probability should be viewed in the context of time, rather than occupation. Ultimately, parts of all occupations can be automated. Thus, the risk reported here is relative, not absolute.

The Blinder study (2009) examined all U.S. occupations similarly and assigned an ordinal level of offshorability of each job according to the description of the O∗NET functions of the job (O∗NET Online, 2019).[1] Later studies largely replicate the original Blinder findings (Blinder & Krueger, 2013; Smith & Rivkin, 2008). As with automation probabilities, it is best to view the level of offshorability as relative, rather than absolute risks of job losses.

Both Frey and Osborne (2017) and Blinder (2009) offer very useful insights into the automation and offshorability of jobs. However, adapting these estimates regionally requires some simplifying assumptions and calculations. The U.S. Bureau of Labor Statistics does not report occupations at the county level, though some states do provide estimates. The American Community Survey (ACS; U.S. Census, 2017), however, provides broad occupation categories at the county level; they are:

1. Management, business, science, and arts occupations
2. Service occupations

[1] See the descriptions of jobs at https://www.onetonline.org.

3. Sales and office occupations
4. Construction, extraction, and maintenance occupations
5. Production, transportation, and material moving occupations

We use these ACS occupational categories which permit us to aggregate the probability of automation to the county level. Occupational categories are aggregated to workers' county of residence, not necessarily to the county in which their job is located. This allows us to collapse both the Blinder and Frey and Osborne studies into a single county level of exposure to either trade or automation. We also converted Blinder's rank of the offshorability of occupations to an index from 1 to 100 so as to offer some comparability with the automation probabilities at the county level.

We first evaluate the occupation-level employment risk by multiplying the probability of relative risk of automation and offshorability for occupations and their respective national employment.

$$\text{Occupation Employment Risk}_{oi} = P_{oi} \times N_{o} \tag{1}$$

where subscripts i is automation or offshorability; o is each occupation. The probability of risk, P, comes from Frey and Osborne (2017) for automation risk or from Blinder (2009) for offshorability risk; N is the number of national employment for each occupation from Bureau of Labor Statistics (2014). We then compute the expected value of this Occupation Employment Risk weighted by the national employment and aggregated at the five broad ACS occupation categories for automation and offshorability risk.

$$\text{ACS Employment Risk}_{\text{ACSi}} = \left[\frac{\sum_{oi} P_{o} \times N}{\sum_{Boi} N} \right]_{\text{ACS}} \tag{2}$$

Subscript ACS represents each of the five broad occupation categories of the American Community Survey, and i is automation or offshorability. We then multiply this weighted share of employment risk to automation and offshorability across each of the five broad ACS occupation employment of all U.S. counties. Subscript c is the county, and i is automation or offshorability.

$$\text{County Employment Risk}_{ci} = \text{ACS Employment Risk}_{\text{ACSi}} \times N_{c} \tag{3}$$

Potential losses due to offshoring and automation should be interpreted carefully. As a workplace is automated, for example, it is unlikely all occupations will be eliminated. Rather, some jobs will be created, some no longer needed, and others will be unaffected. While the automation of an assembly plant might result in the loss of much of the workforce in assembly occupations, it might also result in an increase in the number of workers associated with operating and maintaining the automation equipment. Management occupations may be mostly unaffected. In contrast, a plant that closes due to offshoring of production will lose all occupations within the factory, even if individual occupations are not readily offshorable. This is a particularly relevant problem since the county level ACS data aggregates occupations. So, we cannot differentiate the management of a factory from the management of a hospital, though both face very different offshoring risks.

Note that there is abundant literature on labor shocks due to automation and the role of education (Schultz, 1975). This literature argues that education tends to mitigate labor market shocks. Furthermore, the degree of labor market complementarities of technology shocks is often ignored, while the labor substitution effects are overstated (Autor, 2014, 2015). Better understanding the speed and differential effects of automation-related labor market shocks will emerge later as one of our research recommendations.

Additionally, automation and offshoreability risk from these two studies are estimated across the margin of tasks. Other factors, such as relative price changes of finished goods and the relative costs of capital and labor play a very important role in the decision to offshore or automate a firm. So, these figures should be viewed as a relative risk of job losses due to automation or offshorability. While we are certain that automation will occur, and that centuries of specialization of labor and trade liberalization will continue over the long run, we are highly uncertain of the pace of these events. Still, the existing research allows us to craft maps that highlight the potential employment risks due to automation and offshorability of jobs.

Findings

To better illustrate the occupations we describe, what follows are the ten most and least offshorable jobs and automatable occupations in Tables 1, 2, 3, and 4. These data provide insight into the level of detail of occupations along with the wage and probability of automation. We provide only a representative list of the least offshorable jobs, since 518 of the 819 occupations included are not offshorable directly.

Interpreting these tables does demand some caution. The automation-related jobs offer an easy interpretation; the relative risk measure is essentially a weighted measure of total employment risk. A 0.67 means that two-thirds of jobs are at 100% risk of automation, and the remaining third at 0% risk, or that the average job is at a 67% risk of automation loss. For offshorability, the number represents a weighted share of jobs that could be offshored. For example, in the first county (Aleutians East Borough, Alaska) roughly 31% of jobs are first on the ranking of offshorability, or conversely, all the jobs rank in the 32nd percentile of the Blinder (2009) offshorability measure. See Table 5.

These rankings will no doubt give pause to many communities. Indeed, the authors work in Indiana, a state that can claim 4 of the top 25 automation counties, and 7 of the top 25 offshorable counties in the nation. We wish to reiterate that these are not predictions of job losses, but are merely representations of the relative risk to automation and offshoring-related job losses that may occur in the coming years.

Table 1 Ten most offshorable occupations

SOC Code	Occupation	Number of employees (1000's)	Annual wage
15-1131	Computer programmers	328.6	$ 29,460
43-9021	Data entry keyers	216.8	$ 79,530
17-3012	Electrical and electronics drafters	30.1	$ 59,520
17-3013	Mechanical drafters	65.7	$ 53,520
15-1111	Computer and information research scientists	25.6	$ 80,110
15-2011	Actuaries	24.6	$ 97,070
15-2021	Mathematicians	3.5	$ 111,110
15-2041	Statisticians	30.0	$ 110,620
15-2099	Mathematical science occupations, all other	1.8	$ 66,210
27-4032	Film and video editors	33.5	$ 23,530

Table 2 Ten most automatable occupations

SOC Code	Occupation	Number of employees (1000's)	Annual wage
43-9021	Data entry keyers	216.8	$ 29,460
15-2099	Mathematical science occupations, all other	1.8	$ 66,210
41-9041	Telemarketers	237.9	$ 23,530
13-2053	Insurance underwriters	103.4	$ 65,040
15-2091	Mathematical technicians	1.2	$ 46,600
51-6051	Sewers, hand	12.0	$ 23,640
13-2082	Tax preparers	90.4	$ 36,450
51-9151	Photographic process workers and processing machine operators	28.8	$ 26,590
25-4031	Library technicians	101.8	$ 32,310
49-9064	Watch repairers	2.7	$ 34,750

Tables 1–5 clearly imply a degree of concentration of both automation and offshorability risk, which is visually represented in the maps presented in Fig. 1. In both maps, which show the relative risk of employment changes due to automation of tasks and offshorability of jobs, the red colored regions exhibit a higher relative risk of automation or offshorable job losses. As these maps indicate, we find that a far smaller share of jobs can be offshored than can be automated. The risk for offshorable jobs at the county level ranges from 11% to nearly 22%. While offshoring clearly does represent a significant labor market risk to counties, the risk of job loss due to automation is much higher. Counties with the lowest risk are still looking at the potential for losing 36% of jobs, while counties at the highest risk may see automation-related job loss of over 2/3 (67%).

As is apparent from these maps, there is a great degree of regional variation in the risk of job losses due to offshoring and automation. There are clear clusters of high

Table 3 Ten representatives least offshorable occupations

OES Code	Occupation	Number of employees (1000's)	Annual wage
29-1125	Recreational therapists	18.6	$ 45,890
11-9161	Emergency management directors	10.5	$ 67,330
49-1011	First-line supervisors of mechanics, installers, and repairers	447.1	$ 63,010
21-1023	Mental health and substance abuse social workers	117.8	$ 42,170
29-1181	Audiologists	13.2	$ 74,890
21-1022	Healthcare social workers	160.1	$ 52,380
29-1122	Occupational therapists	114.6	$ 80,150
29-2091	Orthotists and prosthetists	8.3	$ 64,430
29-2099	Health technologists and technicians, all other	102.2	$ 41,260
29-1022	Oral and maxillofacial surgeons	6.8	$ 233,900

Table 4 Ten least automatable occupations

OES Code	Occupation	Number of employees (1000's)	Annual wage
29-1125	Recreational therapists	18.6	$ 45,890
11-9161	Emergency management directors	10.5	$ 67,330
49-1011	First-line supervisors of mechanics, installers, and repairers	447.1	$ 63,010
21-1023	Mental health and substance abuse social workers	117.8	$ 42,170
29-1181	Audiologists	13.2	$ 74,890
21-1022	Healthcare social workers	160.1	$ 52,380
29-1122	Occupational therapists	114.6	$ 80,150
29-2091	Orthotists and prosthetists	8.3	$ 64,430
29-2099	Health technologists and technicians, all other	102.2	$ 41,260
29-2092	Hearing aid specialists	5.9	$ 49,600

risk in the industrialized Midwest, pockets in the Southwest and West, and in several urban places across the country.[2] To extend the spatial analysis, and to inform a forward-looking policy, we offer two related analysis in labor markets beyond counties; we test for both spatial autocorrelation and rural/urban differences in risk level using the USDA's Rural-Urban Continuum Codes (RUCCs). This is formally the population weighted mean of the automation or offshorability measure in adjacent counties. This was calculated through the use of a first order contiguity matrix, $\tilde{W}$, such that the adjacent county is $\tilde{W}y_j$ and gives the value of each in county y_i. We note again that ACS data link occupations to household residence not to their county of employment.

[2] Maps for each major U.S. Census region are available at www.bsu.edu/cber.

Table 5 25 Counties at highest risk of automation and offshoring

	County	Automation risk	County	Offshorability risk
1	Aleutians East Borough, Alaska	0.67	Aleutians East Borough, Alaska	0.31
2	Quitman County, Georgia	0.67	Pontotoc County, Mississippi	0.31
3	Aleutians West Census Area, Alaska	0.65	Tippah County, Mississippi	0.30
4	Buena Vista City, Virginia	0.65	Roseau County, Minnesota	0.30
5	Chickasaw County, Mississippi	0.65	LaGrange County, Indiana	0.30
6	Allendale County, South Carolina	0.65	Los Alamos County, New Mexico	0.30
7	Tyrrell County, North Carolina	0.65	Clinton County, Indiana	0.30
8	Coosa County, Alabama	0.64	DeKalb County, Tennessee	0.30
9	LaGrange County, Indiana	0.64	Chickasaw County, Mississippi	0.30
10	Murray County, Georgia	0.64	Kosciusko County, Indiana	0.30
11	Covington City, Virginia	0.64	Aleutians West Census Area, Alaska	0.30
12	Dillon County, South Carolina	0.64	Whitfield County, Georgia	0.30
13	Switzerland County, Indiana	0.64	Falls Church City, Virginia	0.30
14	Blackford County, Indiana	0.64	Williamson County, Tennessee	0.30
15	Whitfield County, Georgia	0.64	Jackson County, Kentucky	0.30
16	Conecuh County, Alabama	0.64	Moore County, Tennessee	0.30
17	Benton County, Mississippi	0.63	Elkhart County, Indiana	0.30
18	Treutlen County, Georgia	0.63	Blackford County, Indiana	0.30
19	Greene County, Alabama	0.63	Williams County, Ohio	0.30
20	Meigs County, Tennessee	0.63	Hamilton County, Indiana	0.30
21	Pickens County, Alabama	0.63	Arlington County, Virginia	0.30
22	Galax City, Virginia	0.63	Elk County, Pennsylvania	0.30
23	Perry County, Indiana	0.63	DeKalb County, Indiana	0.30
24	Atkinson County, Georgia	0.63	Howard County, Maryland	0.30
25	Estill County, Kentucky	0.63	Dallas County, Iowa	0.30

Testing for spatial autocorrelation allows us to compare the risk of automation and job offshoring in counties and the average exposure to each in their neighboring counties. The notion behind this is that labor markets for individual counties will typically comprise the county itself and adjacent counties. This matters because a low correlation between adjacent counties would suggest lower vulnerability to the risk of automation or offshoring since counties with higher risk might be surrounded by counties of lower risk, and vice versa. A higher positive correlation between the

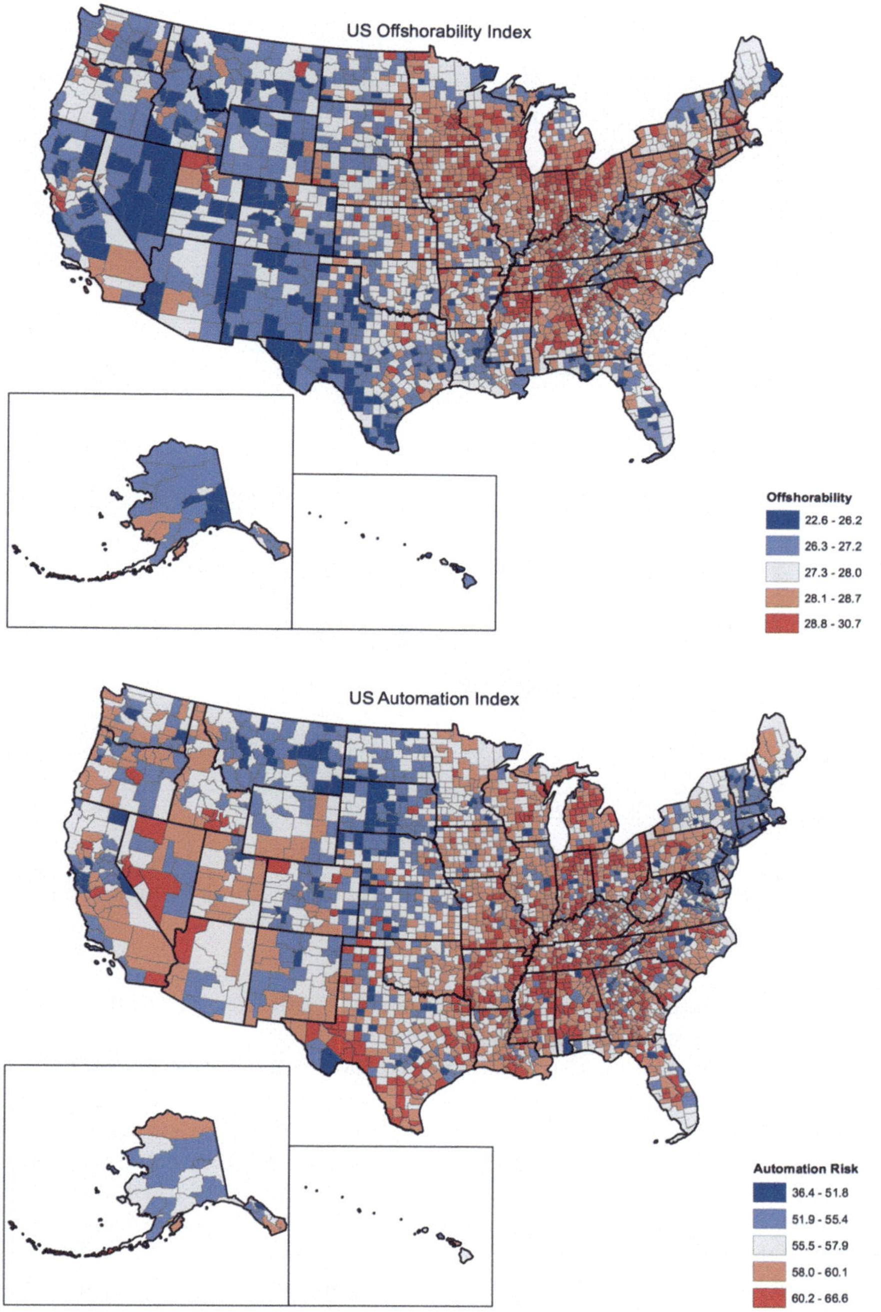

Fig. 1 Relative risk of automation and offshoring job losses by county. Sources: Blinder (2009); Frey and Osborne (2017); authors' calculations

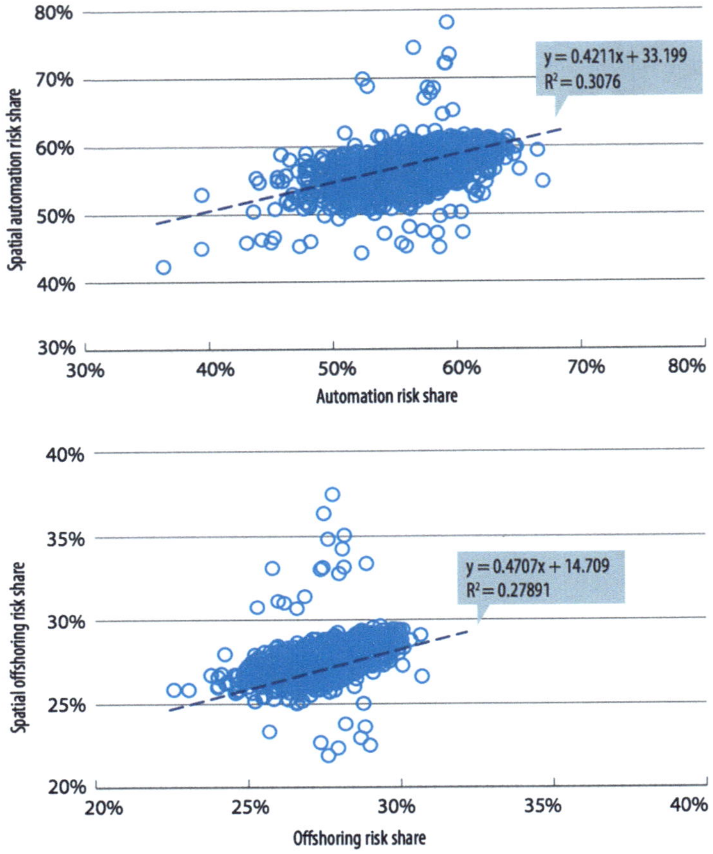

Fig. 2 Automation and offshoring risk share in own county and average of adjacent counties. Sources: Blinder (2009); Frey and Osborne (2017); authors' calculations

two suggests that risk to automation or offshorability are clustered, and that broader labor market regions share similar risks.

Figure 2 shows that the risk of job losses related to automation or offshoring is highly correlated. Counties with low risk are adjacent to lower risk counties, and high-risk counties are adjacent to other high-risk counties. This clustering of risk imposes concerns beyond purely economic considerations. The fiscal consequences of clustered risk are also significant, as few states have adopted fiscal instruments designed for vastly different regional outcomes. This calls for a much deeper exploration of the "new federalism" and the role that state and local governments may play across several margins of automation and offshorable job losses. New federalism refers to centralization of tax collections but decentralization of expenditures through the use of intergovernmental direct transfers (block grants; See Weingast, 2009, for an example on incentives).

We were also interested in the possibility that rural and urban counties experience differential levels of risk of job loss. Higher levels of risk in rural counties could be particularly concerning if those counties are also part of highly concentrated areas of risk of job loss due to automation and offshoring. What we find, as seen in Fig. 3, is that trade or offshorability job risk is more evenly distributed across the rural–urban continuum than is automation risk. Automation risk is lower in highly urbanized and very rural places than it is in more suburban or urban fringe counties.

The implication of the rural/urban differences in automation is that regional variation in potential job losses accrues across several margins. Industrial structure, educational attainment, and the degree of rurality all affect the potential employment risk of increased automation and trade-related job losses. Moreover, the degree to which automation-related job losses are concentrated may significantly influence such factors as local income inequality and intergenerational mobility (Chetty, Hendren, Kline, & Saez, 2014). Spatial concentration may also play a role in agglomeration economies as employment shocks tend to have a disproportionate impact on nonurban areas. One result of this may be the reinforcing of multiple equilibria in economic development; as poor places grow more slowly, more populous, and better-educated regions grow more quickly.

Labor market adjustments under trade and productivity shocks have been unequal at the regional level. Differential exposure to automation and trade clearly play a part in this, but worker differences also matter, as do broader labor market conditions. Job losses in rural places, concentrated in regions, and during periods of cyclical unemployment exacerbate labor market outcomes in both wages and re-employment (Autor, Dorn, & Hanson, 2016; Yagan, 2016). Individual differences in labor market outcomes may also be linked to initial levels of human capital and the likely returns to retraining. Workers who benefit from retraining investments or who are located in larger labor markets may be less likely to experience labor force displacement due to automation (Schultz, 1975). Understanding the duration and magnitude of these shocks as well as policy-related effects on labor market outcomes is needed to develop policy options.

The urgency of this is difficult to overstate. As difficult as labor market adjustments of the past generation may have been, it is likely that the vulnerability of labor markets to differential automation shocks may be much larger than previous experience with trade. To illustrate this, and to answer our second research question, we offer two simple analyses. The first correlates trade and automation exposure at the county level with county level educational attainment (Fig. 4). The second examines these risks correlated with income at the county level (Fig. 5).

As Fig. 4 illustrates, levels of local educational attainment are more closely correlated with a greater relative risk of automation related job losses than with trade-related losses. Even considering that the data from trade adjustments may include many occupations that have already been subject to significant offshoring, the simple correlation between educational attainment and offshoring risk is modest relative to the automation risk. This suggests that the speed of the automation related employment changes could be far more disruptive than those accompanying offshoring.

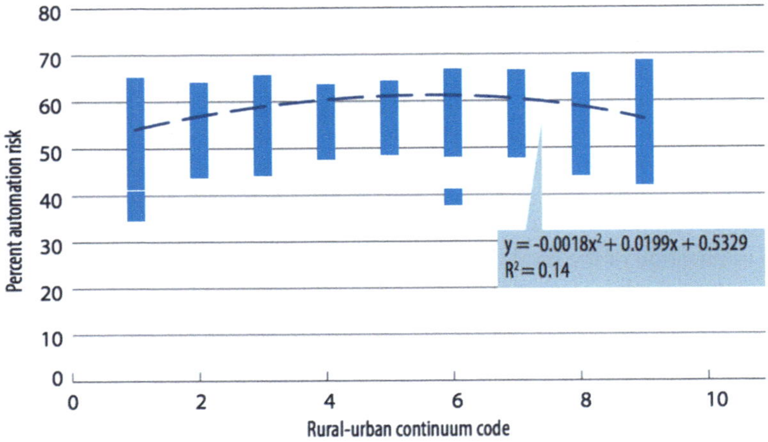

Automation Risk

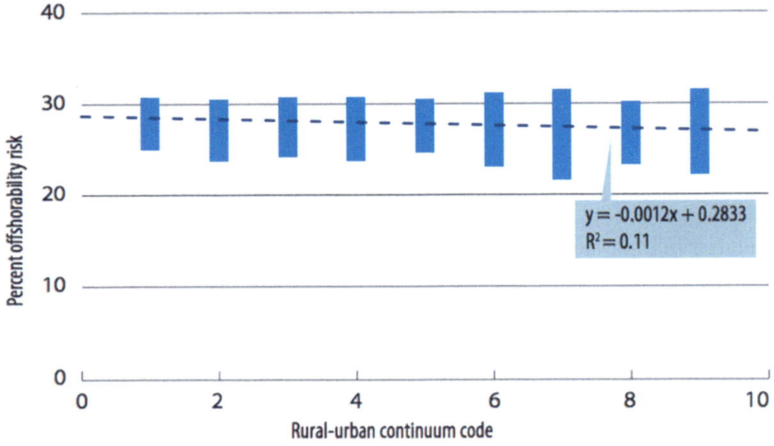

Offshoring Risk

Fig. 3 Automation and offshoring related job risk by rural–urban continuum codes. Sources: Blinder (2009), Frey and Osborne (2017); USDA, 2013; authors' calculations. Note: The USDA Rural Urban Continuum Code measures the degree of urbaneness. The values of one, two, and three represent counties in metro areas of over one million, between 250,000 and one million, and fewer than 250,000, respectively. The values four and five denote counties of more than 20,000 that are adjacent or not adjacent to a larger urban area respectively. Six denotes a location of greater than 25,000 but less than 20,000 adjacent to metro county, and seven is a similarly sized county that is not adjacent to a metro county. The value of nine is for completely rural places with fewer than 2500 residents. See https://www.ers.usda.gov/data-products/rural-urban-continuum-codes.aspx#.U0VBhleG-Hs.

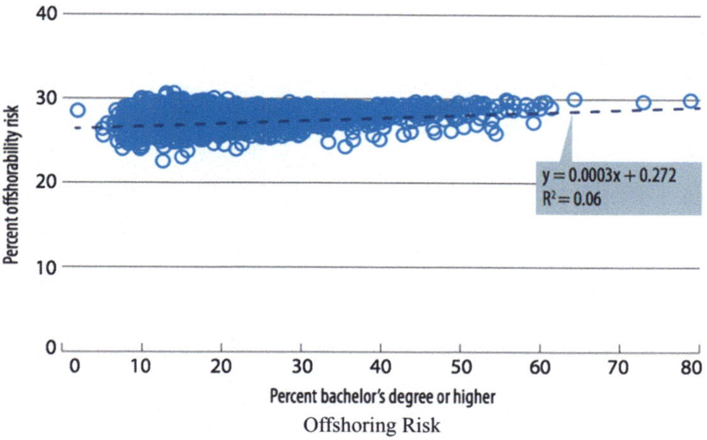

Fig. 4 County-level educational attainment by automation and offshoring risk. Sources: Blinder (2009), Frey and Osborne (2017); authors' calculations

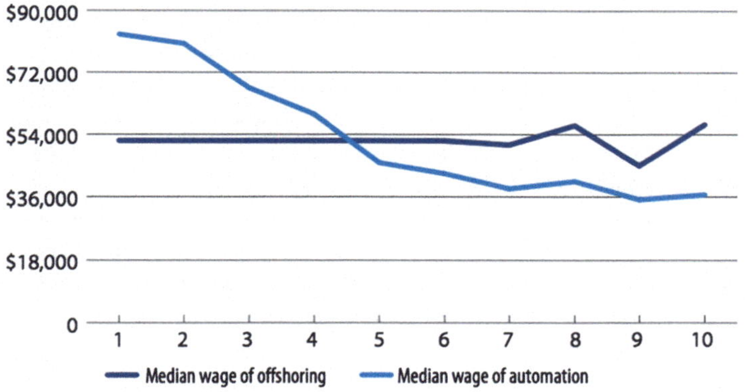

Fig. 5 Automation and offshoring risk by income decile. Sources: Blinder (2009); Bureau of Labor Statistics; Frey and Osborne (2017); authors' calculations

To arrive at Fig. 5, we aggregated occupational median earnings with deciles of relative risks of offshorability and automation. Occupations face roughly equal trade-related risk across income deciles.[3] However, low levels of automation risk are associated with much higher wages. Indeed, occupations in the lowest automation risk decile average more than $80,000 in annual salary, while occupations in the highest decile of automation risk have incomes less than $40,000 per year.

[3] The ninth decile of offshorability occupational median earnings was slightly lower than eighth and tenth decile because the ninth decile mostly include "production, transportation and material moving" occupations and very few "management, professional and related" occupations.

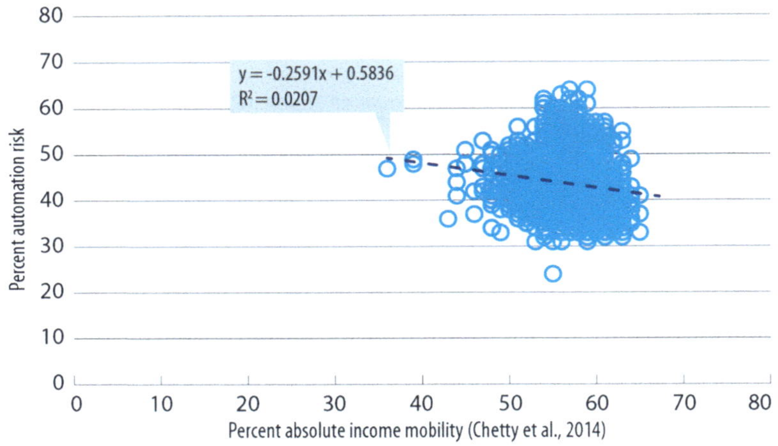

Fig. 6 County-level automation risk and income mobility. Sources: Chetty et al. (2014), Frey and Osborne (2017); authors' calculations

In addition to earnings related clustering of job losses for automation-related jobs, there is a very apparent clustering of intergenerational income mobility and risk of automated job losses. Using analysis of absolute income mobility between generations (Chetty et al., 2014), we plot the simple correlation to automation-related job risk. We observe a correlation between automation risk and lower income mobility at the county level in the U.S. (Fig. 6).

The optimistic result of this correlation is that it argues that employment polarization from automation-related shocks may be less than observed in the past. However, the troubling aspect of this is that employment losses may be concentrated within the most vulnerable households, which might be more geographically concentrated.

Discussion

Although relatively simplistic and descriptive, important potential implications for workers and households emerge from our analysis. As social scientists have long asserted, employment is more than an economic indicator. One's job and its related characteristics, such as prestige and wages, are integral in identity formation and social location. The consequence is that job displacement or involuntary job loss due to nonperformance-based reasons, such as automation or offshoring, not only has direct impacts on the economic well-being of people, families, and communities, but also indirectly impacts health and mortality, well-being, educational attainment, community integration, and upward mobility. It is in the interaction of economic and noneconomic impacts that households and communities will be faced with the greatest challenges if vulnerability to job displacement becomes actual job loss.

Of course, job displacement does have important economic implications that go beyond the period of displacement. Not only do displaced workers tend to experience longer periods of unemployment than do workers who were laid off for other reasons, but they also experience substantial loss of income over their lifetimes (Faber, 2005). The cumulative lifetime loss of income for displaced workers is estimated at around 20%, and income impacts can be observed for 20 years post-displacement (Brand & Wachter, 2013). Moreover, job instability remains elevated for these workers for at least a decade after the original displacement event (Brand, 2014). When displaced workers do find work, they are more likely to work part-time, seasonally, or as contract workers. The jobs they do eventually land are likely to be of lower quality in terms of authority, autonomy, and benefits as compared to their pre-displaced employment and compared to their non-displaced counterparts (Brand, 2006).

On a very basic level, the long-term job instability and depression of wages has a direct impact on economic well-being. Unemployment is associated with higher rates of poverty, lower rates of homeownership, and higher use of government assistance. The impacts of displacement go beyond economics, however. Health, family stability, educational outcomes, and social integration are also impacted at the individual, family, and community levels.

The impact of job displacement on health is seen in the short- and long-term for both mental and physical health. Displacement is associated with higher rates of depression and anxiety, which can be as high as 30% greater than for nondisplaced workers. Displacement is also associated with lower levels of positive psychological assets, such as self-esteem, satisfaction with life, and social supports (Burgard, Brand, & House, 2007). Workers who have experienced displacement have higher rates of mortality for at least 20 years after the original job loss (Sullivan & von Wachter, 2009; von Wachter, 2010). They see an increase in hospitalizations, use of medical services, and disability benefits, and have more disability, cardiovascular disease, medical conditions, self-destructive behaviors, and suicide (Burgard et al., 2007). Many displaced workers also lose their health coverage, making medical care more expensive and less accessible at the very time their medical needs are increasing.

Economic shocks also have the potential to increase family tension and disruption, resulting in an increased risk for divorce and family conflict. The effect of divorce and conflict on children's well-being is well documented. When all else is equal, children from divorced or high-conflict households have worse outcomes than children from intact households and households with little family conflict (Amato & Keith, 1991). Even without divorce or conflict, family stability can suffer due to displacement. Families that experience job loss may need to move for new jobs, which in and of itself creates family stress, school disruptions, and social network disintegration. Highly concentrated automation job losses in rural areas may ultimately exacerbate rural population declines that accompany the growth of cities (Moretti, 2012). Moreover, economic instability makes it more difficult for already disadvantaged families to provide basic necessities, such as education fees, transportation, food, and safe housing (Kalil & Ziol-Guest, 2008).

Unsurprisingly, the impacts of job displacement have a longer term impact on the educational outcomes for the children of displaced parents. Children in homes that have experienced job displacement are more likely to have to repeat a grade, drop out of school, and get suspended or expelled than are children in homes without job displacement (Johnson, Kahlil, & Dunifon, 2012). The children also have lower educational attainment and earn less as adults than do children from homes that do not experience job displacement (Kalil & Wightman, 2011; Page, Stevens, & Lindo, 2009). Downward mobility of parents due to job displacement may also negatively impact how children value education and work in their lives.

Lower educational outcomes are not limited to children from homes with job displacement, however. Researchers have also found indirect effects on peers and teachers in communities with high levels of displacements (Ananat, Gassman-Pines, & Gibson-Davis, 2011). Because individuals and families experience job displacement within a larger societal context, communities themselves are impacted by displacement. Displaced workers are less likely to participate in social organizations such as churches, youth groups, charitable organizations, and informal social events with family, friends, and neighbors (Brand & Burgard, 2008). Adults' and children's social networks are impacted, and the social withdrawal that often accompanies job displacement impacts the broader community.

The findings of direct and indirect impacts of displacement are not homogenous across populations, however. The negative long-term impacts of displacement have been found to be worse for low-skilled, less-educated workers, who are likely to work in more vulnerable jobs, as indicated in Fig. 4. Highly educated and skilled workers in high-wage positions, on the other hand, are not only less vulnerable to displacement, but are more likely to experience *skills transfer* when they are displaced (Faber, 2005). Alternatively, the negative indirect impacts of displacement may create less disruption in low-income households with existing job instability because of the coping strategies previously developed in the face of economic insecurity, whereas professional and white-collar workers may experience more psychological distress due to the untested nature of newfound economic insecurity (Brand, 2014). Households with one income earner, single mother households, and minority households would also be expected to experience these vulnerabilities differently.

Policy Responses

These observations about concentrated regional and worker risks of dislocation through trade and automation motivate a brief discussion of federal, state, and local policies designed to mitigate unequal effects of labor market shocks. We discuss these in turn.

Federal Level

The U.S. maintains a suite of policy interventions designed to assist households and regions affected by trade and automation. The suite of policies aimed at individual workers and households includes Trade Adjustment Assistance (TAA), Unemployment Insurance, Supplemental Assistance for Needy Families (SNAP), Temporary Assistance for Needy Families (TANF), and Medicaid. Despite the seeming flexibility of TAA, the best evidence suggests it plays a modest role in overall worker assistance in the wake of trade-related job displacement (Autor, Dorn, & Hanson, 2016; Baicker & Rehavi, 2004). There is also increasing evidence that workers may use other benefits such as Social Security retirement and disability as a substitute for other assistance programs (David & Duggan, 2006; Duggan, 2003; Krueger & Meyer, 2002). These programs are supplemented by a variety of state and local programs ranging from the federally funded, locally managed training assistance programs, such as the Workforce Investment Act, to local organizations providing food, clothing, and housing assistance.

The suite of efforts designed to help households weather the disruption of job loss and to sustain labor supply are directed at individuals, not regions. Very little regionalization of public or transition assistance is currently available for regions facing structural adjustment. What is available is largely limited in scope and size, such as in enterprise zones, impoverished areas in which incentives (e.g., tax concessions) are offered to encourage business investment and provide jobs for the residents (see Ham, Swenson, İmrohoroğlu, & Song, 2011; Neumark & Kolko, 2010). State and Local governments instead focus on industrial policy at the local level.

State and Local Level

Policy attention to job losses through diverging industrial patterns is not new. State and local governments have long sought to attract businesses and address regional economic divergence through a variety of public policies, including tax abatements and incentives, large infrastructure development efforts, changes to labor market policies (i.e., Right to Work), and regulatory policy designed to attract economic activity to a state or region. A broad scholarly debate over the usefulness of these policies has engaged scholars for more than two decades. There is an emerging consensus that the scale and focus of many policies at the state and local level have rendered disappointing results. Still, in 2017 most local economic development efforts remained narrowly focused on attracting and retaining businesses in their region. These policies are more apparent outside large urban places, suggesting a more immediate research concern for smaller urban centers and rural communities. Efforts concentrate on "footloose" firms that can locate their production or headquarters without worry about local demand for their goods or services.

Even in places where alternative strategies have begun to influence local economic development efforts, resources are primarily focused on activities to attract new businesses to the community. The most recent survey by the International City/County Management Association (ICMA) reports a mean municipal expenditure on economic development at $1.3 million per year with traditional business attraction services comprising most of the expenditures.

Among the more notable contribution to research on local and state economic development policies include Gabe and Kraybill (2002), who evaluated tax incentives on over 350 firms in Ohio from 1993 through 1995. Employing data on recipients and non-recipients, the authors reported that the firms that did not receive incentives outperformed the recipient firms in growth expectations. In a review of the impact of Michigan's Economic Growth Authority (MEGA) incentives on county employment growth in manufacturing, wholesale, and construction, no discernible effect on employment in these sectors was found (Hicks & LaFaive, 2011). Both studies influenced subsequent changes to incentives in Ohio and Michigan. These studies cast doubt on the ability of communities to effectively manage business location decisions through the narrow application of development incentives as well as the benefit of capturing firm relocation on local economies. More broad analysis of the suite of local economic development incentives reports a very small impact on overall outcomes of these efforts (Reese, 2013). Surprisingly, no more than one in ten dollars spent on development have any effect (Fisher & Peters, 1998).

A supply-side view of economic development efforts is offered by Hicks (2016). He argues that most research has focused on evaluating the demand side elements of firm relocation, while the availability of "footloose" jobs has shrunk dramatically over the past several decades. In Fig. 7, Hicks (2016) calculates the total net employment growth from 1969 to 2015 in the U.S., across two types of industries:

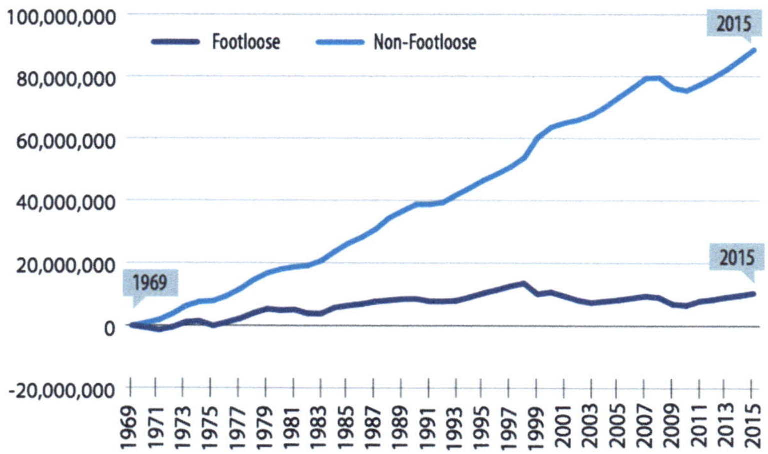

Fig. 7 Cumulative growth in footloose and non-footloose jobs in the U.S. (1969–2015). Source: Bureau of Economic Analysis; Hicks, 2016

footloose and non-footloose. Footloose jobs are those that export their goods or services outside a region and can therefore make location choices about where to produce. Non-footloose jobs are those that require a specific local context. In this calculus, all manufacturing and warehousing/wholesaling jobs, non-site-specific business services (such as the motion picture industry), and all nonlocal financial services are footloose. The remaining jobs are in industries that are dependent upon local consumption. This measure is imperfect; it does not, for example, count the small share of corporate headquarters positions which could conceivably locate anywhere. Still, the marked growth in non-footloose jobs versus the nearly static growth of footloose jobs offers a very distinct visualization of the local economic development problem; communities are chasing job growth that largely does not exist. Indeed, all the net growth in footloose jobs was in financial services, while nearly all the local and state incentives focus on manufacturing firms. Simply stated, incentives focused on attracting manufacturing firms are likely to be unsuccessful; communities should instead consider alternative economic and community development, such as amenities, to attract and retain population.

Despite significant research on the impact of federal, state, and local policy, the potential for historically large labor market shocks is an argument for an update to much of the existing literature. This leads us to consider a number of implications for research and policy analysis.

Future Research and Policy Analysis

In light of the varied impacts of job displacement, there are a number of areas where research is warranted. This work should seek to determine both the relationship between displacement and impacts and the appropriate policy response to mitigate negative impacts to individuals, families, and communities.

Improved measurements of automation and offshorability risks is obviously an essential area of research. Frey and Osborne (2017) and Blinder (2009) have set a high bar, but retrospective examinations of risk may better inform projections about the speed and magnitude of employment changes as well as adjustment costs. In particular, it is important to understand the impact of industrial structure on the role automation plays as either a substitute or complement to labor. Automation that is a complement for labor should increase employment, while automation that is a substitute will reduce employment. Any effective policy intervention will have to understand this nuanced effect of automation.

There is limited research that investigates the correlation between displacement and broader community effects. Given the importance of community on long-term economic outcomes, family formation and disruption, and intergenerational mobility, this relationship deserves more attention (see Chetty et al., 2016; Kalil & Wightman, 2011; Page et al., 2009). This is an especially urgent problem outside large urban areas where less research attention has been focused in recent years, and where socioeconomic and demographic conditions might exacerbate these vulnerabilities. Many nonmetropolitan and rural areas are, for example, aging rapidly. An older workforce closer to retirement age may increase the likelihood of a proliferation of nontransferable skills while also limiting the efficacy of policies aimed at retraining, ultimately requiring a different policy strategy than in communities with a younger workforce.

Similarly, both the research and policy communities would benefit from multilevel analysis that examines the interactions between community conditions and family or individual level characteristics. Whether job-loss risk due to automation is in fact higher among already vulnerable workers living in highly vulnerable communities, as our findings suggests, has important implications for our future society and potential policy responses. Highly vulnerable populations absorbing much of the risk of automation has the potential to deepen existing inequalities for generations, and should be a top research and policy priority in the future.

What characterizes individual, family, and community resilience to economic shocks, such as job displacement, can also be a productive area of research. The Great Recession has provided an important test case for the efficacy of expanding some government benefits, such as unemployment insurance and skills retraining programs. Evaluating the costs and benefits of support services to individuals, families, and communities now may allow for the adoption of these institutions prior to large labor market shocks in the future. Additionally, understanding how families cope with economic shocks, make ends meet in the face of economic insecurity, and do or do not return to pre-displacement socioeconomic positions will give researchers and policy makers better information about how to support continued upward mobility in an era of widespread economic vulnerability. Intergenerational effects are important, both for individual households and for regions. The persistence of shocks relative to the magnitude of policy responses will continue to be a fruitful area of research.

Individual, household, and community healthcare outcomes resulting from widespread employment shocks will also be a fruitful path of research. This research should evaluate both supply and demand issues related to healthcare, focusing on the context of recent and ongoing federal policy changes. This, too, is an especially urgent problem for rural areas where market power in healthcare markets may exacerbate access issues for households.

The interactions between automation and offshoring risk matter also to the distribution of wage and employment gains at the occupation and regional level. So, too, do labor market conditions unrelated to trade and automation. For example, we recommend a better understanding of the role of agglomerations, particularly labor market thickness, in buffering the effects of automation and offshoring. The degree of connectedness between rural places and urban labor markets is important in understanding the distributional effects of job losses.

Infrastructure differentials between regions and the impact on the fiscal structure, re-employability, and population change will be important in offering insights into appropriate policy responses. In particular, the role of broadband and other telecommunications infrastructure, roads, and transportation services in community sustainability in the wake of employment shocks should figure into the policy discussion. In this context, the role of transportation infrastructure in defining labor market size, especially for rural and micropolitan places will be important for evaluating spending priorities.

The role of public finance in mitigating economic shocks related to trade and automation should also be considered as a key component to any regional strategy. Likewise, a better understanding of the efficacy of regional industrial policy is important moving forward.

Limitations

The potential research and policy directions highlighted above also indicate some limitations of our study. Primarily, data limitations restricted our analysis to descriptives and disallowed us from examining interactions between geographic and socioeconomic concentration of job risk. Although one can make educated inferences based on other related research, statistically knowing the degree to which *both* geographic and socioeconomic concentration are correlated with potential job losses due to automation and offshoring could identify vulnerable communities and people.

Additionally, while this analysis provides an overview of potentially vulnerable places in which people live and work, it cannot tell us when these job disruptions will occur, nor does it speak to the net benefit of trade or technology-related productivity growth. Trade and technology-related productivity growth are undoubtedly positive over the long run. What is at issue are the distributional effects, which are likely to be significant. Moreover, this analysis cannot speak to the potential response by entrepreneurs and households that might find significant opportunities resulting from technology and trade-related changes. However, from this analysis we can offer additional analyses pointing toward much that is unknown about the potential distributional impact should automation or offshoring job losses continue at their recent pace or accelerate in years to come.

Summary

In the preceding pages, we have combined existing research into the likelihood of job automation and the risk of job offshorability and applied these analyses to counties in the U.S. Acknowledging that the past two decades have been ones of enormous economic and social anxiety associated with this phenomenon, we argue that the potential for an even more disruptive period lies in the immediate future. Importantly, the extreme political and social discontent of the past few years accompanied net job growth and a reasonably mild trade and automation disruption of less than 5% of total employment. The evidence outlined above suggests a much higher share of jobs are susceptible to automation and offshorability in the immediate future than in the recent past.

We cannot know the pace or depth of automation and offshorability, but it is clear that large swathes of the U.S. economy are likely to face these changes. Moreover, the risk, especially to job automation, is concentrated across labor markets, and income and educational attainment levels. Thus, the net impacts are likely to differ substantially from the distributional impacts of labor market changes due to automation and offshoring.

We do not wish to be alarmist. Both trade and automation-related economic growth are hallmarks of a vibrant economy. But, as we noted above, workers living in places with high concentrations of similar workers suggests labor market shocks may be increasingly concentrated across geographies. Together, these factors risk increasing political polarization and divergent regional economic outcomes. This warrants effort to better understand the geographic and labor market risks, especially as they involve differential levels of educational attainment and occupational and geographic concentration.

Our goal then is to highlight the relative risk that shocks from automation and trade play on the unequal labor market outcomes across workers and places. We also outline the impact of these labor market shocks across different margins: wage, employment, fiscal stability, social, and health concerns. We also appreciate the significant ongoing research on these phenomena as well as a lengthy history of analysis on the policy role for federal, state, and local governments. The public concern over these issues has occurred at a time of rising employment, no doubt partly due to labor complementarities of recent technological change (see Autor, 2014). However, more rapid or geographically concentrated labor market shocks may not accompany equally robust labor markets. If the social and political discomfort of the past decade and a half occurred during one of the largest labor market expansions in history, less robust economic conditions offer a much more disquieting forecast.

References

Acemoglu, D., & Autor, D. (2010). Skills, tasks and technologies: implications for employment and earnings. In O. Ashenfelter & D. Card (Eds.), *Handbook of labor economics* (Vol. vol. 4, 1st ed., pp. 1043–1171). Amsterdam: Elsevier.

Acemoglu, D., Autor, D., Dorn, D., Hanson, G. H., & Price, B. (2016). Import competition and the great US employment sag of the 2000s. *Journal of Labor Economics, 34*(S1), S141–S198. https://economics.mit.edu/files/9811

Amato, P. R., & Keith, B. (1991). Parental divorce the well-being of children: A meta-analysis. *Psychological Bulletin, 110*(1), 26–46. https://doi.org/10.1037/0033-2909.110.1.26

Ananat, E. O., Gassman-Pines, A., & Gibson-Davis, C. M. (2011). The effects of local employment losses on children's educational achievement. In G. J. Duncan & R. J. Murname (Eds.), *Whither opportunity: Rising inequality, schools, and children's life chances* (pp. 299–313). New York: Russell Sage Foundation.

Arntz, M., Gregory, T., & Zierahn, U. (2016). *The risk of automation for jobs in OECD countries: a comparative analysis*. Paris: OECD Publishing. https://doi.org/10.1787/5jlz9h56dvq7-en. (Report No. 189). OECD Social, Employment, and Migration Working Papers.

Autor, D. H. (2014). *Polanyi's paradox and the shape of employment growth* (Report No. 20485). Cambridge, MA: National Bureau of Economic Research. https://www.nber.org/papers/w20485

Autor, D. H. (2015). Why are there still so many jobs? The history and future of workplace automation. *The Journal of Economic Perspectives, 29*(3), 3–30.

Autor, D. H., & Dorn, D. (2013). The growth of low-skill service jobs and the polarization of the U.S. labor market. *The American Economic Review, 103*(5), 1533–1597.

Autor, D. H., Dorn, D., & Hanson, G. H. (2016). The China shock: learning from labor-market adjustment to large changes in trade. *Annual Review of Economics, 8*, 205–240. https://doi.org/10.1146/annurev-economics-080315-015041

Autor, D. H, Dorn, D., Hanson, G. H., & Majlesi, K. (2016). *Importing political polarization? The electoral consequences of rising trade exposure* (Working Paper No. 22637). Cambridge, MA: National Bureau of Economic Research. https://www.nber.org/papers/w22637

Baicker, K., & Rehavi, M. M. (2004). Policy watch: Trade adjustment assistance. *The Journal of Economic Perspectives, 18*(2), 239–255.

Blinder, A. S. (2006). Offshoring: The next industrial revolution? *Foreign Affairs, 85*(2), 113.

Blinder, A. S. (2009). How many U.S. jobs might be offshorable? *World Economics, 10*(2), 41–78.

Blinder, A. S., & Krueger, A. B. (2013). Alternative measures of offshorability: A Survey approach. *Journal of Labor Economics, 31*(1), 97–128.

Bowles, J. (2014). *The computerisation of European jobs*. Brussels: Bruegel. http://bruegel.org/2014/07/the-computerisation-of-european-jobs/

Brand, J. E. (2006). The effects of job displacement on job quality: Findings from the Wisconsin Longitudinal Study. *Research in Social Stratification and Mobility, 24*(3), 274–298. https://doi.org/10.1016/j.rssm.2006.03.001

Brand, J. E. (2014). *The far-reaching impact of job loss and unemployment.* (Working Paper No. PWP-CCPR-2014-011). Los Angeles, CA: California Center for Population Research (CCPR) at UCLA.

Brand, J. E., & Burgard, S. A. (2008). Job displacement and social participation over the life course: Findings for a cohort of joiners. *Social Forces, 87*(1), 211–242.

Brand, J. E., & von Wachter, T. (2013). *The economic and social consequences of job loss and unemployment* [webinar]. Population Reference Bureau (PRB) Available from http://www.prb.org/multimedia/video/2013/job-loss-webinar.aspx.

Brynjolfsson, E., & McAfee, A. (2014). *The second machine age: Work, progress, and prosperity in a time of brilliant technologies*. New York, NY: W. W. Norton & Company.

Bureau of Economic Analysis (BEA), Regional Economic Information Systems. (2017). GDP and Personal Income. https://apps.bea.gov/iTable/index_regional.cfm.

Burgard, S. A., Brand, J. E., & House, J. S. (2007). Toward a better estimation of the effect of job loss on health. *Journal of Health and Social Behavior, 48*(4), 369–384. https://doi.org/10.1177/002214650704800403

Chetty, R., Hendren, N., & Katz, L. F. (2016). The effects of exposure to better neighborhoods on children: New evidence from the Moving to Opportunity Experiment. *The American Economic Review, 106*(4), 855–902.

Chetty, R., Hendren, N., Kline, P., & Saez, E. (2014). Where is the land of opportunity? The geography of intergenerational mobility in the United States. *The Quarterly Journal of Economics, 129*(4), 1553–1623.

David, H., & Duggan, M. G. (2006). The growth in the Social Security Disability rolls: A fiscal crisis unfolding. *The Journal of Economic Perspectives, 20*(3), 71–96.

Duggan, M. G. (2003). The rise in the Disability rolls and the decline in unemployment. *The Quarterly Journal of Economics, 118*(1), 157–206.

Economic Innovation Group (EIG). (2016, May). *The new map of economic growth and recovery.* Washington, DC. https://eig.org/wp-content/uploads/2016/05/recoverygrowthreport.pdf

Faber, H. S. (2005). What do we know about job loss in the United States? Evidence from the Displaced Workers Survey, 1984–2004. *Economic Perspectives, 29*(2), 13–28.

Fisher, P. S., & Peters, A. H. (1998). Industrial incentives: competition among American States and Cities. *Employment Research Newsletter, 5*(2), 1,. 3-4. https://doi.org/10.17848/1075-8445.5(2)-1
Frey, C. B., & Osborne, M. A. (2017). The future of employment: How susceptible are jobs to computerisation? *Technological Forecasting and Social Change, 114C*, 254–280. http://www.sciencedirect.com/science/article/pii/S0040162516302244
Frey, C. B., Osborne, M. A., & Holmes, C. (2016). *Technology at work v2.0: The future is not what it used to be*. Citi Global Perspectives & Solutions. https://www.oxfordmartin.ox.ac.uk/downloads/reports/Citi_GPS_Technology_Work_2.pdf
Gabe, T. M., & Kraybill, D. S. (2002). The effect of state economic development incentives on economic growth of establishments. *Journal of Regional Science, 42*(4), 703–730.
Ham, J. C., Swenson, C., İmrohoroğlu, A., & Song, H. (2011). Government programs can improve local labor markets: Evidence from state enterprise zones, federal empowerment zones and federal enterprise community. *Journal of Public Economics, 95*(7–8), 779–797.
Hicks, M. J. (2016). *Why have local economic development efforts been so disappointing?* Muncie IN: Center for Business and Economic Research, Ball State University. https://projects.cberdata.org/reports/DisappointingEconDevt-20160620.pdf
Hicks, M. J., & Devaraj, S. (2015). *The myth and the reality of manufacturing in America*. Muncie, IN: Center for Business and Economic Research, Ball State University. https://projects.cberdata.org/reports/MfgReality-20170428.pdf
Hicks, M. J., & LaFaive, M. (2011). The influence of targeted economic development tax incentives on county economic growth: Evidence from Michigan's MEGA credits. *Economic Development Quarterly, 25*(2), 193–205.
Houseman, S., Kurz, C., Lengermann, P., & Mandel, B. (2011). Offshoring bias in U.S. manufacturing. *The Journal of Economic Perspectives, 25*(2), 111–132. https://doi.org/10.1257/jep.25.2.111
Johnson, R. C., Kahlil, A., & Dunifon, R. E. (2012). Employment patterns of less-skilled workers: Links to children's behavior and academic progress. *Demography, 49*(2), 747–772. https://doi.org/10.1007/s13524-011-0086-4
Kalil, A., & Wightman, P. (2011). Parental job loss and children's educational attainment in black and white middle-class families. *Social Science Quarterly, 92*(1), 57–78.
Kalil, A., & Ziol-Guest, K. M. (2008). Parental employment circumstances and children's academic progress. *Social Science Research, 37*(2), 500–515. https://doi.org/10.1016/j.ssresearch.2007.08.007
Krueger, A. B., & Meyer, B. D. (2002). Labor supply effects of social insurance. In A. J. Auerbach & M. Feldstein (Eds.), *Handbook of public economics* (Vol. 4, pp. 2327–2392). Amsterdam: Elsevier.
Manyika, J., Lund, S., Chui, M., Bughin, J., Woetzel, J., Batra, P., … Sanghci, S. (2017). *Jobs lost, jobs gained: Workforce transitions in a time of automation*. New York, NY: McKinsey & Company. https://www.mckinsey.com/~/media/mckinsey/featured%20insights/Future%20of%20Organizations/What%20the%20future%20of%20work%20will%20mean%20for%20jobs%20skills%20and%20wages/MGI-Jobs-Lost-Jobs-Gained-Report-December-6-2017.ashx
Moretti, E. (2012). *The new geography of jobs*. Boston, MA: Houghton Mifflin Harcourt.
Neumark, D., & Kolko, J. (2010). Do enterprise zones create jobs? Evidence from California's enterprise zone program. *Journal of Urban Economics, 68*(1), 1–19.
O∗NET Online (2019). Occupational Information Network. https://www.onetonline.org/
Page, M., Stevens, A. H., & Lindo, J. (2009). Parental incomes shocks and outcomes of disadvantaged youth in the United States. In J. Gruber (Ed.), *The problems of disadvantaged youth: An economic perspective* (pp. 213–235). Chicago, IL: University of Chicago Press.
Pierce, J. R., & Schott, P. K. (2016). The surprisingly swift decline of U.S. manufacturing employment. *The American Economic Review, 106*(7), 1632–1662.
Reese, L. A. (2013). If all you have is a hammer: Finding economic development policies that matter. *The American Review of Public Administration, 44*(6), 627–655. https://doi.org/10.1177/0275074013483166

Ricardo, D. (1817). *On the principles of economy and taxation*. London: John Murray. Albemarle Street. Retrieved from The Library of Economics and Liberty. http://www.econlib.org/library/Ricardo/ricP.html

Schultz, T. W. (1975). The value of the ability to deal with disequilibria. *Journal of Economic Literature, 13*(3), 827–846.

Smith, T. D., & Rivkin, J. W. (2008). *A replication study of Alan Blinder's 'how many U.S. jobs might be offshorable?'* (Working Paper No. 08-104). Cambridge, MA: Harvard Business School. https://www.hbs.edu/faculty/Pages/item.aspx?num=32566

Sullivan, D., & von Wachter, T. (2009). Job displacement and mortality: An analysis using administrative data. *Quarterly Journal of Economics, 124*(3), 1265–1306. https://doi.org/10.1162/qjec.2009.124.3.1265

Von Wachter, T. (2010, April 29). *Long-term unemployment: Causes, consequences, and solutions*. Hearing before the Joint Economic Committee of the U.S. Congress. https://www.jec.senate.gov/reports/111th%20Congress/Long-Term%20Unemployment%20-%20Causes,%20Consequences,%20and%20Solutions%20(1878).pdf

Weingast, B. R. (2009). Second generation fiscal federalism: The implications of fiscal incentives. *Journal of Urban Economics, 65*(3), 279–293.

Yagan, D. (2016). *The enduring employment impact of your great recession location* (Working Paper No. 108-16). Berkeley, CA: Institute for Research on Labor and Employment. https://escholarship.org/uc/item/12d0w9bs

Opioid Crisis in the Rural U.S.

Shannon M. Monnat

One would be hard pressed to scroll through the daily news feed and not see a headline about the U.S. opioid epidemic these days. (Opioids refers to all-natural, semisynthetic, and synthetic opioids, including prescription opioids, heroin, and various fentanyls.) Over the last two decades, opioid use disorders and fatal overdose rates have increased dramatically to become a major public health crisis. In 2017, more than 72,000 people living in the U.S. died from drug overdoses, a 329% increase since 1999. Opioids were involved in a startling 68% (49,068) of these deaths (National Institute on Drug Abuse, 2019). Since the mid-2000s, rates of opioid-related emergency department (ED) and inpatient hospital admissions increased by 99% and 64%, respectively (Weiss et al., 2017).

A common narrative surrounding the U.S. opioid crisis is that it has disproportionately affected rural communities. Headlines such as *Rural America in Crisis: The Changing Opioid Overdose Epidemic* (Noonan, 2017), *What's Behind the Addiction Crisis in Rural America?* (van Vlaanderen, 2018), and *Why is the Opioid Epidemic Hitting Rural America Especially Hard?* (Runyon, 2017) paint a nearly monolithic picture of a rural America in crisis. To be sure, this coverage has contributed much-needed attention and resources to downtrodden rural areas, but it also misrepresents the geography of opioid overdoses and ignores the vast heterogeneity in the severity of the problem across different rural areas.

Accordingly, this chapter describes geographic trends in opioid mortality, discusses these trends within the broader contexts of U.S. *deaths of despair* and declining rural health, elucidates explanations for the emergence and perpetuation of the opioid crisis and its geographic variation, summarizes the consequences of the crisis for rural families and communities, and proposes some promising strategies for addressing the opioid crisis and other substance problems in the hardest-hit rural

S. M. Monnat (✉)
Syracuse University, Syracuse, NY, USA
e-mail: smmonnat@maxwell.syr.edu

J. E. Glick et al. (eds.), *Rural Families and Communities in the United States*,
National Symposium on Family Issues 10, https://doi.org/10.1007/978-3-030-37689-5_5

communities. Ultimately, the information presented in this chapter dispels the myth that the opioid crisis is disproportionately rural, demonstrates that the magnitude of the problem varies considerably across different rural areas, and urges us to view the U.S. opioid problem from within the larger context of economic, family, health, and social problems occurring along the rural–urban continuum.

Geographic Trends in Opioid Mortality

Although metro counties have consistently had higher opioid mortality rates than nonmetro counties, the aggregate rate has increased more in nonmetro areas over the past two decades. (Throughout the chapter, metropolitan status categories are based on the 2013 National Center for Health Statistics (NCHS) Urban-Rural Scheme for Counties.) In 2016, the age-adjusted opioid mortality rate for metro counties nationally was 14.6 per 100,000 population, up from 3.6 in 1999 (306% increase). The rate for nonmetro counties was 12.6 in 2016, up from 1.5 in 1999 (563%). Of course, deaths alone do not capture the full extent of the problem. More than 2 million Americans have a prescription opioid use disorder (OUD), and nearly 950,000 are current heroin users (Substance Abuse and Mental Health Services Administration, 2016). Nationally representative studies on rural–urban differences in heroin and prescription opioid misuse find higher rates in urban areas or no significant difference (Lenardson, Gale, & Ziller, 2016; Rigg & Monnat, 2015; Weiss et al., 2017). However, rates of opioid misuse are higher among specific vulnerable rural populations, including: American Indians, military veterans, and individuals with disabilities (Havens, Young, & Havens, 2011; Keyes, Cerda, Brady, Havens, & Galea, 2014; Rigg & Monnat, 2015; Van Gundy, 2006), and rates of babies born dependent on opioids (neonatal abstinence syndrome) are higher in rural than in urban areas (Ko et al., 2016; Villapiano, Winkelman, Kozhimannil, Davis, & Patrick, 2017).

Much of the research on rural–urban differences in opioid mortality does not distinguish trends in the types of opioids that have contributed to these deaths. Understanding these differences is important because the effectiveness of particular interventions at quelling the overdose surge will likely vary depending on the type of opioid contributing to most deaths. For example, prescription drug monitoring programs, physician training, and opioid prescribing limits will be less effective at reducing overdoses in places where heroin or fentanyl are the primary contributors to overdose deaths.

As shown in Fig. 1, as of the mid-2000s, mortality rates from prescription opioids have been higher among nonmetro counties than metro counties. Moreover, prescription opioid mortality rates continued to grow in nonmetro counties throughout the 2010s, while beginning to level off in metro counties. In metro counties, rates from heroin deaths surpassed those for prescription deaths in 2015, and heroin remains a larger contributor to metro overdoses than to nonmetro overdoses. Synthetic opioids, like fentanyl, are 50–100 times more potent than morphine and

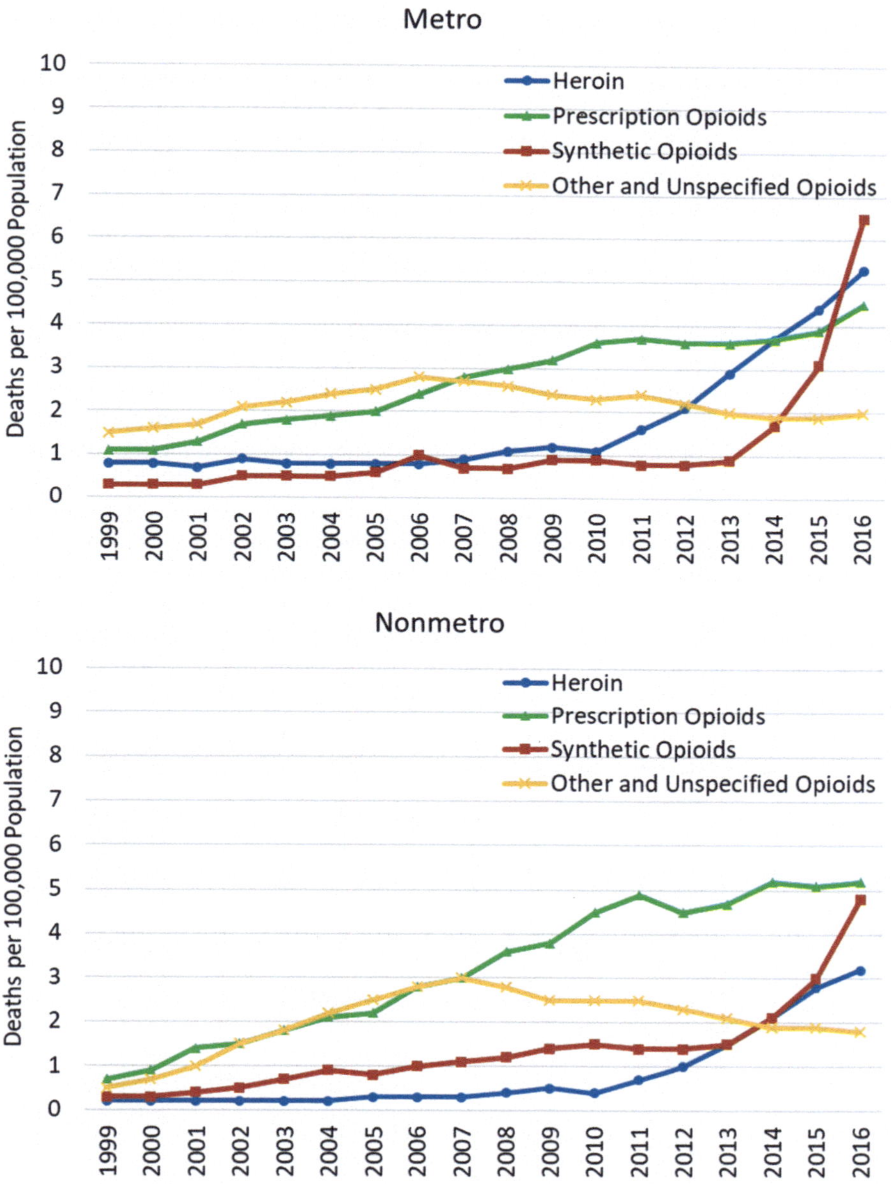

Fig. 1 Fatal opioid overdose rates by type of opioid for metro and nonmetro counties, 1999–2016. Note: Rates are age adjusted. Source: National Center for Health Statistics, CDC, 2018a, 2018b

are increasingly mixed (both intentionally and non-intentionally) with heroin, cocaine, and other substances, drastically increasing the risk of overdose. Synthetic opioid deaths have surged since 2014 in both metro and nonmetro counties, particularly in the northeastern region of the U.S. As of 2016, synthetic opioids are the primary contributor to overdoses in metro areas, and trends suggest that synthetic opioids are likely to become the main contributor to overdoses in nonmetro areas in the coming years.

The aggregate mortality rates discussed thus far mask considerable regional variation in opioid deaths and variation across gradations of metropolitan status. Rates of opioid-related hospital admissions and emergency department (ED) visits are high in some predominantly rural areas, including Appalachia, New England, and the Mountain West, but rates have remained relatively low in other predominantly rural areas, such as the Delta South and upper Great Plains (Keyes et al., 2014).

As shown in Fig. 2, opioid mortality rates are highest and have risen most sharply among Midwestern large central metro counties (i.e., counties in metropolitan statistical areas with populations of 1 million or more). In the northeast, rates have been highest outside of large central metro counties, with comparable rates between large fringe metro, medium/small metro, and nonmetro counties. Large increases in rates since the early 2010s in northeastern and midwestern counties are largely attributable to fentanyl and other synthetic opioids. Rates are comparatively lower in the South and West, with the lowest rates found among large metro counties in the West. Only in the western U.S. do nonmetro counties have higher opioid mortality

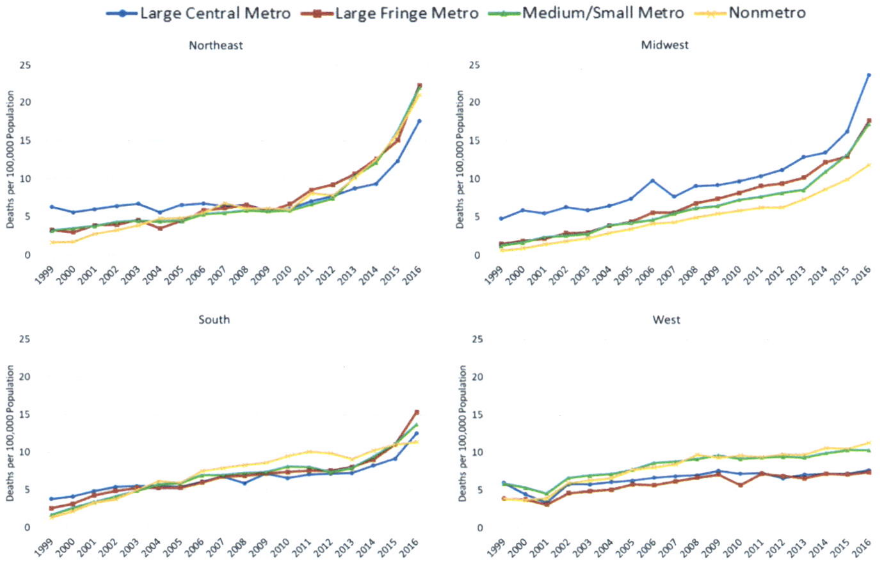

Fig. 2 Fatal opioid overdose rates by region and metro status. Note: Rates are age adjusted. Source: National Center for Health Statistics, CDC, 2018a, 2018b

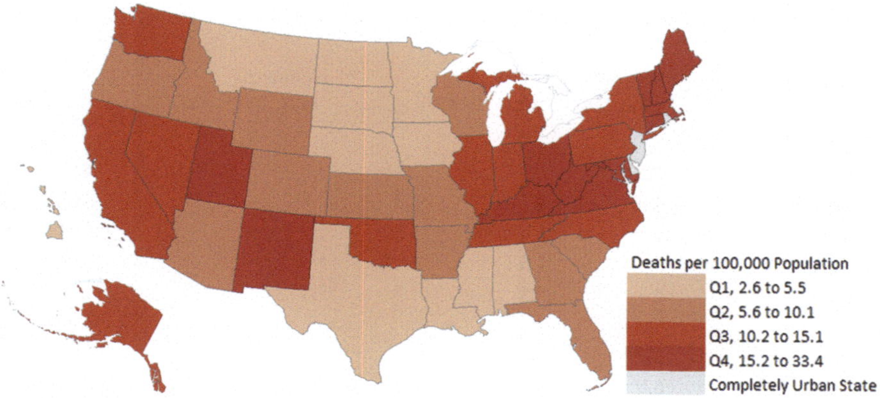

Fig. 3 Fatal opioid overdose rates for nonmetro counties, 2014–16 (age adjusted). Source: National Center for Health Statistics, CDC, 2018a, 2018b

rates than metro counties, yet nonmetro rates in the West remain lower than nonmetro rates in the other three regions.

There is also substantial *within-region* variation in nonmetro opioid mortality rates. Figure 3 shows rates only for nonmetro counties in each state, 2014–16. Nonmetro opioid mortality rates were highest in West Virginia (33.4 per 100,000), Connecticut (26.5), New Hampshire (24.2), Massachusetts (22.4), and Ohio (21.6). Rates were substantially lower among the nonmetro counties in Nebraska (2.6), Alabama (3.2), South Dakota (3.6), Louisiana (4.1), and Texas (4.4). Harrison County, KY has the highest fatal drug overdose rate in the country. Most of the counties in the top 100 are within the heart of Appalachia, but also include many tribal communities—places with intergenerational poverty and little opportunity for upward mobility. I will return to the economic context of the U.S. opioid crisis later in the chapter.

Demographic Differences in Opioid Mortality

Substantial media and scholarly attention has been paid to the fact that fatal opioid overdose rates are highest and have risen most sharply among middle-aged non-Hispanic whites (particularly without a four-year college degree) over the past two decades (Case & Deaton, 2015, 2017; Monnat, 2017). Table 1 shows demographic differences in fatal opioid overdose rates across metro and nonmetro counties. In both metro and nonmetro counties, rates are highest among non-Hispanic whites and American Indians, males, and individuals aged 25–54 years. Several other key findings are worth highlighting. First, fatal opioid overdose rates are much lower among nonmetro blacks compared to metro blacks, a difference that partly explains why fatal opioid overdose rates are comparatively lower in many southern states,

Table 1 Fatal opioid overdose rates by demographic group and metro status, 2000–02 and 2014–16

	Metro			Nonmetro		
	2000–2002	2014–2016	% change	2000–2002	2014–2016	% change
Race/ethnicity						
NH White	4.5	16.0	255.6	3.0	13.0	333.3
NH Black	4.6	8.7	89.1	0.8	3.3	312.5
NH American Indian	4.6	15.3	232.6	2.7	12.4	359.3
Asian/Pacific Islander	0.4	1.3	225.0	NA	2.1	NA
Hispanic	3.4	5.5	61.8	2.5	5.2	108.0
Sex						
Female	2.3	7.8	239.1	1.8	8.7	383.3
Male	6.0	16.0	166.7	3.6	13.6	277.8
Age group						
15–24	2.7	8.2	203.7	2.0	5.7	185.0
25–34	5.4	21.7	301.9	4.1	20.9	409.8
35–44	9.6	20.4	112.5	6.5	22.2	241.5
45–54	8.6	20.0	132.6	4.7	19.7	319.1
55–64	2.6	15.3	488.5	1.5	11.7	680.0
65+	0.8	3.5	337.5	0.4	2.5	525.0

Notes: Rates are age adjusted; *NA* rate suppressed by CDC (<10 deaths in this group over this time period); *NH* non-Hispanic
Source: National Center for Health Statistics, CDC (2018a, 2018b)

where virtually all the nation's rural blacks reside (U.S. Census, 2015). Second, whereas metro males have higher fatal opioid overdose rates than nonmetro males, the reverse is true for females; nonmetro females had a mortality rate of 8.7 per 100,000 in 2014–16, compared to 7.8 for metro females. Moreover, the nonmetro female opioid mortality rate increased by 383% between 2000 and 2016, a much larger increase than for metro females or metro and nonmetro males. Third, although working-age adults (in both metro and nonmetro counties) continue to have higher fatal opioid overdose rates than younger and older adults, the largest increase in mortality rates since the early 2000s has been among nonmetro individuals aged 55 years or older.

Opioid Crisis in the Broader Rural Health Context

It is important to consider the current opioid problem within the context of rural health more generally. After decades of lower or nearly comparable all-cause mortality rates in rural than in urban areas, a rural mortality penalty emerged in the 1980s and has grown in each subsequent decade (Cosby et al., 2008). This trend reversal was due in part to smaller improvements in heart disease mortality in rural than in urban areas (Cossman, James, Cosby, & Cossman, 2010), but increases in drug and alcohol deaths and suicides (the so-called *deaths of despair*) in rural areas have also contributed to the growing gap (Fontanella et al., 2015; Singh & Siahpush, 2014).

Table 2 shows age-adjusted rates for all-cause mortality and for specific major causes of death in the U.S. for 2000–2002 and 2014–2016 for metro and nonmetro counties and by region among nonmetro counties. Nonmetro counties have higher all-cause mortality rates and have experienced smaller declines in all-cause mortality than metro counties over this period. Nationally, declines in all-cause mortality since the early 2000s have been driven by declines in mortality from heart disease (the largest contributor to death), cancer, stroke, and diabetes. However, declines in mortality from these causes have been smaller in nonmetro than in metro counties. Moreover, as with opioid mortality, rates and changes in rates for these major chronic causes of death vary substantially across regions. Among nonmetro counties, mortality rates from heart disease, cancer, chronic obstructive pulmonary disease (COPD), stroke, and diabetes are highest in the south. Nonmetro counties in the west have comparatively lower rates of mortality from heart disease, cancer, and diabetes, despite having higher rates of death from suicide and alcohol-induced causes (primarily cirrhosis of the liver and alcoholic liver disease).

Although opioids have received significant media and political attention of late, the U.S. is really facing a triple set of epidemics—drugs, alcohol, and suicide—constituting three of the most serious public health crises of the century. Over 2 million people have died from drug overdoses, alcohol, and suicides since 2000, and life expectancy among NH whites in the U.S. declined two years in a row, due almost entirely to these three causes (Case & Deaton, 2017). Rates of death from two of these causes (alcohol and suicide) are significantly higher and have increased more in rural areas (see Table 2; also see Fontanella et al., 2015; Ivey-Stephenson, Crosby, Jack, Haileyesus, & Kresnow-Sedacca, 2017; Kegler, Stone, & Holland, 2017; Nestadt, Triplett, Fowler, & Mojtabai, 2017). The nonmetro West has particularly high rates of mortality from suicide and alcohol, whereas the nonmetro Northeast and Midwest have particularly high rates of drug poisoning.

Despite the recent surge in opioid mortality, substance use problems are not new to rural areas. Indeed, many rural parts of the U.S. have long struggled with alcohol use disorders and the production and use of illicit substances like methamphetamine. Moreover, smoking prevalence is higher in rural than in urban areas, even after adjusting for demographic and psychosocial differences, and the rural smoking disparity has widened over the past decade (Doogan et al., 2017).

Methamphetamine use has long been a problem in many rural areas (Reding, 2009). An often-ignored reality is that methamphetamine is affecting rural communities that have remained relatively immune to the opioid crisis, including communities in Iowa and Nebraska. Local anecdotal reports suggest that methamphetamine may be overtaking heroin as the predominant drug problem in some places (Hernandez & Radnovich, 2018; Rezvani, 2018; Robles, 2018). Domestic production of methamphetamine has declined each year since 2010, but inbound seizures of meth from Mexico have increased (Drug Enforcement Administration, 2017). Although methamphetamine kills far fewer people than

Table 2 Mortality rates for major causes of death by metro status, 2000–2002 and 2014–2016

			Nonmetro only			
	Metro	Nonmetro	Northeast	Midwest	South	West
All-cause mortality						
2000–02	849.7	914.6	856.5	853.1	1000.7	846.4
2014–16	707.9	838.8	762.6	792.4	924.1	746.5
% change	−16.7	−8.3	−11.0	−7.1	−7.7	−11.8
Drug poisoning (accidental and unknown intent)						
2000–02	6.0	4.5	3.7	3.0	5.3	6.4
2014–16	15.4	15.4	20.0	13.9	15.5	15.4
% change	156.7	242.2	440.5	363.3	192.5	140.6
Drug poisoning (intentional)						
2000–02	1.3	1.2	1.1	1.1	1.2	1.8
2014–16	1.5	1.6	2.0	1.5	1.4	2.4
% change	15.4	33.3	81.8	36.4	16.7	33.3
Suicide (other than drug induced)						
2000–02	9.0	12.1	10.4	10.9	12.1	16.6
2014–16	11.0	15.9	13.8	14.8	15.4	21.6
% change	22.2	31.4	32.7	35.8	27.3	30.1
Alcohol						
2000–02	12.3	12.0	10.0	9.4	12.9	17.5
2014–16	13.7	16.2	12.7	13.5	16.2	25.0
% change	11.4	35.0	27.0	43.6	25.6	42.9
Heart disease						
2000–02	254.1	272.3	266.7	254.0	305.2	218.0
2014–16	168.7	203.2	187.0	190.0	230.5	163.8
% change	−33.6	−25.4	−29.9	−25.2	−24.5	−24.9
Cancer						
2000–02	192.9	202.7	200.0	196.4	213.6	186.8
2014–16	152.6	174.7	168.3	172.2	185.7	152.3
% change	−20.9	−13.8	−15.9	−12.3	−13.1	−18.5
COPD						
2000–02	42.7	49.3	48.7	46.0	51.5	52.2
2014–16	38.3	53.6	45.9	51.6	59.0	48.0
% change	−10.3	8.7	−5.7	12.2	14.6	−8.0
Stroke						
2000–02	57.6	64.1	53.9	60.4	71.3	59.4
2014–16	36.3	41.3	33.3	38.9	47.0	36.3
% change	−37.0	−35.6	−38.2	−35.6	−34.1	−38.9
Diabetes						
2000–02	24.9	27.4	24.9	26.1	29.9	24.9
2014–16	20.2	25.5	22.2	24.0	28.4	22.5
% change	−18.9	−6.9	−10.8	−8.0	−5.0	−9.6

Source: National Center for Health Statistics, CDC (2018a, 2018b)

Note: Rates are age adjusted and represent deaths per 100,000 population; % change is based on author's calculations opioids, it has devastating impacts on the physical and mental health of users, including anxiety, confusion, insomnia, hallucinations, paranoia, violent behavior, and severe tooth decay and skin sores (National Institute on Drug Abuse, 2013). The impact on families and local communities is also substantial and includes criminal activity, family/child neglect, poor work performance, and environmental contamination (Donnermeyer & Tunnell, 2007).

As shown in Fig. 4, since the mid-2000s, the fatal overdose rate from benzodiazepines (a class of psychoactive prescription drugs used to treat anxiety, insomnia, epilepsy, and alcohol dependence) has been higher in nonmetro versus metro counties. Rates of fatal overdose from psychostimulants (predominantly methamphetamine) have been higher in nonmetro than metro counties since the early 2010s. Importantly, over half of drug overdoses involve more than one drug (Rigg, Monnat, & Chavez, 2018). Although the concurrent use of opioids with benzodiazepines and the lacing of cocaine with fentanyl have contributed to increases in overdose rates from these drugs, the fact that rates from cocaine and benzodiazepines continue to rise is evidence that the problem is bigger than opioids.

That the geographic patterns for drug, alcohol, and suicide mortality vary from those for the chronic diseases presented in Table 2 suggests that the forces contributing to geographic variation in chronic disease may vary somewhat from the forces contributing to geographic variation in drug, alcohol, and suicide mortality. I now turn to a discussion of the causes of the opioid crisis and potential explanations for geographic variation in drug mortality rates.

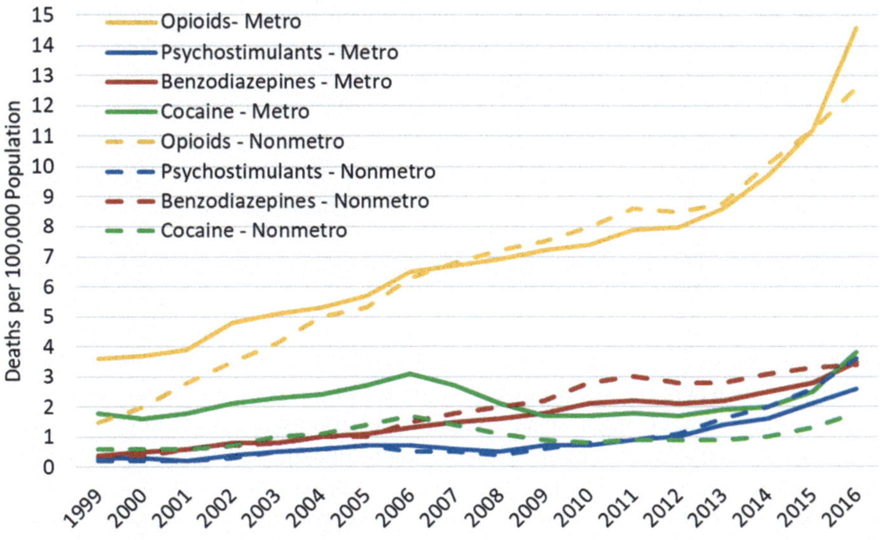

Fig. 4 Mortality rates for specific drugs, by metro status, 1999–2016 (age adjusted). Source: National Center for Health Statistics, CDC (2018a, 2018b)

What Caused the Opioid Crisis? The Spark versus the Kindling

The Spark: Pills, Pills, and More Pills

For good reason, substantial criticism has been levied against the major pharmaceutical companies who manufactured and aggressively marketed prescription opioids and the physicians who overprescribed them (Kolodny et al., 2015; Van Zee, 2009). Opioids were not always widely prescribed for everyday chronic pain. They were once reserved primarily for traumatic injury victims and terminal cancer patients. Beginning in the 1990s, however, pain advocates in the U.S. pushed to get pain recognized as the *fifth vital sign*. They argued that pain is just as important to measure as body temperature, pulse, respiration, and blood pressure. Physicians were encouraged to ask patients about their pain and medicate them for it.

In 1996, pharmaceutical company Purdue Pharma introduced an extended-release oxycodone product to the market—OxyContin®. Purdue capitalized on the pain advocacy campaign of the 1990s and heavily marketed OxyContin® for everyday pain in a way that was unprecedented for a Schedule 2 drug (Quinones, 2015; Van Zee, 2009). Purdue claimed OxyContin® was less addictive than other opioid products and did not provoke withdrawal symptoms because its time-release formula allowed for delayed drug absorption. This made physicians comfortable in prescribing it for a wide range of chronic ailments, from back pain to headaches to menstrual cramps, and for minor surgeries such as wisdom teeth extraction. However, not only was OxyContin® far more potent than other opioid painkillers, but people with addictions quickly learned they could crush, liquefy, and inject the tablets to experience the full dose at once.

Purdue encouraged their sales reps to aggressively market OxyContin® to physicians, especially in places where other opioids were already heavily prescribed (Van Zee, 2009). Representatives from Purdue and other pharmaceutical companies targeted the lowest hanging fruit—the injured and jobless and people on disability with Medicaid, particularly in Appalachia's rural communities (Quinones, 2015; Van Zee, 2009). Although some physicians remained skeptical about using opioids to treat chronic pain and fearful of the addiction risk, others prescribed liberally. Still others viewed the increased demand for prescription opioids as an entrepreneurial opportunity. Enter high-volume prescribing pain clinics (i.e., pill mills)—establishments where physicians doled out prescriptions for OxyContin® and other opioids, often without much or any diagnosis or follow-up. As Quinones (2015) illustrates in his book, *Dreamland*, patients would line up, pay cash, and leave with hundreds of pills, some of which they used themselves but most of which they would sell. These clinics first popped up in the most economically depressed regions of Ohio, Kentucky, and West Virginia in the late 1990s and then spread across the country (Quinones, 2015). In the late 1990s, in some states with large rural populations, such as Maine, West Virginia, eastern Kentucky, southwestern Virginia, and Alabama, hydrocodone and oxycodone (non-OxyContin) were prescribed at a rate

2.5-5 times the national average. By 2000 in these same places, OxyContin® prescribing rates were 5-6 times higher than the national average (Van Zee, 2009). It is no coincidence that these were the first areas to experience widespread increases in opioid misuse, diversion, overdose, and demand for substance abuse treatment.

As physicians, state health officials, and policymakers caught on to the surge in prescription opioid addiction and diversion, prescription opioids became much more expensive and difficult to obtain. Sam Quinones (2015) describes how small cells of poor rural farm boys from the tiny Mexican town of Xalisco, Nayarit expanded their heroin business from California to small cities and towns throughout the U.S. in the 1990s and 2000s. The dispersion of Hispanics to new destinations across the U.S. in the 1990s (Kandel & Parrado, 2005) enabled the Xalisco boys to blend in and expand to small cities like Nashville, Columbus, Charlotte, and Omaha. Poverty, the desire to escape grueling farm labor, and dreams of prosperity were what brought these young rancheros to the U.S. in the first place. Recognizing the demand created by reductions in the prescription opioid supply, the Xalisco boys headed east to capitalize on the demand from small cities and rural towns already made vulnerable by economic turbulence and OxyContin®.

The Xalisco drug network and the cartels that followed illustrate a "*new rural order*, characterized by dramatic and rapid transformations in American rural life that are, in part, a consequence of growing economic interdependencies with urban centers" (Burton, Lichter, Baker, & Eason, 2013, p. 1129). These growing interdependencies between rural and urban areas (Lichter & Ziliak, 2017) have implications for narcotics distribution. Heroin was once largely an urban problem, but it is now routinely sold in many parts of the rural U.S. where it had been absent, due in large part to fluid and shifting boundaries between rural and urban areas.

Some economists argue that the opioid crisis has been driven entirely by changes to drug environments—namely the surge in prescription opioids—rather than economic or other social conditions (Currie, Jin, & Schnell, 2018; Ruhm, 2018). To be sure, the emergence and widespread availability of powerful and incredibly addictive prescriptive opioids was an essential spark for the opioid epidemic. But you cannot start a fire without kindling. I now turn to a discussion of that kindling.

The Kindling: Economic, Family, and Social Distress

It is not a coincidence that the pharmaceutical companies targeted and widespread opioid prescribing first emerged in places considered to be among the most economically vulnerable in the U.S. Thanks to economic restructuring and 40+ years of federal deregulation, devolution, and disinvestments in education and the social safety net (Lobao, 2014), many places in the U.S. were primed to be vulnerable to opioids–drugs that numb both physical and psychological pain. Although overdose rate increases over the past two decades have been largely driven by a surge in opioid overdoses, deaths involving other drugs, alcohol, and suicides also increased over this period (Monnat, 2017). Supply-side factors cannot explain these trends.

Drug, alcohol, and suicide deaths are not a random collection; they often derive from depression, hopelessness, and chronic pain (Cheatle, 2011; Russ et al., 2015), leading some to refer to them as *deaths of despair* (Case & Deaton, 2017; Monnat, 2016). Especially striking is that rates for all three increased during a period of declining mortality for other major causes of death, including heart disease and cancer, as shown in Table 2.

Geographic differences in population health are driven by complex interactions between economic and political structures, human capital, and the relative vulnerability of residents (Brown & Swanson, 2003; Lobao, 2004; Lobao & Saenz, 2002; Lobao, Zhou, Partridge, & Betz, 2016). Therefore, we cannot fully understand the widespread geographic and demographic variation in opioid misuse and mortality without considering its social and economic determinants (Dasgupta, Beletsky, & Ciccarone, 2018). Social determinants of health are the structural conditions in which people live, work, and socialize that influence stress, health behaviors, and mortality, including economic resources, social relationships, and labor markets (Solar & Irwin, 2010). Slow-moving stressors that manifested over the past 40 years (e.g., industrial transformation, wage stagnation, rising income inequality) and short-term economic and policy shocks (e.g., the Great Recession, austerity, federal safety net policy changes) have had disproportionally negative effects on rural communities. The effects are due to greater concentrations of low-SES residents in rural communities, less diversified labor markets, thinner and weaker institutions, and state and local fiscal decisions (Bailey, Jensen, & Ransom, 2014; Lobao, Hooks, & Tickamyer, 2007). Over the past 40 years, employment restructuring led to the movement of many livable-wage production jobs out of rural areas and the concentration of high-wage high-skill service, finance, and technology-based employment in urban cores (Bailey et al., 2014; Brown & Swanson, 2003; Lobao, 2014; Peters, 2013; Smith & Tickamyer, 2011). This has resulted in wage polarization (Peters, 2012) with fewer, lower wage, and less secure employment opportunities for rural residents (Burton et al., 2013; Slack, 2014).

Selective out-migration of the "best and brightest" (Carr & Kefalas, 2009) intensified the disproportionate geographic clustering of multigenerational economic distress in many rural areas. Research from both urban and rural sociology demonstrates that concentrated and multigenerational economic disadvantage can contribute to collective frustration and hopelessness, lower tax bases, community disinvestments, infrastructural decay, family disintegration, crime, and substance misuse (Brown & Swanson, 2003; Carr & Kefalas, 2009; McLean, 2016; Sampson & Groves, 1989; Smith & Tickamyer, 2011). As a result, a growing body of evidence suggests there are strong associations between macro-level economic distress and poor mental health, suicide, and substance abuse (Frasquilho et al., 2016; Hempstead & Phillips, 2015; Kaplan et al., 2015; Kerr et al., 2017).

It may come as no surprise then, that fatal opioid overdose rates are highest and have increased the most in nonmetro counties with economies dependent on the mining industry (see Fig. 5). Counties dependent on industries like mining and manufacturing have suffered substantial employment downturns and wage stagna-

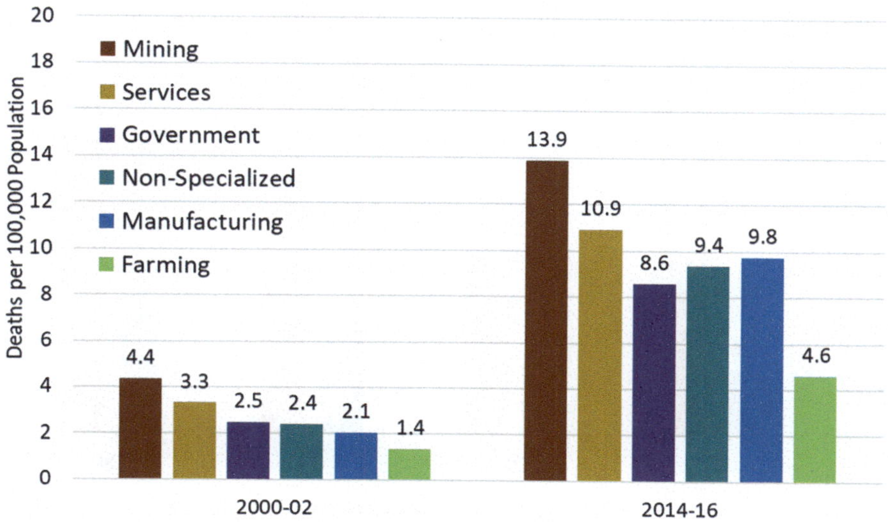

Fig. 5 Average county fatal opioid overdose rate by economic dependence type, 2000–02 and 2014–16 (Nonmetro counties only). Source: Author's calculations from National Center for Health Statistics, National Vital Statistics System, restricted-access mortality micro data, 2000-2016. Notes: Means are adjusted for the following county-level variables from the 2000 U.S. Census: percent non-Hispanic black, American Indian, veterans, and aged 65 years or older; Economic dependency categories are based on the USDA Economic Research Service County Typology codes for 2004

tion in recent decades, making them high-risk environments for substance misuse (Keyes et al., 2014; McLean, 2016). Moreover, as previously explained, OxyContin® and other strong opioids were heavily marketed in mining-dependent Appalachian communities long before they spread across the rest of the U.S. (Keyes et al., 2014; Quinones, 2015). In fact, with such close ties to this region, OxyContin® was once referred to as "hillbilly heroin" (Inciardi, Surratt, Cicero, & Beard, 2009). In old factory and mining towns where good-paying jobs disappeared long ago, and in places where strong manufacturing employment was replaced by low-paying and nonsecure service occupations, opioids became the only currency (Macy, 2018; Quinones, 2015); selling them was one of the only ways to make money (Jonas, Young, Oser, Leukefeld, & Havens, 2012). The differential distribution of overdose rates across communities with different industrial structures can lend insights about how economic conditions from decades ago may be contributing to today's drug problems.

Figure 6 shows average county-level fatal opioid overdose rates and rates from overdoses involving any drug in 2014-16 for nonmetro counties at each quartile of economic distress in 2000. I measure economic distress using a factor-weighted index (Cronbach's alpha=0.83) composed of standardized (z-scored) U.S. Census 2000 values for county-level percent poverty, percent unemployed, percent not in

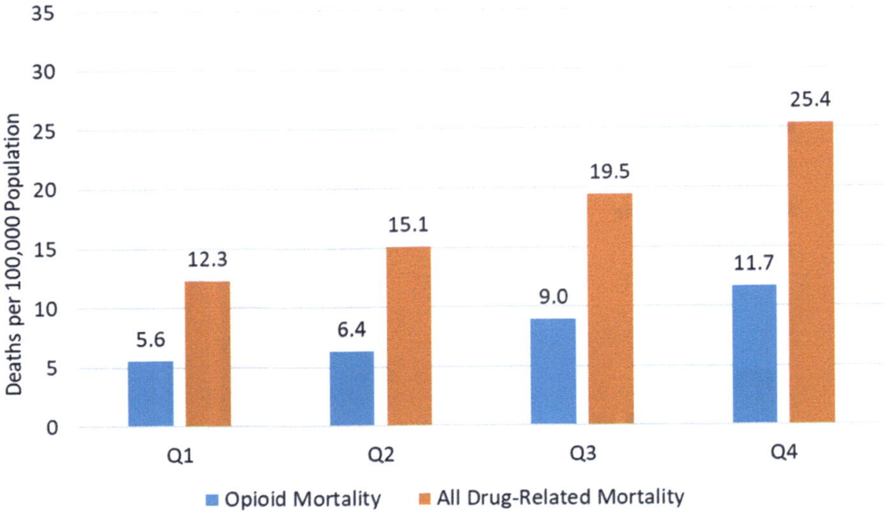

Fig. 6 Average fatal overdose rates in 2014–16 by the level of economic distress in 2000 (Nonmetro counties only). Note: Rates are age adjusted. Source: Author's calculations from National Center for Health Statistics, National Vital Statistics System, restricted-access mortality micro data, 2014–2016

the labor force, percent age 25+ years with less than a four-year college degree, percentage of households receiving public assistance, and the ratio of state-to-county median household income. I use measures from the 2000 U.S. Census rather than more recent estimates from the American Community Survey (ACS) to minimize reverse causality bias and allow for a lagged effect of economic distress on mortality. Means are adjusted for county percent black, American Indian, foreign-born, veterans, and residents aged 65 years and older to account for compositional differences across quartiles of economic distress.

For both opioid overdose specifically, and all-drug overdoses more generally, average rates are higher at higher levels of economic distress. For example, compared to counties in the lowest quartile of economic distress, counties in the highest quartile have an average of 13.1 more drug deaths per 100,000 population per year. This equates to approximately 1,750 excess deaths annually among nonmetro counties in the highest versus lowest quartile of economic distress. Importantly, it is not just one specific component of the economic distress index driving these differences. The pattern holds for each of the economic indicators that comprise the index; higher levels of distress equate with higher average drug mortality rates. The past-decade surge in opioid (and other self-harm) deaths corresponds with significant economic challenges, including long-term deindustrialization, growing income inequality, and increased geographic concentration of poverty (Iceland & Hernandez, 2017; Saez & Zucman, 2016). Moreover, economic disadvantage has emerged in once prosperous middle- and working class communities (Alexander,

2017; Quinones, 2015; Thiede, Kim, & Valasik, 2018), where residents long accustomed to financial security and feelings of control over their destinies—fundamental social determinants of health (Syme, 1989; Whitehead et al., 2016)—suddenly find themselves powerless (Chen, 2015; Newman, 1999). Economic insecurity, including poverty and joblessness, can threaten individual identity, leading to unmet expectations, barriers to desired role attainment, and social and economic exclusion (Catalano & Dooley, 1983; Whitehead et al., 2016). For example, prime-age men who are not in the labor force experience notably lower levels of emotional well-being, derive relatively little meaning from their daily activities, and are more likely than working men to feel pain and take pain medication daily (Krueger, 2017), all of which may explain increased rates of substance abuse and overdose (Ahmedani et al., 2017).

Economic distress is often accompanied by family distress, like marital disintegration and multiple partner fertility (Burton et al., 2013), which are important distal risk factors for substance abuse (Ananat, Gassman-Pines, Francis, & Gibson-Davis, 2017; Frasquilho et al., 2016; Olfson et al., 2017). Despite the myth of stronger families and more traditional family values in rural areas, the past two decades have been witness to increases in single-parent households, nonmarital cohabitation, and multiple partner fertility in rural areas (Burton et al., 2013), and a greater share of births are to unmarried mothers in rural than in urban areas (Livingston, 2018). The disadvantages associated with these family structures can undermine health behaviors and often manifest themselves in poor health outcomes (Burton et al., 2013).

Differences in fatal overdose rates between counties in the lowest versus highest quartiles of family distress are shown in Fig. 7. Family distress is measured with U.S. Census 2000 values for county-level percentage of families with children headed by a single parent and percent divorced or separated. As with economic distress, counties characterized by higher levels of family distress in 2000 had higher average opioid mortality rates and drug mortality rates overall in 2014-16 than counties with less family distress, net of controls for county racial/ethnic, veteran, and age composition.

The economic and family factors contributing to geographic variation in opioid and other drug mortality are universal along the rural–urban continuum (Monnat, 2018). However, the relationship between both economic and family distress and drug mortality rates is stronger in rural counties; differences in average rates between the lowest and highest quartiles of economic and family distress and mortality rates are larger in rural counties.

As sociologist Emile Durkheim (Durkheim, 1897/1966) argued over 120 years ago, social integration is a key factor in explaining self-harm behaviors. During periods of serious social or economic upheaval, social cohesion declines, risk of disconnection (anomie) increases, and self-harm behaviors, such as suicide, increase (Durkheim, 1897/1966). Along these lines, hopelessness and dislocation may be the ties that bind distressed economic and family conditions to increases in opioid misuse and mortality.

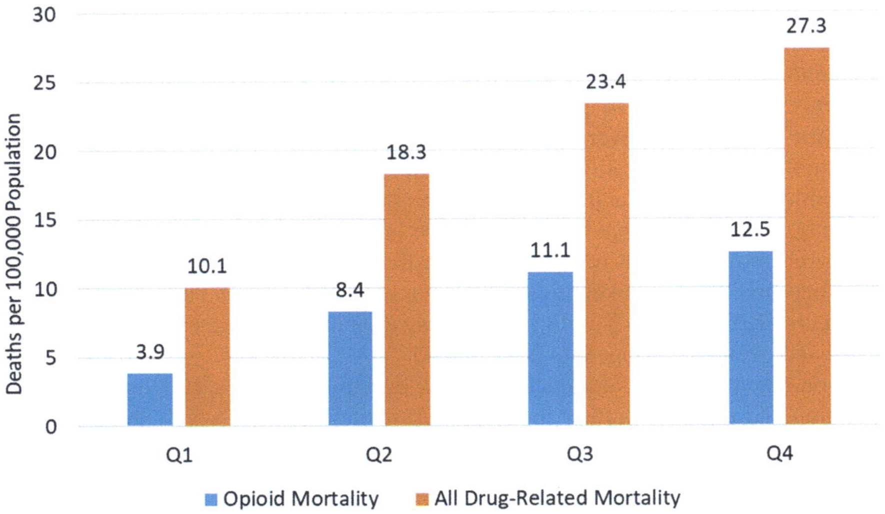

Fig. 7 Average mortality rates in 2014–16 by the level of family distress in 2000 (Nonmetro Counties Only). Note: Rates are age adjusted. Source: Author's calculations from National Center for Health Statistics, National Vital Statistics System, restricted-access mortality micro data, 2014–2016

Special Rural Challenges

Despite the fact that the opioid crisis is not disproportionately worse, on average, in rural than in urban areas, several features of rural communities have exacerbated the problem and have made addressing drug addiction and other health problems more difficult in rural areas, especially those that have been hardest hit. First, rural areas are home to disproportionate shares of populations who are at risk of substance misuse, including American Indians, military veterans, the elderly, the disabled, individuals who suffer from chronic pain, manual laborers, and the poor (Havens et al., 2011; Keyes et al., 2014; Rigg & Monnat, 2015; Van Gundy, 2006).

Second, adequately addressing and preventing addiction requires addressing structural needs, such as secure employment, affordable housing, and physical and mental health care, all of which are in short supply in many rural communities. Access to primary health care may facilitate preventive health interventions that protect against injury risk or long-term chronic pain and disability for which opioids are commonly prescribed. Access to mental health care may facilitate necessary substance abuse treatment. However, physical and mental health care, substance use treatment, and harm reduction programs tend to be more limited in rural areas, have a more limited range of services, and require longer travel distances (Borders & Booth, 2007). Even when such services are available, lack of privacy and stigma may be a greater barrier to treatment use among rural than urban residents (Pullen & Oser, 2014). Due to further distance to providers in rural areas, emergency medical responses to overdoses take longer, reducing the odds of survival (Hancock et al., 2017).

Third, an unintended consequence of the crackdown on opioid prescribing has been chronic pain patients reporting difficulty getting the opioids they need to manage pain. As chronic pain is more prevalent among rural than among urban residents (Day & Thorn, 2010), lack of access to opioid pain medication among those who need it for legitimate pain is having a disproportionate impact in rural communities (Stone, 2018).

Fourth, opioid addiction has led to significant increases in drug arrests, incarceration, and jail overcrowding in rural areas (Levin & Haugen, 2018). Although urban counties have higher drug arrest rates, rural counties have experienced larger increases in drug arrests since 2013. By and large, rural communities do not have the infrastructure, including beds, pretrial services, supervisory staff, and substance treatment case managers, to absorb these large increases. Based on current trends, the backlog of drug cases in rural communities will continue to mount, meaning that more individuals struggling with addiction will languish in jail without treatment while they await pretrial sentencing.

Finally, as discussed in more detail later, the opioid crisis has led to increases in child protective service reports and foster care placements (National Advisory Committee on Rural Health and Human Services, 2016), thereby exacerbating already-existing service shortages in many rural communities.

Consequences of the Opioid Crisis in the Rural U.S.

The mortality data presented earlier represent only a tiny fraction of those suffering from substance abuse disorders, and the effects ripple beyond those who die to include families, friends, first responders, service providers, and employers. Nationally, the cost of the opioid crisis, including health care, criminal justice, lost productivity, and value of lives lost is now estimated at $504 billion annually, representing 2.8% of GDP (Council of Economic Advisors, 2017). In terms of employment, we have come full circle with the opioid crisis. High rates of unemployment and job displacement fueled the despair and hopelessness that gave way to widespread opioid addiction. Now employers report having a difficult time finding employees who can pass a drug test. Widespread drug abuse hinders the growth of industry and makes it difficult for communities to attract new residents. This has severe long-term implications for rural economic development.

Beyond these material impacts, there are additional costs to families, children, and communities. The opioid crisis has major implications for changing family forms in rural areas. Substance misuse contributes to serious family trauma, including conflicts between partners, physical, verbal, and emotional abuse, and adverse health and development risks for children. Although comprehensive research is sparse, emerging evidence suggests that opioid addiction is exacerbating and complicating the already high prevalence of domestic violence in rural areas (Davidov et al., 2017). In addition to more domestic violence incidents involving an addicted party, shelters are experiencing increased demand from more domestic violence victims struggling with opioid addiction (Driscoll, 2017).

The opioid crisis is also having direct impacts on children. Children exposed to parental substance misuse have increased emotional and behavioral problems and difficulties establishing attachments and trusting relationships (Smith, 2018). Adverse childhood experiences, such as abuse, witnessing parental domestic violence, and parental incarceration and death place children at higher risk of developing substance abuse and mental health disorders in adulthood (Monnat & Chandler, 2015). In addition to the emotional trauma, the death or incarceration of a parent due to drugs often results in the residential displacement of children. State child welfare systems have reported increases in substance abuse problems among the families who are brought to their attention (National Advisory Committee on Rural Health and Human Services, 2016).

Parental drug addiction and overdose have led to a record number of children entering the foster care system. In West Virginia, the state with the highest overdose rate, foster care placements have increased by 42% since 2014, and placements are up by over 30% in Alabama, Alaska, California, Idaho, Minnesota, and New Hampshire (Birnbaum & Lora, 2018). In both North Carolina (Gebelein, 2018) and New Hampshire (Smith, 2018), drugs were listed as a factor in over half of all out-of-home placements in 2016. Just as with the urban crack-cocaine epidemic of the 1980s and 1990s, more rural grandparents are now raising their grandchildren than at any point in recent history because their own children are addicted to drugs, incarcerated, or have died from overdose. In 2005, 2.5 million children were living with custodial grandparents. By 2015, that number had increased to 2.9 million (Wiltz, 2016). This has important implications for rural communities, where economic resources and housing for older populations are already limited.

Other health crises have unfolded as a manifestation of opioid addiction. A record high percentage of children are born with neonatal abstinence syndrome (NAS; Smith, 2018), a condition that can lead to extended hospital stays, risk of complications, and delays in child development (Bradley, 2018). Between 2000 and 2012, the percentage of babies born with NAS in the U.S. increased fivefold (Patrick, Davis, Lehman, & Cooper, 2015), and the incidence of maternal opioid use and NAS are disproportionately higher in rural versus urban counties (Ko et al., 2016; Villapiano et al., 2017). The opioid crisis is also facilitating the spread of infectious diseases. In 2015, an HIV infection outbreak spread through a network of persons who inject drugs (PWID; mostly young and white) in a small rural community in Scott County, Indiana. Out of a population of 4,200, at least 194 people were infected, and nearly 95% were also infected with Hepatitis C Virus (HCV). The CDC has identified another 220 counties across the U.S. that are vulnerable to the rapid spread of HIV and HCV due to larger networks of PWID (National Advisory Committee on Rural Health and Human Services, 2016). This and similar events represent a major shift in the geography of HIV; since the beginning of the U.S. HIV epidemic, most injection drug users who became infected were middle aged or older black men living in urban areas. Outbreaks like these strain local public health systems that, in rural areas, may already be struggling to serve residents' needs.

Promising Strategies for Addressing the Opioid Crisis

Many of the strategies for successfully addressing the opioid crisis are not specific to rural areas; they are universal to communities along the rural–urban continuum. Other efforts must pay particular attention to the unique population, economic, political, and social challenges in rural communities (Rigg et al., 2018; Rigg & Monnat, 2015). The most effective strategies will be those that consider treatment, recovery, harm reduction, and prevention, and that encompass both downstream and upstream approaches. The National Rural Health Association (Hancock et al., 2017), Rural Health Information Hub (2018), Centers for Disease Control and Prevention (2018), and United States Department of Agriculture (2018) have all developed prevention and treatment recommendations for how to combat substance use problems in rural communities and describe several national and local rural responses to the opioid crisis.

Many of the commonly recommended strategies include increasing availability of and access to treatment, particularly Medication Assisted Treatment (MAT), making Naloxone (the opioid antagonist used to reverse opioid overdoses, sold under the brand name, Narcan®) widely available, funding research on the development of new pain treatments, increasing adherence to evidence-based prescribing practices, and universal use of prescription drug-monitoring programs. Moreover, there is widespread acknowledgment among public health experts that repealing provisions of the Affordable Care Act will take away health insurance coverage from people who need mental health and substance abuse treatment and have disproportionate impacts on residents of rural communities.

Although many of the above recommendations are laudable, to date, interventions along these lines have been largely ineffective, as evidenced by the continued increase in opioid and increasingly other drug overdose rates. How to tackle the opioid crisis depends on exactly what problem we are trying to solve. Are we simply trying to save lives right now, or are we interested in dealing with the underlying causes that got us here in the first place? The biggest problem with U.S. public health is that we invest most of our resources in tackling problems after they emerge rather than investing in prevention. This explains why we spend more money on health care than any other advanced country and have less-than-mediocre results to show for all of that spending. We have disinvested in the very types of institutions that help build strong societies–including education and community. Thus far, interventions, recommendations, and the funding allocated to tackle the opioid crisis have disproportionately targeted downstream mechanisms, while upstream strategies that address prevention and promote opportunities for people to live happy and healthy lives have largely been ignored. As demonstrated throughout this chapter, our problem is bigger than opioids. Our problem is bigger than drugs altogether.

Until we deal with the underlying causes of despair, isolation, disconnection, and lack of opportunity and meaning, we will remain vulnerable to future drug epidemics. I highlight some promising upstream solutions below.

First, prevention programs can help reduce substance abuse in rural and urban communities alike, particularly when focused on adolescents. Programs using evidence-based strategies, such as the PROSPER Program (Iowa State University, 2018), that involve parents within schools and churches have been shown to build resilience and pro-social skills and reduce the risk of substance misuse, criminal behavioral, and teenage pregnancy.

Second, promoting opportunities for social interaction through churches, community associations, and sports and recreational centers can facilitate personal and community linkages, trust, goodwill, belonging, and social cohesion, which may buffer against isolation, depression, boredom, and substance misuse (Putnam, 2000; Yen & Syme, 1999). In previous research, I have shown that counties with a larger presence of social capital promoting institutions, such as churches and sports establishments, have lower average drug overdose rates (Monnat, 2018). Overall, rural communities may be advantaged by their comparatively higher community attachment and social capital, but there is a wide divergence in social capital across the U.S., with Midwestern farming-dependent counties having much greater comparative social capital than other rural regions (Rupasingha, Goetz, & Freshwater, 2006).

Third, insofar as federal economic and pharmaceutical regulatory policies have gotten us into this mess, the federal government has a role to play in addressing the crisis. Given the findings in this chapter related to economic distress and drug overdose rates, the most effective upstream solutions may well be a massive revitalization of the depressed economies of many rural communities and small cities. It is no coincidence that overdose rates are highest in places with the most depressed economies and labor markets that have hemorrhaged decent-paying and secure jobs over the past three decades. The U.S. unemployment rate is at its lowest point since before the Great Recession of 2007–2009. Yet, this official figure masks high rates of disgruntled and underemployed workers and working-age adults who are out of the labor force due to disability. Good economic policy is good public health policy. Real adjustment and forward-looking policy would mean offering practical training in the types of trades and skills that will be needed over the next couple of decades and working with companies to enact better transition programs for employees for when labor needs change or jobs are eliminated based on economic ebbs and flows. Corporations that shut down or relocate factories or downsize their workforces by replacing people with automation have not historically provided these kinds of transition services.

Revitalizing the U.S. economy for a wide swath of the U.S. population rather than just those living in fast-growing urban hubs may require something akin to the Marshall Plan. The Marshall Plan was a post-World War II initiative wherein the U.S. provided over $12 billion in aid to Western Europe (equivalent to $100 billion in current U.S. dollars) to rebuild war-torn regions, modernize industry, and improve prosperity. Although the U.S. is not currently recovering from the devastation of a World War, the long-term effects of economic restructuring, globalization, and government disinvestment–economic distress, family breakdown, loss of community cohesion, infrastructural decay–can be thought of as akin to the effects of war. A new Marshall Plan may seem like a radical proposal, but the opioid crisis and declining U.S. life expectancy more generally are radical problems. We did not get here overnight, and quick and easy fixes are not going to reverse this problem. This far-upstream approach is likely to have positive effects on not only reversing the opioid crisis, but on improving health and well-being more generally.

Although the federal government certainly has an essential role to play in reversing the opioid crisis and promoting public health more broadly, the solutions cannot be entirely federal government driven. Across the country, small grassroots efforts have emerged to fight back against addiction. These groups and task forces, composed of family members, first responders, law enforcement, the medical community, and public health professionals are coming together to build harm reduction programs, increase treatment access, and spread prevention information. Something bigger is happening, though; neighbors are meeting each other, coming together toward a common goal, and strengthening community cohesion. This cohesion is an important buffer against future problems. As Quinones (2015) so eloquently states in *Dreamland,* "The antidote to heroin is not Narcan. The antidote to heroin is community".

Conclusion

The countervailing cliché, used for the laudable aim of promoting sympathy about those affected by opioids, is that addiction does not discriminate. Technically this is true. It is not as though there is some magic immunity from addiction. The upside of the message is that it forces us to come to grips with the fact that addiction is not due to individual pathologies or the cultural problems of inner cities (as was the faulty perception during the crack-cocaine epidemic). However, it is also true that drug addiction and overdose rates are much higher among certain demographic groups and in certain geographic areas than in others. The risk of repeating the cliché that "addiction does not discriminate" is that resources and intervention efforts may not be appropriately targeted at the places with the greatest need.

The opioid addiction and overdose crisis is occurring within a larger context of other health problems and economic and family breakdown. Despite widespread media and political attention on opioids, we cannot lose sight of the fact that heart disease remains the largest killer in rural and urban areas alike. Moreover, the combined rate from alcohol-induced deaths and suicides remains higher than the rate for drug overdoses. In the current frenzy to get a tourniquet on the opioid crisis, we must not lose sight of these other major contributors to rural mortality.

As I have argued in this chapter, we cannot fully understand the widespread geographic and demographic variation in opioid misuse and mortality without considering its social and economic determinants. The opioid problem reflects economic and social conditions that prevailed decades ago with the dynamics playing out now.

References

Ahmedani, B. K., Peterson, E. L., Hu, Y., Rossom, R. C., Lynch, F., Lu, C. Y., … Simon, G. E. (2017). Major physical health conditions and risk of suicide. *American Journal of Preventive Medicine, 53*(3), 308–315. https://doi.org/10.1016/j.amepre.2017.04.001

Alexander, B. (2017). *Glass house: The 1% economy and the shattering of the all-American town*. New York: St. Martin's Press.

Ananat, E. O., Gassman-Pines, A., Francis, D. V., & Gibson-Davis, C. M. (2017). Linking job loss, inequality, mental health, and education. *Science, 356*(6343), 1127–1128. https://doi.org/10.1126/science.aam5347

Bailey, C., Jensen, L., & Ransom, E. (Eds.). (2014). *Rural America in a globalizing world: Problems and prospects for the 2010s*. Morgantown, WV: West Virginia University Press.

Birnbaum, E., & Lora, M. (2018, June). *Opioid crisis sending thousands of children into foster care*. The Hill. Retrieved from http://thehill.com/policy/healthcare/393129-opioid-crisis-sending-thousands-of-children-into-foster-care?userid=50245.

Borders, T. F., & Booth, B. M. (2007). Research on rural residence and access to drug abuse services: Where are we and where do we go? *Journal of Rural Health, 23*(S1), 79–83. https://doi.org/10.1111/j.1748-0361.2007.00128.x

Bradley, R. (2018). *Prenatal substance exposure and associated factors: Inequality housing, financial problems, domestic violence, foster care, adoption, living arrangements* (Undergraduate honors thesis). The Ohio State University. Retreived from https://kb.osu.edu/handle/1811/84914

Brown, D. L., & Swanson, L. E. (2003). *Challenges for rural America in the twenty-first century*. University Park, PA: Pennsylvania State University Press.

Burton, L. M., Lichter, D. T., Baker, R. S., & Eason, J. M. (2013). Inequality, family processes, and health in the "new" rural America. *American Behavioral Scientist, 57*(8), 1128–1151. https://doi.org/10.1177/0002764213487348

Carr, P. J., & Kefalas, M. (2009). *Hollowing out the middle: The rural brain drain and what it means for America*. Boston, MA: Beacon Press.

Case, A., & Deaton, A. (2015). Rising morbidity and mortality in midlife among white non-Hispanic Americans in the 21st century. *Proceedings of the National Academy of Sciences, 112*(49), 15078–15083. https://doi.org/10.1073/pnas.1518393112

Case, A., & Deaton, A. (2017). *Morbidity and mortality in the 21st century*. Washington, DC: The Brooking Institution. Retrieved from https://www.brookings.edu/bpea-articles/mortality-and-morbidity-in-the-21st-century/

Catalano, R., & Dooley, D. (1983). Health effects of economic instability: A test of economic stress hypothesis. *Journal of Health and Social Behavior, 24*(1), 46–60.

Centers for Disease Control and Prevention (CDC). (2018a). *Multiple cause of death 1999–2017*, CDC WONDER Online Database, released December, 2017. Retrieved September 7, 2018, from https://wonder.cdc.gov/

Centers for Disease Control and Prevention (CDC). (2018b). *Preventing opioid overdoses among rural Americans* (Opioid Overdoses Policy Brief). Retrieved September 10, 2018, from https://www.cdc.gov/ruralhealth/drug-overdose/policybrief.html

Cheatle, M. D. (2011). Depression, chronic pain, and suicide by overdose: On the edge. *Pain Medicine, 12*(Suppl. 2), S43–S48. https://doi.org/10.1111/j.1526-4637.2011.01131.x

Chen, V. T. (2015). *Cut loose: Jobless and hopeless in an unfair economy*. Oakland: University of California Press.

Cosby, A. G., Neaves, T. T., Cossman, R. E., Cossman, J. S., James, W. L., Feierabend, N., … Farrigan, T. (2008). Preliminary evidence for an emerging nonmetropolitan mortality penalty in the United States. *American Journal of Public Health, 98*(8), 1470–1472. https://doi.org/10.2105/ajph.2007.123778

Cossman, J. S., James, W. L., Cosby, A. G., & Cossman, R. E. (2010). Underlying causes of the emerging nonmetropolitan mortality penalty. *American Journal of Public Health, 100*(8), 1417–1419. https://doi.org/10.2105/AJPH.2009.174185

Council of Economic Advisors (CEA). (2017). *The underestimated cost of the opioid crisis*. Washington, DC: Executive Office of the President. Retrieved from https://www.whitehouse.gov/briefings-statements/cea-report-underestimated-cost-opioid-crisis/

Currie, J., Jin, J.Y., & Schnell, M. (2018, March). *U.S. employment and opioids: Is there a connection?* (NBER Working Paper No. 24440). Washington, DC: National Bureau of Economic Research. Retrieved Sept. 8, 2018, from http://www.nber.org/papers/w24440

Dasgupta, N., Beletsky, L., & Ciccarone, D. (2018). Opioid crisis: No easy fix to its social and economic determinants. *American Journal of Public Health, 108*(2), 182–186.

Davidov, D. M., Davis, S. M., Zhu, M., Afifi, T. O., Kimber, M., Goldstein, A. L., ... Stocks, C. (2017). Intimate partner violence-related hospitalizations in Appalachia and the non-Appalachian United States. *PLoS ONE, 12*(9), e0184222. https://doi.org/10.1371/journal.pone.0184222

Day, M. A., & Thorn, B. E. (2010). The relationship of demographic and psychosocial variables to pain-related outcomes in a rural chronic pain population. *Pain, 151*(2), 467–474.

Donnermeyer, J. F., & Tunnell, K. (2007). In our own backyard: Methamphetamine manufacturing, trafficking and abuse in rural America. *Rural Realities, 2*(2). https://www.ruralsociology.org/assets/docs/rural-realities/rural-realities-2-2.pdf

Doogan, N. J., Roberts, M. E., Wewers, M. E., Stanton, C. A., Keith, D. R., Gaalema, D. E., ... Higgins, S. T. (2017). A growing geographic disparity: Rural and urban cigarette smoking trends in the United States. *Preventive Medicine, 104*, 79–85. https://doi.org/10.1016/j.ypmed.2017.03.011

Driscoll, K. (2017, November). Opioid crisis compounds rising domestic violence cases. *Dayton Daily News*. Retrieved from https://www.daytondailynews.com/business/opioid-crisis-compounds-rising-domestic-violence-cases/oprLmgFPyiwBx09TWnqbjI/.

Drug Enforcement Administration. (2017). *DEA releases 2017 National Drug Threat Assessment* [Press release]. Retrieved from https://www.dea.gov/press-releases/2017/10/23/dea-releases-2017-national-drug-threat-assessment

Durkheim, E. (1897/1966). *Suicide*. New York: The Free Press.

Fontanella, C. A., Hiance-Steelesmith, D. L., Phillips, G. S., Bridge, J. A., Lester, N., Sweeney, H. A., & Campo, J. V. (2015). Widening rural-urban disparities in youth suicides, United States, 1996–2010. *JAMA Pediatrics, 169*(5), 466–473. https://doi.org/10.1001/jamapediatrics.2014.3561

Frasquilho, D., Matos, M. G., Salonna, F., Guerreiro, D., Storti, C. C., Gaspar, T., & Caldas-de-Almeida, J. M. (2016). Mental health outcomes in times of economic recession: A systematic literature review. *BMC Public Health, 16*, 115. https://doi.org/10.1186/s12889-016-2720-y

Gebelein, M. (2018, May). Opioid epidemic inundating public health, foster care systems. *North Carolina Health News*. Retrieved from https://www.northcarolinahealthnews.org/2018/05/16/opioid-epidemic-inundating-public-health-foster-care-systems/.

Hancock, C., Mennenga, H., King, N., Andrilla, H., Larson, E., & Schou, P. (2017). *Treating the rural opioid epidemic (Policy Brief)*. Washington, DC: National Rural Health Association. Retrieved from https://www.ruralhealthweb.org/NRHA/media/Emerge_NRHA/Advocacy/Policy%20documents/Treating-the-Rural-Opioid-Epidemic_Feb-2017_NRHA-Policy-Paper.pdf

Havens, J. R., Young, A. M., & Havens, C. E. (2011). Nonmedical prescription drug use in a nationally representative sample of adolescents: Evidence of greater use among rural adolescents. *Archives of Pediatrics & Adolescent Medicine, 165*(3), 250–255.

Hempstead, K. A., & Phillips, J. A. (2015). Rising suicide among adults aged 40-64 years: The role of job and financial circumstances. *American Journal of Preventive Medicine, 48*(5), 491–500. https://doi.org/10.1016/j.amepre.2014.11.006

Hernandez, L., & Radnovich, C. (2018, February). Oregon meth-related deaths higher than ever. *U.S. News & World Report*. Retrieved from https://www.usnews.com/news/best-states/oregon/articles/2018-02-24/oregon-meth-related-deaths-higher-than-ever.

Iceland, J., & Hernandez, E. (2017). Understanding trends in concentrated poverty: 1980–2014. *Social Science Research, 62*, 75–95. https://doi.org/10.1016/j.research.2016.09.001
Inciardi, J. A., Surratt, H. L., Cicero, T. J., & Beard, R. A. (2009). Prescription opioid abuse and diversion in an urban community: The results of an ultrarapid assessment. *Pain Medicine, 10*(3), 537–548. https://doi.org/10.1111/j.1526-4637.2009.00603.x
Iowa State University. (2018). *Prosper partnerships*. Ames, IA: Partners in Prevention Science Institute. http://helpingkidsprosper.org/
Ivey-Stephenson, A. Z., Crosby, A. E., Jack, S. P. D., Haileyesus, T., & Kresnow-Sedacca, M. J. (2017). Suicide trends among and within urbanization levels by sex, race/ethnicity, age group, and mechanism of death—United States, 2001–2015. *Morbidity and Mortality Weekly Report Surveillance Summaries, 66*(SS-18), 1–16. https://doi.org/10.15585/mmwr.ss6618a1
Jonas, A. B., Young, A. M., Oser, C. B., Leukefeld, C. G., & Havens, J. R. (2012). OxyContin as currency: OxyContin use and increased social capital among rural Appalachian drug users. *Social Science & Medicine, 74*(10), 1602–1609.
Kandel, W., & Parrado, E. A. (2005). Restructuring of the US meat processing industry and new Hispanic migrant destinations. *Population and Development Review, 31*(3), 447–471. https://doi.org/10.1111/j.1728-4457.2005.00079.x
Kaplan, M. S., Huguet, N., Caetano, R., Giesbrecht, N., Kerr, W. C., & McFarland, B. H. (2015). Economic contraction, alcohol intoxication and suicide: Analysis of the National Violent Death Reporting System. *Injury Prevention, 21*(1), 35–41. https://doi.org/10.1136/injuryprev-2014-041215
Kegler, S. R., Stone, D. M., & Holland, K. M. (2017). Trends in suicide by level of urbanization—United States, 1999–2015. *Morbidity and Mortality Weekly Report, 66*(10), 270–273.
Kerr, W. C., Kaplan, M. S., Huguet, N., Caetano, R., Giesbrecht, N., & McFarland, B. H. (2017). Economic recession, alcohol, and suicide rates: Comparative effects of poverty, foreclosure, and job loss. *American Journal of Preventive Medicine, 52*(4), 469–475. https://doi.org/10.1016/j.amepre.2016.09.021
Keyes, K. M., Cerda, M., Brady, J. E., Havens, J. R., & Galea, S. (2014). Understanding the rural-urban differences in nonmedical prescription opioid use and abuse in the United States. *American Journal of Public Health, 104*(2), E52–E59. https://doi.org/10.2105/Ajph.2013.301709
Ko, J. Y., Patrick, S. W., Tong, V. T., Pate, R., Lind, J. N., & Barfield, W. D. (2016). Incidence of neonatal abstinence syndrome-28 states, 1999–2013. *Morbidity and Mortality Weekly Report, 65*(31), 799–802.
Kolodny, A., Courtwright, D. T., Hwang, C. S., Kreiner, P., Eadie, J. L., Clark, T. W., & Alexander, G. C. (2015). The prescription opioid and heroin crisis: A public health approach to an epidemic of addiction. *Annual Review of Public Health, 36*(1), 559–574. https://doi.org/10.1146/annurev-publhealth-031914-122957
Krueger, A. B. (2017). *Where have all the workers gone? An inquiry into the decline of U.S. labor force participation. Brookings Papers on Economic Activity*. Washington, DC: The Brookings Institite. Retrieved https://www.brookings.edu/wp-content/uploads/2017/09/1_krueger.pdf
Lenardson, J. D., Gale, J. A., & Ziller, E. C. (2016). *Rural opioid abuse: Prevalence and user characteristics* (Research & Policy Brief No. PB-63-1). Maine Rural Health Research Center. Retrieved from http://muskie.usm.maine.edu/Publications/rural/Rural-Opioid-Abuse.pdf
Levin, M., & Haugen, M. (2018). *Open roads and overflowing jails: Addressing high rates of rural pretrial incarceration*. Austin, TX: Center for Effective Justice, Texas Public Policy Foundation. Retrieved from https://files.texaspolicy.com/uploads/2018/08/16104511/2018-04-RR-Rural-Pretrial-Incarceration-CEJ-Levin-Haugen-1.pdf
Lichter, D., & Ziliak, J. P. (2017). The rural-urban interface: New patterns of spatial interdependence and inequality in America. *The Annals of the American Academy of Political and Social Science, 672*(1), 6–25.
Livingston, G. (2018, June). Family life is changing in different ways across urban, suburban, and rural communities in the U.S. *Pew Research Center, Fact Tank*. Retrieved from https://www.pewresearch.org/fact-tank/2018/06/19/family-life-is-changing-in-different-ways-across-urban-suburban-and-rural-communities-in-the-u-s/

Lobao, L. (2004). Continuity and change in place stratification: Spatial inequality and middle-range territorial units. *Rural Sociology, 69*(1), 1–30. https://doi.org/10.1526/003601104322919883

Lobao, L. (2014). Economic change, structural forces, and rural America: Shifting fortunes across communities. In C. Bailey, L. Jensen, & E. Ransom (Eds.), *Rural America in a globalizing world: Problems and prospects for the 2010s* (pp. 543–555). Morgantown, WV: West Virginia University Press.

Lobao, L., & Saenz, R. (2002). Spatial inequality and diversity as an emerging research area. *Rural Sociology, 67*(4), 497–511. https://doi.org/10.1111/j.1549-0831.2002.tb00116.x

Lobao, L., Zhou, M., Partridge, M., & Betz, M. (2016). Poverty, place, and coal employment across Appalachia and the United States in a new economic era. *Rural Sociology, 81*(3), 343–386. https://doi.org/10.1111/ruso.12098

Lobao, L. M., Hooks, G., & Tickamyer, A. R. (Eds.). (2007). *The sociology of spatial inequality*. Albany, NY: State University of New York Press.

Macy, B. (2018). *Dopesick: Dealers, doctors, and the drug company that addicted America*. New York: Little, Brown, and Company.

McLean, K. (2016). "There's nothing here": Deindustrialization as risk environment for overdose. *International Journal on Drug Policy, 29*, 19–26. https://doi.org/10.1016/j.drugpo.2016.01.009

Monnat, S. M. (2016). *Deaths of despair and support for Trump in the 2016 presidential election* (Research Brief 12/04/16). University Park, PA: The Pennsylvania State University, Department of Agricultural Economics, Sociology, and Education Retrieved from http://aese.psu.edu/directory/smm67/Election16.pdf

Monnat, S. M. (2017). *Drugs, alcohol, and suicide represent growing share of U.S. mortality* (National Issue Brief #112). Durham, NH: University of New Hampshire Carsey School of Public Policy.. Retrieved from https://carsey.unh.edu/publication/drugs-alcohol-suicide

Monnat, S. M. (2018). Factors associated with county-level differences in U.S. drug-related mortality rates. *American Journal of Preventive Medicine, 54*(5), 611–619.

Monnat, S. M., & Chandler, R. F. (2015). Long-term physical health consequences of adverse childhood experiences. *The Sociological Quarterly, 56*(4), 723–752.

National Advisory Committee on Rural Health and Human Services. (2016, July). *Families in crisis: The human service implications of rural opioid misuse* (Policy Brief). Rockville, MD, Retrieved from https://www.hrsa.gov/advisorycommittees/rural/publications/opioidabuse.pdf

National Institute on Drug Abuse. (2013, September). *What are the long-term effects of methamphetamine abuse?* Retrieved from https://www.drugabuse.gov/publications/research-reports/methamphetamine/what-are-long-term-effects-methamphetamine-abuse.

National Institute on Drug Abuse. (2019, January). *Overdose death rates*. Retrieved from https://www.drugabuse.gov/related-topics/trends-statistics/overdose-death-rates

Nestadt, P. S., Triplett, P., Fowler, D. R., & Mojtabai, R. (2017). Urban-rural differences in suicide in the state of Maryland: The role of firearms. *American Journal Public Health, 107*(10), 1548–1553. https://doi.org/10.2105/ajph.2017.303865

Newman, K. S. (1999). *Falling from grace: Downward mobility in the age of affluence*. Berkeley, CA: University of California Press.

Noonan, R. (2017, November). Rural America in crisis: The changing opioid overdose epidemic [Public Health Matters Blog post]. Centers for Disease Control and Prevention. Retrieved from https://blogs.cdc.gov/publichealthmatters/2017/11/opioids/

Olfson, M., Blanco, C., Wall, M., Liu, S.-M., Saha, T. D., Pickering, R. P., & Grant, B. F. (2017). National trends in suicide attempts among adults in the United States. *JAMA Psychiatry, 74*(11), 1095–1103. https://doi.org/10.1001/jamapsychiatry.2017.2582

Patrick, S. W., Davis, M. M., Lehman, C. U., & Cooper, W. O. (2015). Increasing incidence and geographic distribution of neonatal abstinence syndrome: United States, 2009–2012. *Journal of Perinatology, 35*(8), 650–655.

Peters, D. J. (2012). Income inequality across micro and meso geographic scales in the midwestern United States, 1979–20091. *Rural Sociology, 77*(2), 171–202. https://doi.org/10.1111/j.1549-0831.2012.00077.x

Peters, D. J. (2013). American income inequality across economic and geographic space, 1970–2010. *Social Science Research, 42*(6), 1490–1504. https://doi.org/10.1016/j.ssresearch.2013.06.009
Pullen, E., & Oser, C. (2014). Barriers to substance abuse treatment in rural and urban communities: A counselor perspective. *Substance Use & Misuse, 49*(7), 891–901. https://doi.org/10.3109/10826084.2014.891615
Putnam, R. D. (2000). *Bowling alone: The collapse and revival of American community*. New York, NY: Simon and Schuster.
Quinones, S. (2015). *Dreamland: The true tale of America's opiate epidemic*. New York, NY: Bloomsbury Press.
Reding, N. (2009). *Methland: The death and life of an American small town*. New York: Bloomsbury.
Rezvani, A. (writer). (2018, June). A new wave of meth overloads communities struggling with opioids [Radio program]. In R. Martin & D. Hajek (Host) *Health News from NPR*. National Public Radio. Retrieved from https://www.npr.org/sections/health-shots/2018/06/20/619929939/a-new-wave-of-meth-overloads-communities-struggling-with-opioids.
Rigg, K. K., & Monnat, S. M. (2015). Urban vs. rural differences in prescription opioid misuse among adults in the United States: Informing region specific drug policies and interventions. *International Journal of Drug Policy, 26*(5), 484–491. https://doi.org/10.1016/j.drugpo.2014.10.001
Rigg, K. K., Monnat, S. M., & Chavez, M. N. (2018). Opioid-related mortality in rural America: Geographic heterogeneity and intervention strategies. *International Journal of Drug Policy, 57*, 119–129. https://doi.org/10.1016/j.drugpo.2018.04.011
Robles, F. (2018, February). Meth, the forgotten killer, is back. And it's everywhere. *New York Times.*. Retrieved from https://www.nytimes.com/2018/02/13/us/meth-crystal-drug.html
Ruhm, C. (2018). *Deaths of despair or drug problem?* (Working Paper No. 24188). Cambridge, MA: National Bureau of Economic Research. Retrieved from http://www.nber.org/papers/w24188
Runyon, L. (Writer). (2017, January). Why is the opioid epidemic hitting rural America especially hard? [Radio program] *Weekend All Things Considered*. Illinois: National Public Radio. Retrieved from http://www.nprillinois.org/post/why-opioid-epidemic-hitting-rural-america-especially-hard#stream/0.
Rupasingha, A., Goetz, S. J., & Freshwater, D. (2006). The production of social capital in US counties. *The Journal of Socio-Economics, 35*(1), 83–101. https://doi.org/10.1016/j.socec.2005.11.001
Rural Health Information Hub. (2018). *Substance abuse in rural areas*. Retrieved from https://www.ruralhealthinfo.org/topics/substance-abuse
Russ, T. C., Kivimaki, M., Morling, J. R., Starr, J. M., Stamatakis, E., & Batty, G. D. (2015). Association between psychological distress and liver disease mortality: A meta-analysis of individual study participants. *Gastroenterology, 148*(5), 958–966.e4. https://doi.org/10.1053/j.gastro.2015.02.004
Saez, E., & Zucman, G. (2016). Wealth inequality in the United States since 1913: Evidence from capitalized income tax data. *The Quarterly Journal of Economics, 131*(2), 519–578. https://doi.org/10.1093/qje/qjw004
Sampson, R. J., & Groves, W. B. (1989). Community structure and crime: Testing social-disorganization theory. *American Journal of Sociology, 94*(4), 774–802.
Singh, G. K., & Siahpush, M. (2014). Widening rural-urban disparities in life expectancy, U.S., 1969–2009. *American Journal of Preventive Medicine, 46*(2), e19–e29. https://doi.org/10.1016/j.amepre.2013.10.017
Slack, T. (2014). Work in rural America in the era of globalization. In C. Bailey, L. Jensen, & E. Ransom (Eds.), *Rural America in a globalizing world: Problems and prospects for the 2010s* (pp. 573–590). Morgantown, WV: West Virginia University Press.
Smith, K. (2018, Spring). *Parental substance use in New Hampshire: Who cares for children?* (Regional Brief #53). Durham, NH: Carsey School of Public Policy, University of New Hampshire. Retrieved from https://carsey.unh.edu/publication/parental-substance-nh

Smith, K. E., & Tickamyer, A. R. (2011). *Economic restructuring and family well-being in rural America*. University Park, PA: The Pennsylvania State University Press.

Solar, O., & Irwin, A. (2010). *A. conceptual framework for action on the social determinants of health*. Geneva, Switzerland: WHO. Retrieved from http://www.who.int/sdhconference/resources/ConceptualframeworkforactiononSDH_eng.pdf

Stone, W. (Writer). (2018, January). In rural Arizona, some doctors worry tighter opioid regulations could backfire. [Radio program] Phoenix: 91.5 KJZZ. Retrieved from https://kjzz.org/content/596974/rural-arizona-some-doctors-worry-tighter-opioid-regulations-could-backfire

Substance Abuse and Mental Health Services Administration. (2016). *National survey on drug use and health*. Rockville, MD: Center for Behavior Health Statistics and Quality. https://pdas.samhsa.gov/#/

Syme, S. L. (1989). Control and health: A personal perspective. In A. Steptoe & A. Appels (Eds.), *Stress, personal control, and health*. New York, NY: Wiley.

Thiede, B., Kim, H., & Valasik, M. (2018). The spatial concentration of America's rural poor population: A postrecession update. *Rural Sociology, 83*(1), 109–144. https://doi.org/10.1111/ruso.12166

U.S. Census Bureau. (2015). *American Community Survey, 2010–14*. Washington, DC. Retrieved from https://factfinder.census.gov/faces/nav/jsf/pages/index.xhtml

United States Department of Agriculture (USDA). (2018). *Opioid misuse in rural America*. Washington, DC. Retrieved from https://www.usda.gov/topics/opioids

Van Gundy, K. T. (2006). Substance abuse in rural and small town America. *Reports on rural America, 1*(2). Durham, NH: Carsey Institute, University of New Hampshire Retrieved from https://scholars.unh.edu/cgi/viewcontent.cgi?article=1006&context=carsey

van Vlaanderen, Zoe. (2018, January). What's behind the addiction crisis in rural America? [Blog post] Addiction Medicine Update, National Council on Alcoholism and Drug Dependence Inc. Retrieved from https://www.ncadd.org/blogs/addiction-update/what-s-behind-the-addiction-crisis-in-rural-america

Van Zee, A. (2009). The promotion and marketing of OxyContin: Commercial triumph, public health tragedy. *American Journal of Public Health, 99*(2), 221–227. https://doi.org/10.2105/AJPH.2007.131714

Villapiano, N. L. G., Winkelman, T. N. A., Kozhimannil, K. B., Davis, M. M., & Patrick, S. W. (2017). Rural and urban differences in neonatal abstinence syndrome and maternal opioid use, 2004–2013. *JAMA Pediatrics, 171*(2), 194–196.

Weiss, A. J., Elixhauser, A., Barrett, M. L., Steiner, C. A., Bailey, M. K., & O'Malley, L. (2017). *Opioid-related inpatient stays and emergency department visits by state, 2009–2014*. (Statistical Brief #219). Rockville, MD: Healthcare Cost and Utilization Project (HCUP). Retrieved from https://www.hcup-us.ahrq.gov/reports/statbriefs/sb219-Opioid-Hospital-Stays-ED-Visits-by-State.jsp

Whitehead, M., Pennington, A., Orton, L., Nayak, S., Petticrew, M., Sowden, A., & White, M. (2016). How could differences in 'control over destiny' lead to socio-economic inequalities in health? A synthesis of theories and pathways in the living environment. *Health & Place, 39*(Suppl. C), 51–61. https://doi.org/10.1016/j.healthplace.2016.02.002

Wiltz, T. (2016, November). Why more grandparents are raising children. *PEW Stateline*. Retrieved from https://www.pewtrusts.org/en/research-and-analysis/blogs/stateline/2016/11/02/why-more-grandparents-are-raising-children

Yen, I. H., & Syme, L. S. (1999). The social environment and health: A discussion of the epidemiologic literature. *Annual Review of Public Health, 20*, 287–308. https://doi.org/10.1146/annurev.publhealth.20.1.287

Demographic Components of Aging in the Nonmetropolitan U.S., 1980–2017

John Cromartie

Population aging is arguably the most significant demographic transformation of the twenty-first century with implications for all aspects of society, including family composition, intergenerational ties, health and well-being, the supply of workers, and the demand for housing, transportation, and many other goods and services. The number of persons 60 years and older (the United Nation's threshold) is expected to more than triple by 2100, rising from 962 million in 2017 to 2.1 billion in 2050 and 3.1 billion in 2100 (United Nations, 2015). In the U.S., the population 65 years and older is expected to double from roughly 50 to 100 million between now and 2060; to increase as a percentage of the population from 15% to 24%; and to become much more racially and ethnically diverse, with non-Hispanic whites declining from 78% to 55% of older Americans (Mather, Jacobsen, & Pollard, 2015).

Aging is a hallmark of the modern age, the inevitable outcome of a human success story extending back more than 200 years (Kinsella & Phillips, 2005). Increased longevity and declining fertility are the historical engines of aging globally, together defining the well-known demographic transition. However, explanations for their timing and geographic variations are scale dependent (Phillips & Feng, 2017). At regional and national levels, the timing and speed of the demographic transition and the aging that invariably results—has varied with improvements in the food supply, nutrition, sanitation, socioeconomic status, and national population policies. Differences in the timing of these advances explain why more developed countries experienced earlier aging transitions and today have much older population structures.

Disclaimer Required Because Author is a U.S. Government Employee: The findings and conclusions in this publication are those of the author and should not be construed to represent any official USDA or U.S. Government determination or policy.

J. Cromartie (✉)
United States Department of Agriculture, Economic Research Service, Kansas City, MO, USA
e-mail: John.Cromartie@usda.gov

J. E. Glick et al. (eds.), *Rural Families and Communities in the United States*, National Symposium on Family Issues 10, https://doi.org/10.1007/978-3-030-37689-5_6

At more local levels, migration and the aging-in-place caused by migration play a dominant role in explaining the geography of aging (Fuguitt & Heaton, 1995). Population growth rates for older age groups are typically higher in urban areas, and the majority of older people in most countries live in urban areas. However, population aging usually refers to an increase in the proportion of a population in older age groups in a given area. In this sense, rural spaces across the globe are leading the trend, and age-specific patterns of migration between urban and rural areas are the dominant demographic triggers. Population aging is a global phenomenon that is manifesting itself first in rural communities.

In the U.S., 18% of the nonmetropolitan (nonmetro) population is 65 years or older compared with 14% in metropolitan (metro) areas. Over 75% of "older-age" counties—defined here as counties with 20% or more of their population age 65 years and older—are nonmetro counties (Cromartie, 2018). In the first 7 years of this decade alone, the number of nonmetro older-age counties more than doubled, from 446 to 920. The dominant demographic component explaining current county-level aging is not migration but the aging-in-place of the baby boom cohort as they began to age past 65 years in 2011. Past migration trends helped shape geographic variation in the timing and extent of aging across different types of nonmetro and metro counties.

Previous research shows that rural aging is largely attributable to two major migration trends: (1) out-migration of young adults leading to accelerated aging-in-place, such as in regions historically dependent on farming, forestry and mining; and (2) older-age retirement or near-retirement in-migration, primarily to amenity-rich destinations (Fuguitt & Beale, 1993; Glasgow & Brown, 2012; Lichter, Fuguitt, Heaton, & Clifford, 1981; Nelson, 2013). At the same time, researchers have pointed beyond the dichotomy, describing the underlying demographic processes as "intricate and varied" (Lichter et al., 1981) or "nuanced" (Glasgow & Brown, 2012). An analysis of nonmetro older-age counties (those with 20% or more residents 65 years and older) cross-classified with ERS county typologies both reinforces and points beyond the "two sides" narrative of rural aging (Cromartie, 2018). One-third of nonmetro older-age counties are also counties with persistent population loss, indicating chronic out-migration of young adults. Another third are retirement destinations or have recreation-based economies. That leaves one-third that do not fall into these contrasting categories, suggesting the need to have more direct and precise measures of the demographic impacts on aging. Some of these unclassified regions may be affected by both processes simultaneously or have undergone transitions over time from young-adult out-migration and aging-in-place to older-age in-migration. What is needed is a method to directly measure the demographic components of aging, to help identify the diversity of aging environments in the rural U.S.

In this chapter, I examine nonmetro aging in the U.S., focusing on how different demographic processes contribute to aging in different parts of the country. I begin by describing the changing geography of rural aging in the U.S. since 1980 and highlight differences in the type of older-age counties appearing before and after 2010. I then measure the impact of demographic components (e.g., natural change, net migration) on the change in the percent of the population 65 years and older since 1980, using a previously established decomposition method (Fuguitt & Beale, 1993; Lichter et al., 1981). Findings are reported for nonmetro areas as a whole (as currently defined) and for six case-study regions.

Rural counties age in different ways and it is important to have precise measures of the demographic components of aging as they vary over time and space. Young-adult out-migration and retirement in-migration are dominant components of rural aging, but their relative importance has shifted over time. There may be undetected geographic overlap or transition areas in their otherwise distinct geographic footprints. Other demographic trends may be contributing in smaller ways to the aging process. It is particularly important that we have such a tool as the current aging process intensifies and expands geographically with the aging of the baby boom generation. Aging is beginning to happen in areas that are more racially diverse and more challenged by economic circumstances.

This chapter is intended to contribute to an applied research agenda on rural aging that is relevant to rural development policy-making at USDA and to the research and service needs of its land-grant partners. Given that spatial heterogeneity of demographic processes and outcomes is a critical message of policy-oriented research (i.e., one size does not fit all), the focus here is on building a research strategy to map and explain the spatial diversity in rural aging processes. Aging research conducted across disciplines has clearly demonstrated that geographic context is central to the aging process and to policy responses to aging challenges (Glasgow & Berry, 2013; Golant, 2015; Nelson, 2014; Skinner, Andrews, & Cutchin, 2018). This case-study analysis contributes to an expanding literature focused on rural aging that seeks to develop theory and models to explain how demography, rurality, and community interact at different levels to facilitate outcomes for older adults (Winterton et al., 2016).

Nonmetropolitan Aging Trends, 1980–2017

In 1982, the U.S. Senate Special Committee on Aging convened a hearing to gather "...information about the true status of rural older Americans and offer a clearer indication of where our legislative efforts should be focused in the future, in order to best provide for the[ir] needs...to see if there are differences that we need to be aware of as policymakers" (Pressler, 1982, p. 2).

At this hearing, USDA demographer Calvin Beale reported that close to 12% of the rural population was over 65 years old compared with 10% of the urban population, but went on to highlight growing geographical disparities in older-age distribution (Beale, 1982). His map (approximately reproduced in Fig. 1) highlighted counties with one in six residents aged 65 years and older (16.7%) and those with 1 in 5 older residents (20%). The number of rural counties with more than one-sixth older age residents had grown from 125 to more than 500 between 1970 and 1980. The primary cause of rural aging at the time was clear from the map: Counties were highly concentrated in the Great Plains and Corn Belt, where agricultural restructuring and lack

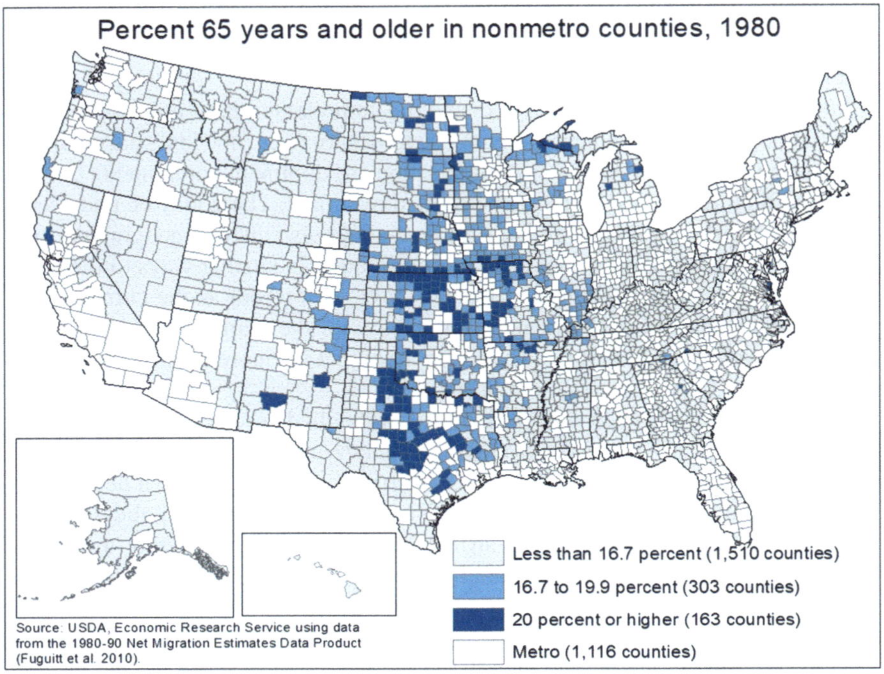

Fig. 1 Source: USDA, Economic Research Service using data from the 1980–1990 Net Migration Estimates Data Product (Fuguitt et al., 2010)

of alternative employment had caused out-migration of younger people, leaving behind an older aging-in-place population.

Beale went on to describe a newer demographic trend beginning to noticeably affect rural aging. Net in-migration of older people in rural areas was increasing during the 1970s, adding roughly 45,000 people per year during that decade. A second map of counties with relatively high in-movement of people 65 years or older (not reproduced here) showed that destinations were dispersed widely throughout the country. It was no longer a Sun Belt phenomenon but now encompassed parts of New England, northern Michigan, the Sierra Nevadas, and the Puget Sound region.

Two of Beale's insights regarding the trend foreshadow themes of this chapter. First, some of these in-migration growth areas had already advanced to the state of having high older-age proportions. Affected areas visible in Fig. 1 include the upper Great Lakes, the Ozarks, and the central Texas Hill Country. Second, older people who move to rural areas tend to be wealthier and better educated than the local older population.

Fast forward 30 years and the same map shows that both young-adult out-migration and older-age in-migration had greatly expanded the geographical reach of rural aging (Fig. 2). The number of nonmetro counties (as currently defined) with 20% or more of the population at older ages increased from 303 in 1980 to 446 in 2010. Two very different trends with significantly different (though not completely

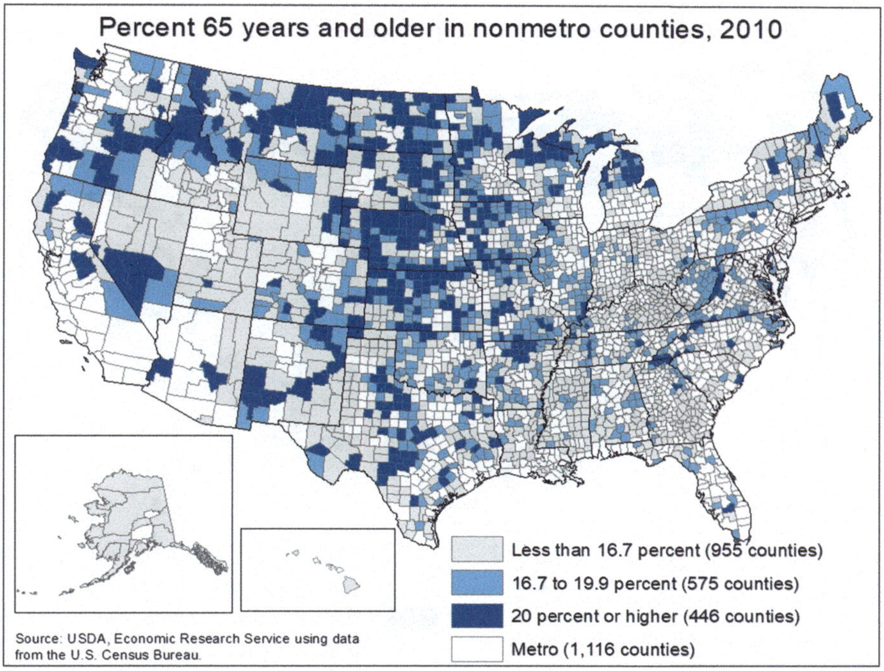

Fig. 2 Source: USDA, Economic Research Service using data from the U.S. Census Bureau

separate) spatial outcomes were now contributing equally to rural aging. Older-age counties increased in relatively scenic areas in the upper Great Lakes and the Ozarks, and new areas emerged in other high-amenity regions such as the southern Appalachians, northern Rockies, and Pacific Coast. Most counties in these regions had attracted increasing numbers of older-age migrants, especially during the 1990s, while others were aging due to younger out-migration or a combination of both. Aging-in-place leading to older-age counties in out-migration regions also increased, especially in the northern Great Plains and northwest Iowa.

With older baby boomers beginning to age past 65 years, the number of nonmetro older-age counties more than doubled in just the first 7 years of this decade, from 446 to 920 (Fig. 3). Much of the expansion occurred in or adjacent to already established older-age regions, such as in the northern Rockies, the northern Great Plains and Corn Belt, and the southern Appalachians. What is striking is the expansion into regions with different socioeconomic profiles and many more counties that may not easily fit into the two primary types of older-age counties. Such regions include the Rio Grande Valley, New England, the southern Coastal Plains, and along the Virginia–North Carolina border. Most nonmetro counties in Indiana, Ohio, and Kentucky, many of them located in manufacturing and mining regions undergoing significant economic dislocations, increased to above the 16.7% threshold during 2010–2017.

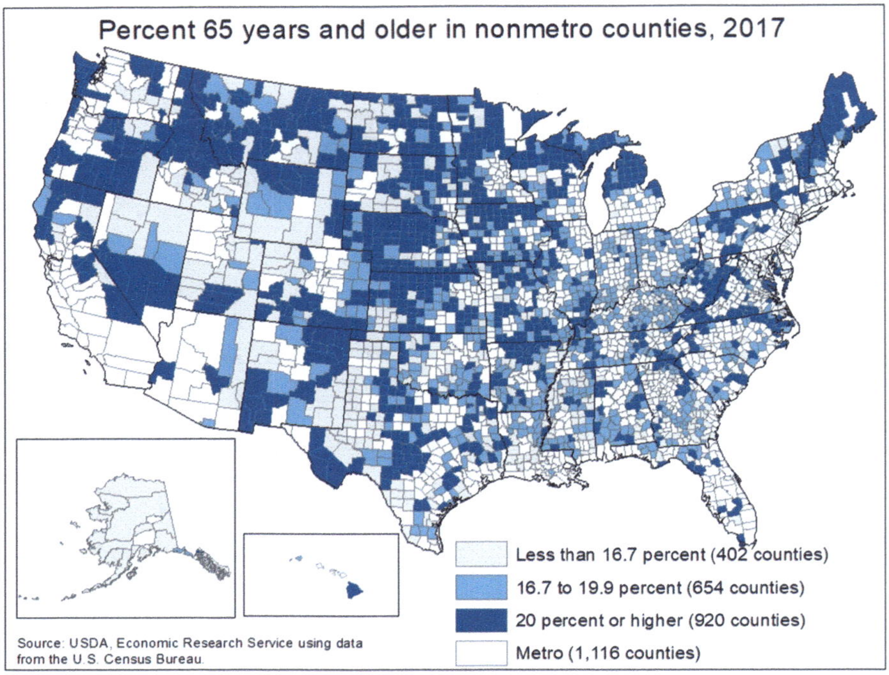

Fig. 3 Source: USDA, Economic Research Service using data from the U.S. Census Bureau

Table 1 compares socioeconomic indicators among three nonmetro county groups: older-age counties appearing before 2010, new older-age counties, and counties still below the 20% threshold. Older-age counties of both types are less racially diverse, show higher education levels and per capita income, and have lower rates of poverty. Interestingly, older-age counties had similar unemployment levels in 2010 and lower rates of employment recovery since then. The biggest differences are between previously established older-age counties and younger counties. Non-Hispanic whites make up 86% of the population in the former group and 75% in the latter. Per capita incomes are $3000 higher in the previously established older-age counties. Newer older-age counties fall somewhere in between the other two groups on some indicators. Compared with previously established older-age counties, they include a higher share of non-Hispanic blacks, slightly lower levels of education and income, and higher poverty rates.

Differences are small but they do suggest that older-age counties are beginning to expand into areas with greater economic challenges and fewer resources needed to support older residents. As older-age counties diversify in this manner, it is likely harder to describe rural aging in terms of just two dominant migration-related narratives. What follows is an analysis of changes in demographic processes underlying aging in nonmetro areas as a whole since 1980 and in six case study regions chosen to represent different types of rural aging scenarios.

Table 1 Comparative profile of nonmetro counties by timing of aging

	Population 65 years and older:		
	Became 20% or higher:		
	Before 2010	After 2010	Still below 20% in 2017
Number of counties	440	480	1056
Percent by race/ethnicity, 2017			
Hispanic	6.6	6.2	9.9
Non-Hispanic black	2.9	5.9	9.8
Non-Hispanic white	86.1	83.5	74.9
Percent with a college degree, 5-year average, 2012–2016	29.3	28	26.9
Per capita income, 5-year average, 2012–2016 ($$$)	25,718	24,360	22,641
Percent in poverty, 5-year average, 2012–2016	14.3	16.6	19.1
Percent unemployed, 2010	9.7	10.2	9.8
Percent employment change, 2010–2017	1.5	1.5	3.2

Source: Economic Research Service, USDA, using data from the U.S. Census and the Bureau of Labor Statistics

Data and Methods

County-level age-specific population and components-of-change estimates were obtained from files for the 1980s (Fuguitt, Beale, & Voss, 2010), for the 1990s (Voss, McNiven, Hammer, Johnson, & Fuguitt, 2004), and for the 2000s (Winkler, Johnson, Cheng, Voss, & Curtis, 2013). These data are the most recent in a series of USDA-sponsored population estimates produced following each decennial census since 1960 (Winkler, Johnson, Cheng, Beaudoin, Voss, & Curtis, 2013). Net migration estimates were derived using the residual method, subtracting measures of natural change based on intercensal birth and death records from population change during a given decade. Errors in measuring natural change and in census enumerations (e.g., undercounts and overcounts) effect estimates derived from the residual method, and results shown here should be interpreted with that in mind. Adjustments were made to base populations each decade to account for estimated enumeration errors. Thus, populations and percentages for the same decennial census year differ slightly from one set to the next. These data are not yet available for the current decade but we have included a limited analysis based on age-specific population estimates for 2010–2017 from the U.S. Census Bureau's Population Estimates Program.

For each decade 1980–2000 and for 2010–2017, change in the percent 65 years and older is decomposed into two demographic components: the change due to population change of people younger than 65 years and those 65 years and older. For 1980–2000, each of these components is further decomposed into the contributions

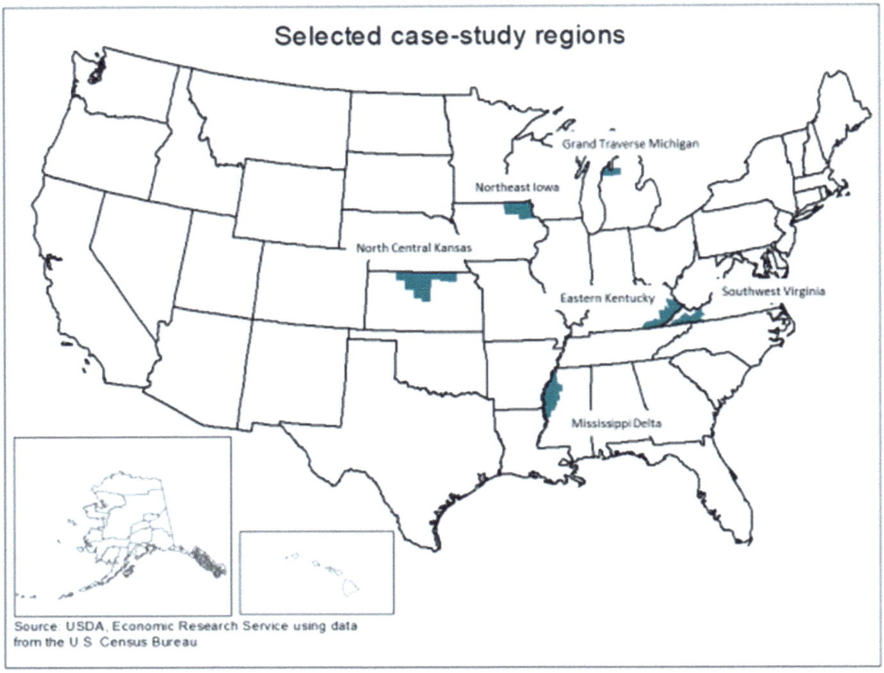

Fig. 4 Source: USDA, Economic Research Service using data from the U.S. Census Bureau

from net migration and natural change (not yet available for 2010–2017). Natural change for people younger than 65 years consists of births minus deaths minus people aging out. Natural change for those 65 years and older consists of those aging into the age group minus deaths. Results are reported for nonmetropolitan areas as a whole and for six case study regions chosen to cover diverse aging environments (Fig. 4). Two were chosen as examples of chronic out-migration areas (North Central Kansas and Northeast Iowa), and one serves as an example of a long-established retirement destination (Grand Traverse Michigan). Three others (Southwest Virginia, Mississippi Delta, and Eastern Kentucky) were chosen to explore other possible aging scenarios and to include newly aging nonmetropolitan regions with markedly different socioeconomic profiles.

A procedure patterned after the analysis of variance is used to decompose the change in percent 65 years and older into changes due to four demographic components. It was used to study nonmetro aging trends prior to 1990 but has not yet been applied to more recent decades (Fuguitt, 1980; Fuguitt & Beale, 1993; Lichter et al., 1981). The contribution from a given component is estimated as the average of outcomes having various demographic components present or absent. In the simple case of having just two components of change, *a* and *b*, there are 2^2 or four possible outcomes: *ab* (presence of *a* and *b*, the actual outcome); *a* (presence of *a* only); *b* (*b* only); and *l* (absence of both *a* and *b*). The change effect of the first factor *a* is

½[(*ab*–*b*) + (*a*–*l*)]. This is the average of two differences: the difference between the outcome with *a* present and *a* absent when *b* is present, and the difference in the outcome with *a* present and *a* absent when *b* is absent. Similarly, the effect of the second factor *b* is ½[(*ab*–*a*) + (*b*–*l*)]. With four components of change, such as in the components-of-change decomposition done here, there are 2^4 or 16 possible outcomes, so the effects are averages of 8 possible differences (see Fuguitt, 1980 for more details).

Findings

Overall Nonmetro Trends

Figure 5 summarizes the changing aging trends for nonmetro areas during four decades. Walking through one example, the upper left diagram shows that the percent 65 years and older increased 1.6 points from 13.2% to 14.8%. The decomposition partitions that change into the amount attributable to change in population younger than 65 years (0.06, on the left) and the amount attributable to change in the population 65 years and older (1.5 on the right). These changes are further partitioned into the amounts attributable to natural increase and net migration. For the younger population, the 0.06 effect is the balance between a −0.49 decline in percent older due to natural change and a 0.56 increase from net migration. It must be kept in mind that signs are reversed on the left side for younger ages: the 0.56 *increase* in percent older stemming from net migration indicates a *decrease* in population from younger net migration.

Results for nonmetro counties as a whole show extensive variation in aging across decades, ranging from decline in the 1990s to a nearly 3-point increase in percent older in the current decade. Aging is most often associated with population decline while population growth (other than in retirement destinations) tends to slow aging, so it is not surprising to see an acceleration of aging during this current decade and a decline in aging during the rural rebound in the 1990s. Net migration rates among younger groups switched from −5% in the 1980s to 4% in the 1990s and, as a result, change in the percent ages 65 years and older shifted from 0.6 to −0.5. But size differences of birth cohorts contributed equally to the decline in aging during the 1990s. Natural change for older residents dipped from 630,000 to 217,000 between the 1980s and 1990s as people born during 1925–1935 (a period of reduced fertility) began turning 65 years. The contribution to aging decreased from 1.44 to 0.64. Components-of-change statistics are not yet available for the current decade but will likely show a similar combination of factors in opposing directions: a decline in aging from lower net migration and accelerated aging from the entrance of baby boomers into older ages.

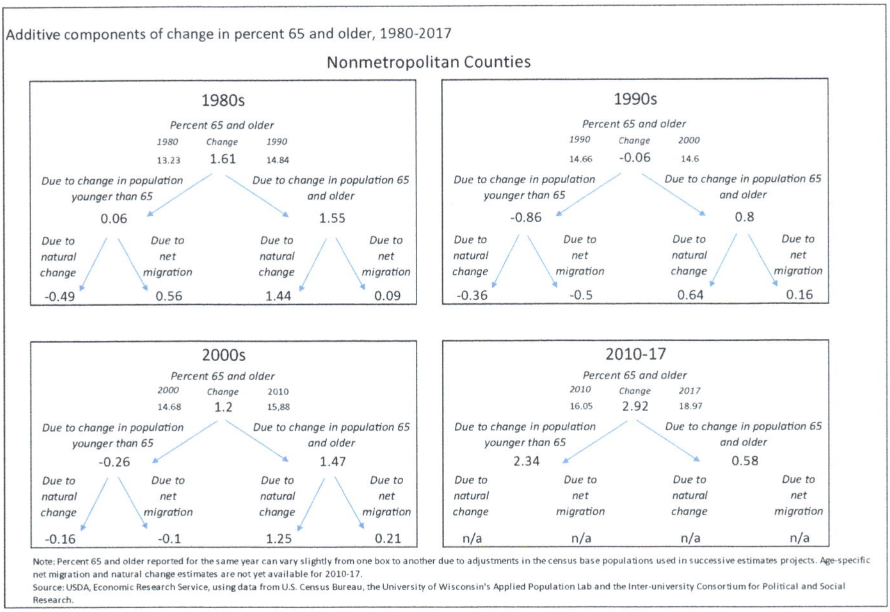

Fig. 5 Source: USDA, Economic Research Service, using data from the U.S. Census Bureau, the University of Wisconsin's Applied Population Lab and the Inter-university Consortium for Political and Social Research

Out-migration Regions

The first region among our case study examples, North Central Kansas, represents the extreme of aging through young-adult out-migration, leading to population decline and overall natural decrease (Fig. 6). The younger population declined by 15,000 from 1980 to 2017 while the older population declined by 3000. North Central Kansas is the only region to appear on the Fig. 1 map as having 20% or more residents in older age groups in 1980. Long-term out-migration dating back to the 1950s and before can be detected in the results here. First, with sustained out-migration comes fewer births, reflected in the switch from positive natural change among younger residents in the 1980s (which lowered aging) to negative natural change, increasing aging in both the 1900s and 2000s. Second, aging halted during the 1990s and 2000s, because the population had already aged to the point of natural decrease among older residents, meaning deaths exceeded the number of people aging in. These are the largest natural decrease impacts seen in the six case study regions. Finally, the rise in aging resumed during this current decade, most likely because of the aging in of the baby boom cohort. However, the 1.3 rise in percent older during 2010–2017 is by far the lowest increase in aging among the six case study regions.

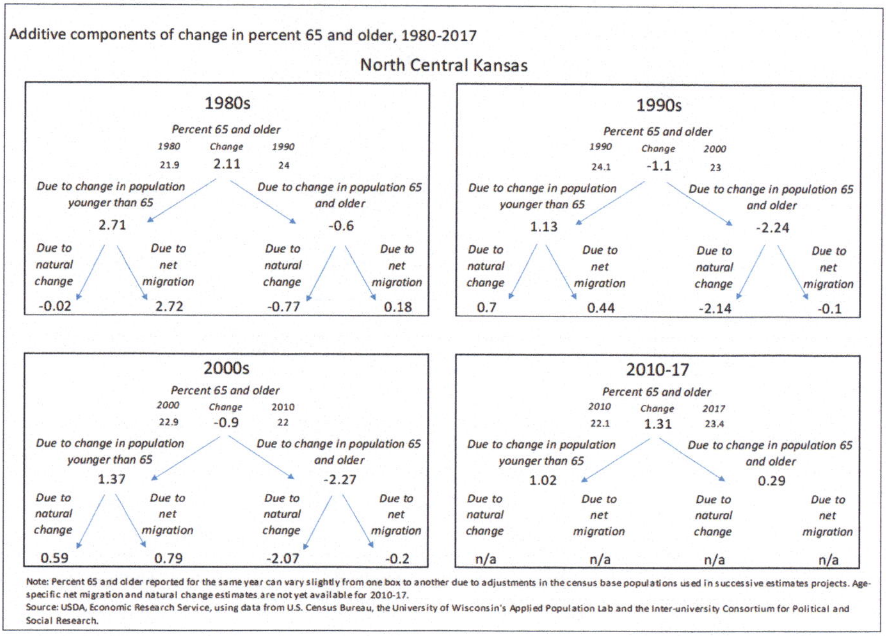

Fig. 6 Source: USDA, Economic Research Service, using data from the U.S. Census Bureau, the University of Wisconsin's Applied Population Lab and the Inter-university Consortium for Political and Social Research

The second example demonstrates that out-migration regions vary in the timing and severity of aging trends (Fig. 7). Northeastern Iowa is less remote and more reliant on a farm sector (dairy) that had been less subject to consolidation forces prior to this period. Results show that the region did not experience the same levels of out-migration early on, and did not reach 20% older until after 2010. During the decades shown here, younger out-migration contributed to aging in a similar manner as in North Central Kansas, but the age structure was still young enough to show natural increase among those 65 years and older in two of the three decades observed. Also, natural change among younger age groups remained positive, likely reflecting a delayed decline in births compared with North Central Kansas.

Older-Age In-migration Regions

North Central Kansas and our third example, the Grand Traverse region, both had roughly 90,000 people in 1980. Today the region centered on Traverse City, Michigan is more than double the size, with over 150,000 people compared with near 70,000 in North Central Kansas. Grand Traverse shows the expected signature

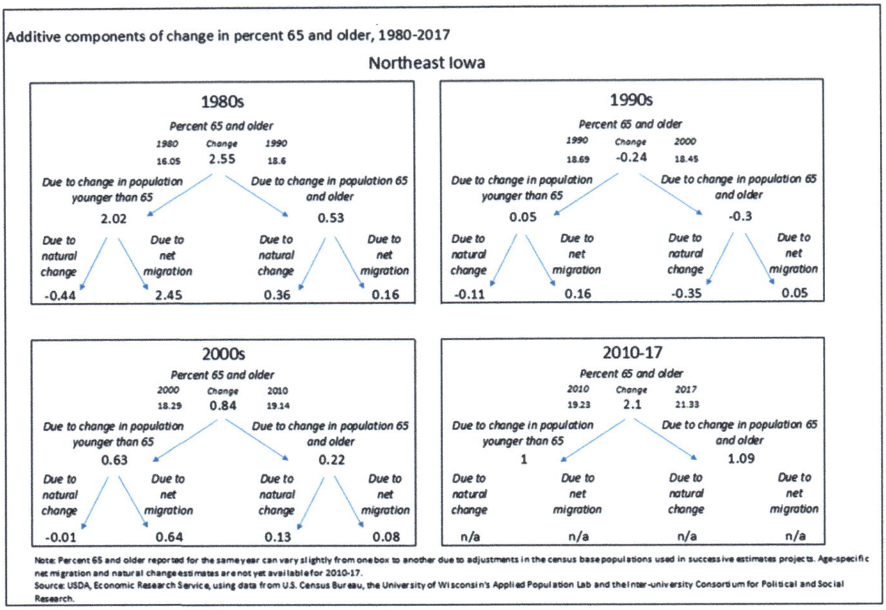

Fig. 7 Source: USDA, Economic Research Service, using data from the U.S. Census Bureau, the University of Wisconsin's Applied Population Lab and the Inter-university Consortium for Political and Social Research

of a rapidly growing, high amenity retirement destination, attracting both young and old alike (Fig. 8). The percent older increased from 12% to 22% during this period, despite the fact that in-migration among younger age groups was having a negative impact on aging up through 2010. Net migration for older age groups averaged close to 20% each decade from 1980 to 2010, while younger in-migration reached only over 15% during the rural rebound of the 1990s. Aging has increased dramatically during the current decade, aided by a decrease in population among younger age groups, a pattern typical of nonmetro post-Recession trends nationwide.

The region in Southwest Virginia recently crossed the 20% threshold marking older-age counties as defined here, but it does not fit into the two primary aging categories based on ERS typologies. It does not qualify as either a persistent population loss county or as a retirement/recreation destination (Cromartie, 2018). Knowledge of the region suggested that it most likely combined elements of both trends, and the results here confirm that suspicion to some degree. The signatures shown in Fig. 9 are closer to that of a region affected by older-age in-migration, at least since 1990. There was a switch to net in-migration of older residents in the 1990s that continued through the 2000s, indicating the increased importance to the region's economy of attracting retirees. But unlike what is seen in Grand Traverse, net migration among younger residents was negative during the 1980s (thus accelerating aging) and close to zero during the 2000s. These trends are indicative of a

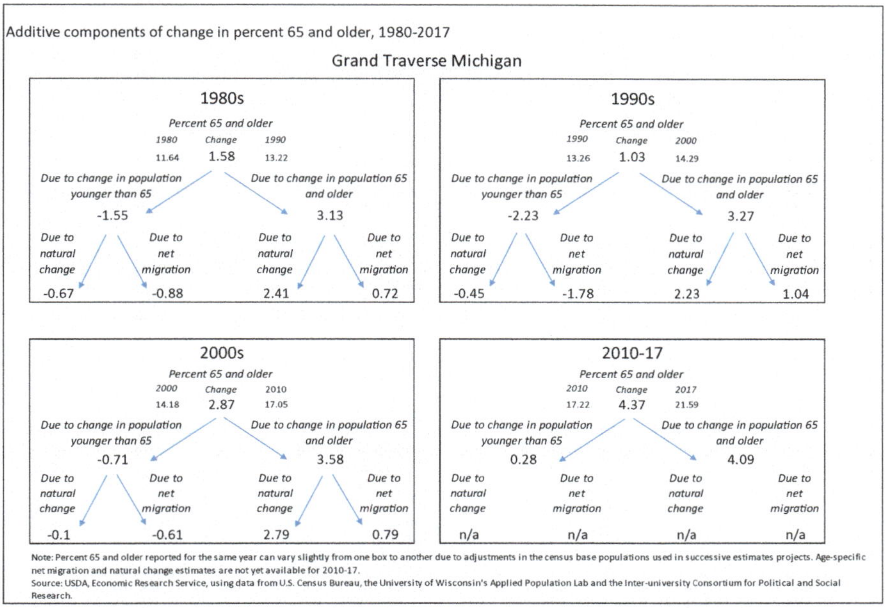

Fig. 8 Source: USDA, Economic Research Service, using data from the U.S. Census Bureau, the University of Wisconsin's Applied Population Lab and the Inter-university Consortium for Political and Social Research

region in transition, still affected by declines in resource-based mining and manufacturing sectors but with increasing job opportunities in recreation and retirement-related service sectors.

Mississippi Delta

The Mississippi Delta is included as an example of the new geography of rural aging emerging this decade. Its demographic profile and socioeconomic conditions stand in sharp contrast to aging regions prior to 2010 (Table 2). Non-Hispanic blacks make up the majority of the population; per capita incomes are half the level found in Grand Traverse; and the unemployment rate in 2010 was three times higher than in North Central Kansas. Despite population decline during each decade 1980–2010 at higher rates than seen in any other case-study region, percent older remained at just under 12% (Fig. 10). Two factors help explain the absence of aging in the presence of depopulation before 2010. First, fertility rates were higher than average during this period, thus the effect of natural change of younger residents on percent older remained much higher than seen in other regions. Second, the region lost the older population through net out-migration during all three decades 1980–2010.

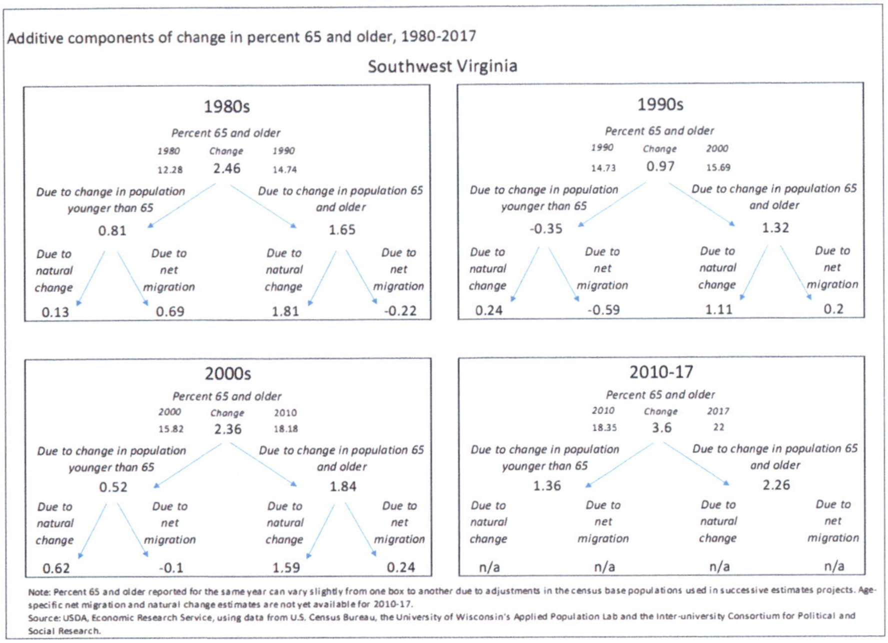

Fig. 9 Source: USDA, Economic Research Service, using data from the U.S. Census Bureau, the University of Wisconsin's Applied Population Lab and the Inter-university Consortium for Political and Social Research

No other region showed this pattern of consistently high, older-age net out-migration. Eastern Kentucky showed net out-migration of older residents in each decade but the effect on aging dropped to nearly zero in the 1990s and 2000s.

After remaining unchanged for 30 years, the percent older in the Mississippi Delta rose nearly 3 points during 2010–2017, to 14.7%. The continuing trend of population decline among young residents contributed roughly half of the increase, with the other half due to the switch from negative to positive growth among older residents. Once available, components-of-change statistics for the decade will likely show the dominant role of aging-in-place of the baby boom cohort in explaining this acceleration here and in similar parts of the rural U.S.

Eastern Kentucky

The Eastern Kentucky region chosen as our final case study region declined in population by 20% between 1980 and 2017. Like the Mississippi Delta, it is a region experiencing severe economic and social distress dating back decades. Fewer than 20% of residents have a college degree, compared with 41% in Grand Traverse, and

Table 2 Socioeconomic characteristics of case study analysis regions

	North Central Kansas	Northeast Iowa	Grand Traverse Michigan	Southwest Virginia	Delta Mississippi	Eastern Kentucky
Number of counties	13	8	4	6	11	14
Percent by race/ethnicity, 2017						
Hispanic	3.3	2.7	3	1.7	2.3	1.2
Non-Hispanic black	1.2	1.1	0.6	2.3	70.6	1.5
Non-Hispanic white	93	94.4	92.7	94.4	25.6	95.7
Percent with a college degree, 5-year average, 2012–2016	30.5	31.0	40.7	22.6	23.8	19.0
Percent in poverty, 5-year average, 2012–2016						
All ages	11.8	10.7	11.6	16.8	35.6	31.6
65 years and older	8.9	8.5	5.6	10.9	19.6	16.9
Percent unemployed, 2010	4.9	6.7	12.1	10.8	14.3	12.2
Percent employment change, 2010–2017	−8.7	0.7	11.4	0.79	−7.9	−12
Per capita income, 5-year avg., 2012–2016 ($$$)	25,424	26,652	29,484	22,024	15,875	17,131

Source: Economic Research Service, USDA, using data from the U.S. Census Bureau and the Bureau of Labor Statistics

poverty rates are close to 3 times higher than in Grand Traverse, for both the total and older populations (Table 2). Unlike in the Mississippi Delta, mortality rates in Eastern Kentucky have risen as a result of the opioid epidemic, which emerged in this region as early as the late 1990s, earlier than most other rural regions. Age shifts in mortality rates caused in large part by increased drug-related deaths can be seen for nonmetro areas as a whole (Fig. 11). The change in nonmetro age-specific mortality rates from 2000 to 2015 shows a rise in mortality among working-age adults but continued declines among older age groups. This trend by itself has accelerated rural aging. A more detailed decomposition of natural change into separate birth, death, and aging components is not yet available, so the exact extent of that impact is not yet known. Preliminary evidence presented here indicates that a measurable mortality-related increase in aging is likely for specific rural regions such as Eastern Kentucky.

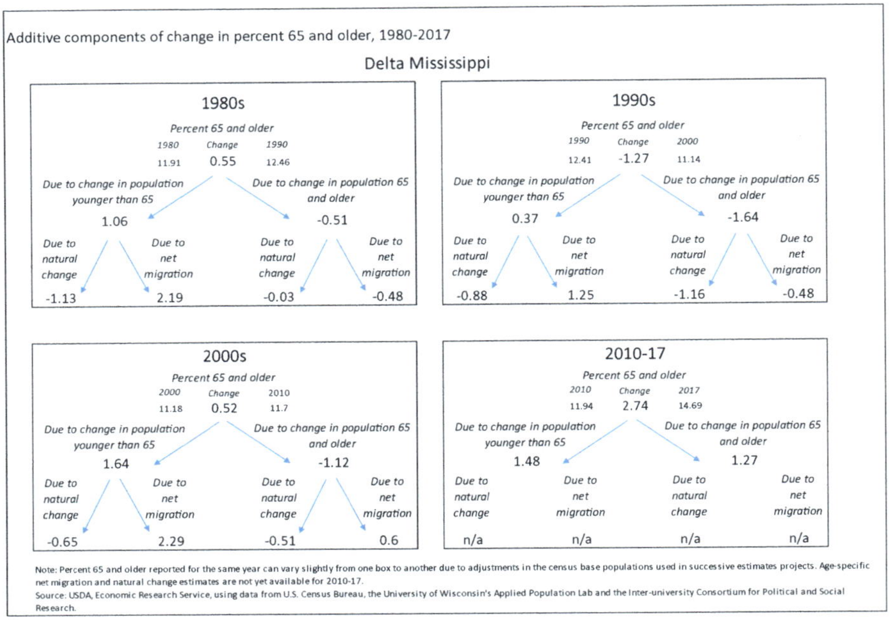

Fig. 10 Source: USDA, Economic Research Service, using data from the U.S. Census Bureau, the University of Wisconsin's Applied Population Lab and the Inter-university Consortium for Political and Social Research

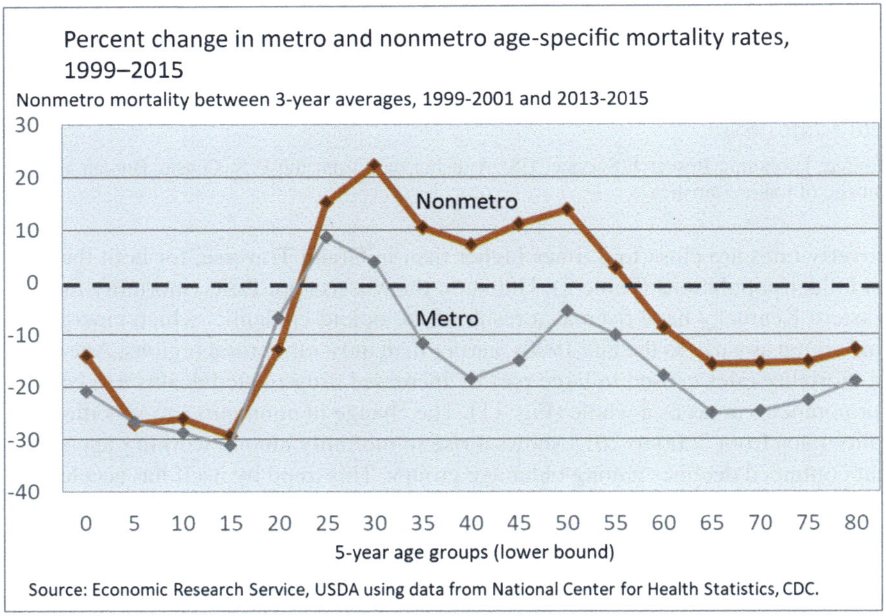

Fig. 11 Reproduced from Cromartie (2017)

Table 3 Mortality trends for younger and older residents of case study analysis regions, 1980–2016

	North Central Kansas	Northeast Iowa	Grand Traverse Michigan	Southwest Virginia	Delta Mississippi	Eastern Kentucky
Age-adjusted death rates (per 100,000)						
15–64 years old						
1990–1998	269	261	256	382	571	475
2000–2009	293	272	220	379	573	518
2010–2016	335	301	234	392	558	588
65 years and older						
1990–1998	4,808	5,009	5,051	5,766	6,031	6,337
2000–2009	5,429	5,075	4,365	5,608	5,879	6,428
2010–2017	5,029	4,807	4,099	5,173	5,717	6,018

Source: Economic Research Service, USDA, using data from the Centers for Disease Control and Prevention

A comparison of changes in age-adjusted death rates from 1990 to 2016, separately for those 15–64 years old and for those 65 years and older, shows the greater prevalence of drug-related mortality in Eastern Kentucky than in other case study regions (Table 3). Three other regions—North Central Kansas, Northeast Iowa, and Southwest Virginia—also show increases in working age mortality, more likely related to the use of methamphetamines than to opioids as in the two Midwest regions. The increase was much higher though in Eastern Kentucky and the decrease in death rates for those 65 years and older was higher there than other regions except for Southwest Virginia.

Changes in causes of aging in Eastern Kentucky are in line with expected changes resulting from these shifts in mortality over the time period covered here, though other factors most likely dominate (Fig. 12). Natural change among younger residents shifted from a positive rate of 4.4% in the 1980s to −0.21% in the 2000s, thus switching from decreasing to accelerating aging in the region. The overall contribution of population change among younger residents to aging increased from 0.7 to 1.43 points between the 2000s and 2010–2017. Most of this change is likely attributable to aging out of the baby boom cohort and to increased net out-migration in the post-Recession era. Drug-related deaths are working in the same direction as these other factors and together they caused a nearly 4% rise in percent older in Eastern Kentucky.

Conclusions

This chapter demonstrates how different demographic trends extending back decades helped shape the timing and geographic variation in aging for nonmetro areas in the U.S. Aging is a global hallmark of this century, transforming urban and

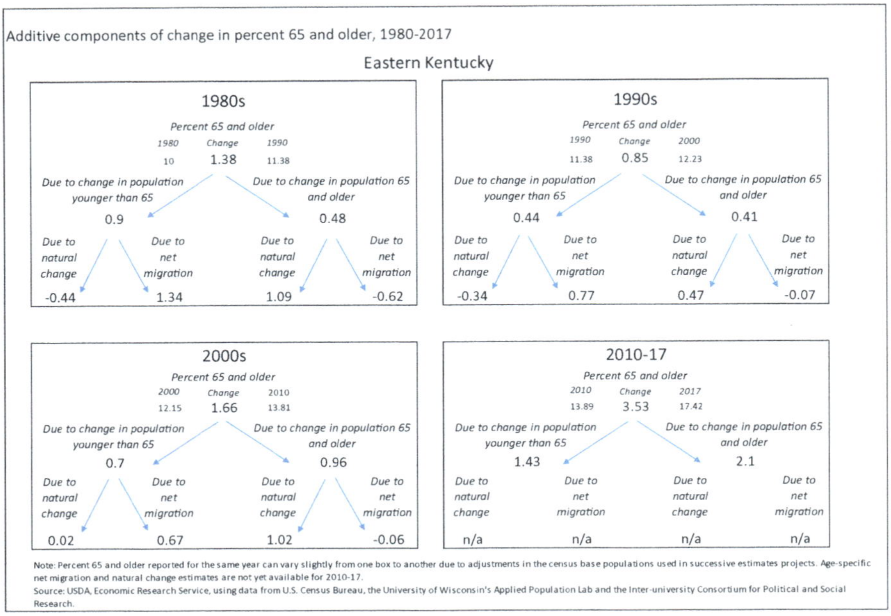

Fig. 12 Source: USDA, Economic Research Service, using data from the U.S. Census Bureau, the University of Wisconsin's Applied Population Lab and the Inter-university Consortium for Political and Social Research

rural areas in developed and developing countries alike in response to long-term reductions in fertility and mortality. But geographic variation in aging is significant at more local levels, where economic conditions and community context play vital roles in determining the health and well-being of older residents. At these scales, particular types of nonmetro areas have been at the forefront of aging trends in the U.S. since the 1970s. Between 1980 and 2010, the number of old-age counties in nonmetro areas increased by 50%, from roughly 300–450. Rural aging has accelerated rapidly during this decade, with the number of "older-age" counties more than doubling to over 900 in just the first 7 years.

Using decomposition techniques, we have measured directly the impacts of two migration trends previously identified through more indirect means as the primary determinants of spatial variation in rural aging. Young-adult out-migration (leading to aging-in-place) and retirement-related in-migration were dominant components of rural aging at the county level during the 1980–2017 period analyzed here. Results for nonmetro areas as a whole show variation in the pace of aging by decade, with aging accelerating during decades with high young-adult out-migration such as the 1980s, and slowing during periods of elevated in-migration such as the Rural Rebound of the 1990s. The pace of aging at any given time is also influenced by the size of the cohort reaching age 65 years, with the relatively small 1930s birth cohort slowing aging in the 1990s and the Baby Boom cohort greatly accelerating the trend during the current decade.

Previous research highlighted the distinct regional distribution of old-age counties linked to different migration patterns. Our case study analysis confirms that aging due to young-adult out-migration is regionally concentrated in remote, farm-dependent regions in the nation's Heartland. Retirement-related in-migration is more typically found in high-amenity destinations with recreation-dependent economies. Findings reported here suggest that the relative importance of these two migration trends has shifted over time, with previously undetected geographic overlap or transition areas in their otherwise distinct geographic footprints. A comparison of two farming-dependent areas shows that out-migration regions can vary in the timing and severity of aging, likely reflecting differences in both relative remoteness and type of farm sector. The components-of-change decomposition helps identify areas such as Southwest Virginia where the two processes seem to overlap.

As baby boomers continue to age past 65 years through 2030, and the number of old-age counties continues to rise rapidly, it is increasingly important to highlight the growing diversity of aging environments. Areas such as the Mississippi Delta and Eastern Kentucky that are not yet old-age counties as defined for this analysis are now on a trajectory to reach that threshold in the near future. They stand in stark contrast to both North Central Kansas and the Grand Traverse regions, with much higher poverty rates, limited human capital resources, and high unemployment linked to high job loss.

Community context matters for rural aging. Previous research documents the influence of geographic and community characteristics on the health and well-being of rural older adults. For instance, access to services in nonmetro areas diminishes as populations age (Thiede, Brown, Sanders, Glasgow, & Kulcsar, 2017). Findings indicate that these circumstances are exacerbated in areas where aging is due to high out-migration among younger adults. Spatial clustering means that services lacking in a given county likely do not exist in neighboring counties either. The type of extreme aging represented by the high out-migration area in North Central Kansas is typical of a broad swath of territory encompassing much of the Great Plains. Thiede and colleagues conclude that these types of areas, with the highest median ages and highest health care needs, are also most likely to lack access to such services in their home and neighboring communities.

Federal and state programs focused on support and service provision in rural communities help fill the needs of a growing older population. As was the case in 1982, policy makers today need "…information about the true status of rural older Americans…in order to best provide for the[ir] needs (Pressler, 1982, p. 2)." Questions asked 38 years ago about "…where to focus legislative efforts…" and "…differences to be aware of..." (Pressler, 1982) are pertinent today and underscore the potential value of the type of spatial demographic research presented here. Understanding the full range of aging scenarios as they developed at different times in different places can help policy making across a range of program areas, including health, nutrition, social security, housing, transportation, and Internet access. For instance, USDA housing programs assist older rural residents with rental support, low-interest guaranteed housing loans, and funding for rehabilitation of older homes. Rental assistance may be needed more in faster growing, more densely settled retirement destinations such as the Grand Traverse region, where housing cost burdens for renters are disproportionately high (Cromartie & Han, 2018). In more sparsely settled regions with aging-in-place populations, access to mortgage credit and housing rehabilitation are likely more pressing concerns. These findings may be useful to program designers and grant managers as they plan for and implement housing support.

Economic development programs that support business retention, promote economic diversity and job growth, and increase incomes for all age groups are likely to reduce out-migration and attract working age newcomers, thus slowing the rate of aging due to younger-age population loss. Such programs include USDA's Business and Industry loans, as well as major investments underway at USDA and elsewhere to expand access to high-speed broadband Internet service. Reliable high-speed Internet provides multiple benefits to older persons living in remote areas of the U.S., addressing medical needs through telehealth and increasing social networks and contacts with family members. Social security, food and nutrition support, and improvements to rural education could contribute to reducing the pace of aging in areas that have begun to age rapidly this decade. Such areas are more diverse racially, with higher poverty rates and lower levels of education.

It is hoped that this case study analysis will stimulate further research to measure and map demographic components of aging at the local level. The increased specificity provided by the decomposition techniques employed here has the potential to extend our understanding of rural aging beyond the two dominant causes of aging: young-adult out-migration and retirement-related in-migration. By continuing to build the case study file and extending the analysis back to the 1950s and 1960s (decades in which rural out-migration peaked), it will be possible to map out a more extensive typology of common aging scenarios. Further refinements to the decomposition could be used to subdivide the natural change component of aging into separate measures for births, aging-in-place, and deaths. Most notably, increasing mortality trends are likely accelerating aging in rural areas affected by the ongoing drug crisis. Such impacts are likely small except in local areas such as Eastern Kentucky with persistently elevated levels of working age mortality. A comprehensive decomposition model of rural aging reflecting the full history of demographic changes affecting today's older residents will likely prove a valuable research tool for the geographic analysis of aging in the years to come.

References

Beale, C. (1982, May 19). *Older rural Americans: Unanswered questions*. Prepared statement before the Special Committee on Aging, United States Senate Ninety-seventh Congress, Second Session. Washington, DC: U.S. Government Printing Office, 15–28. Retrieved July 14, 2018, from https://www.aging.senate.gov/imo/media/doc/publications/5191982.pdf

Cromartie, J. (2017). *Rural America at a glance, 2017 edition*. Economic Information Bulletin (No. EIB-182). Washington, DC: Economic Research Service, U.S. Department of Agriculture. Retrieved from https://www.ers.usda.gov/publications/pub-details/?pubid=85739

Cromartie, J. (2018). *Rural America at a glance, 2018 edition*. Economic Information Bulletin (No. EIB-200). Washington, DC: Economic Research Service, U.S. Department of Agriculture. Retrieved from https://www.ers.usda.gov/publications/pub-details/?pubid=90555

Cromartie, J. B., & Han, P. (2018). What drives spatial variation in housing cost-burden among rural low- and moderate-income renters? In D. E. Albrecht, S. Loveridge, S. Goetz, & R. Welborn (Eds.), *Rural housing and economic development* (pp. 41–59). New York: Routledge.

Fuguitt, G. V. (1980). *Components of change in a proportion* (CDE Working Paper 80-9). Madison, WI: University of Wisconsin-Madison Center for Demography and Ecology. Retrieved from https://www.ssc.wisc.edu/cde/cdewp/80-9.pdf

Fuguitt, G. V., & Beale, C. L. (1993). The changing concentration of the older nonmetropolitan population, 1960–90. *Journal of Gerontology, 48*(6), S278–S288. Retrieved from https://www.ncbi.nlm.nih.gov/pubmed/8228002.

Fuguitt, G. V., Beale, C. L., & Voss, P. R. (2010). *County-specific net migration estimates, 1980-1990* (ICPSR 26761). Ann Arbor, MI: Inter-University Consortium for Political and Social Research. Retrieved from https://www.icpsr.umich.edu/icpsrweb/ICPSR/studies/26761

Fuguitt, G. V., & Heaton, T. B. (1995). The impact of migration on the nonmetropolitan population age structure, 1960-1990. *Population Research and Policy Review, 14*(2), 215–232.

Glasgow, N., & Berry, E. (Eds.). (2013). *Rural aging in the 21st century*. Dordrecht, Netherlands: Springer.

Glasgow, N., & Brown, D. L. (2012). Rural ageing in the United States: Trends and contexts. *Journal of Rural Studies, 28*(4), 422–431. https://doi.org/10.1016/j.jrurstud.2012.01.002

Golant, S. M. (2015). *Aging in the right place*. Baltimore, MD: Health Professionals Press.

Kinsella, K. & Phillips, D. R. (2005). Global aging: The challenge of success. *Population Bulletin*, 60(1), Retrieved August 13, 2018, from https://www.prb.org/wp-content/uploads/2008/07/60.1GlobalAging.pdf

Lichter, D. T., Fuguitt, G. V., Heaton, T. B., & Clifford, W. B. (1981). Components of change in the residential concentration of the elderly population: 1950-1975. *Journal of Gerontology, 36*(4), 480–489. https://doi.org/10.1093/geroni/36.4.480

Mather, M., Jacobsen, L. A., & Pollard, K. M. (2015). Aging in the United States, *Population Bulletin, 70*(2). Washington, DC: Population Reference Bureau. Retrieved August 16, 2018, from https://www.prb.org/wp-content/uploads/2016/01/aging-us-population-bulletin-1.pdf

Nelson, P. (2014). Concentrations of elderly in rural America: Patterns, processes, and outcomes in a neoliberal world. In C. Bailey, L. Jensen, & E. Ransom (Eds.), *Rural American in a globalizing world: Problems and prospects for the 2010s*. Morgantown, WV: West Virginia University Press.

Nelson, P. B. (2013). The geography of rural aging in a regional context, 1990–2008. In N. Glasgow & E. H. Berry (Eds.), *Rural aging in 21st century America* (pp. 37–54). Dordrecht: Springer Netherlands.

Phillips, D. R., & Feng, Z. (2017). Global ageing. In L. Skinner, G. Andrews, & M. Cutchin (Eds.), *Geographical gerontology: Perspectives, concepts, approaches*. New York: Routledge.

Pressler, L. (1982, May 19). *Older rural Americans: Unanswered questions*. Opening Statement before the Special Committee on Aging, United States Senate Ninety-seventh Congress, Second Session. Washington, DC: U.S. Government Printing Office, 1-2. Retrieved July 14, 2018, from https://www.aging.senate.gov/imo/media/doc/publications/5191982.pdf

Skinner, M. W., Andrews, G. J., & Cutchin, M. P. (Eds.). (2018). *Geographical gerontology: Perspectives, concepts, approaches*. New York: Routledge.

Thiede, B. C., Brown, D. L., Sanders, S. R., Glasgow, N., & Kulcsar, L. J. (2017). A demographic deficit? Local population aging and access to services in rural America, 1990–2010. *Rural Sociology, 82*(1), 44–74. https://doi.org/10.1111/ruso.12117

United Nations. (2015). *World population ageing 2015*. Department of Economic and Social Affairs, Population Division. New York: United Nations. Retrieved from https://www.un.org/en/development/desa/population/publications/pdf/ageing/WPA2015_Report.pdf

Voss, P. R., McNiven, S., Hammer, R. B., Johnson, K. M., & Fuguitt, G. V. (2004). *County-specific net migration by five-year age groups, Hispanic origin, race and sex: 1990-2000*. Ann Arbor, MI: Inter-university Consortium for Political and Social Research. Retrieved from https://www.icpsr.umich.edu/icpsrweb/ICPSR/studies/4171

Winkler, R., Johnson, K. M., Cheng, C., Beaudoin, J., Voss, P. R., & Curtis, K. J. (2013). *Age-specific net migration estimates for US counties, 1950–2010*. Applied Population Laboratory, University of Wisconsin-Madison. Retrieved June 30, 2018, from https://netmigration.wisc.edu/

Winkler, R. L., Johnson, K. M., Cheng, C., Voss, P. R., & Curtis, K. J. (2013). *County-specific net migration by five-year age groups, Hispanic origin, race and sex: 2000-2010*. Ann Arbor, MI: Inter-university consortium for Political and Social Research. https://doi.org/10.3886/ICPSR34638.v1

Winterton, R., Warburton, J., Keating, N., Petersen, M., Berg, T., & Wilson, J. (2016). Understanding the influence of community characteristics on wellness for rural older adults: A meta-synthesis. *Journal of Rural Studies, 45*, 320–327. https://doi.org/10.1016/j.jrurstud.2015.12.010

Part III
Family Roles, Well-Being, and Development Pathways in Rural Areas

Rural African Americans' Family Relationships and Well-Being

Velma McBride Murry, Shauna M. Cooper, Marketa Burnett, and Misha N. Inniss-Thompson

I have always believed that hope is that stubborn thing inside us that insists, despite all the evidence to the contrary, that something better awaits us so long as we have the courage to keep reaching, to keep working, to keep fighting.

—President Barack Obama, November 7, 2012

Our chapter is written in a landmark historical context wherein the world witnessed a major event–the election of the first Black president of the United States, Barack Obama. Despite this progress and other achievements since the post-civil rights era, far too many African Americans are disproportionately poor, lack quality education, are under- and unemployed, and are in poor health (Murry & Liu, 2014). Those residing in rural communities are more disadvantaged than their counterparts in urban settings. Increasing poverty and structural economic transformations in rural communities have been likened to Wilson's (1987) characterization of urban economic declined in *The Truly Disadvantaged* (Lee & Singelmann, 2006; Parisi, Grice, Taquino, & Gill, 2005). Rural communities are exposed to an increasing loss of access to health care, as demonstrated by financially distressed medical institutions and the shortage of physicians (Ricketts, 2000). Land is being lost to economic development, and small farm communities are becoming dumping grounds for toxic wastes and sites for prisons, instead of being used to grow food from their land. Consequently, residents of many rural communities lack access to healthy food though the land is rich for farming (Burton, Lichter, Baker, & Eason, 2013). This reduced access to healthy food plays an integral role in health-related outcomes and disparities. These environmental shifts juxtaposed with persistent poverty have resulted in many rural spaces now being labeled as "rural ghettos," where families

V. M. Murry (✉) · M. N. Inniss-Thompson
Vanderbilt University, Nashville, TN, USA
e-mail: velma.m.murry@vanderbilt.edu

S. M. Cooper · M. Burnett
University of North Carolina at Chapel Hill, Chapel Hill, NC, USA

J. E. Glick et al. (eds.), *Rural Families and Communities in the United States*,
National Symposium on Family Issues 10, https://doi.org/10.1007/978-3-030-37689-5_7

reside in areas of "high concentrations of poverty, social isolation, marginal labor force attachment, and social disorganization" (Burton et al., 2013, p. 8).

For African American families, these environmental changes are nested in a context where racism, prejudice, discrimination, oppression, and segregation, relegating them to marginalized social positions, may exacerbate disadvantage. While these conditions take a toll on families and children, many families have the capacity to negotiate and navigate their environment, and are able to be healthy and raise healthy children (Murry, 2019). Yet, the underlying processes that explain how families are able to muster the energy and wherewithal to overcome these challenges are not well understood (Burton et al., 2013). We contend that a full understanding of what goes on inside rural African American families cannot be achieved without careful consideration of both contextual and social risks, as well as assets and resources relevant to fostering positive relationships and well-being in families (Murry, Butler-Barnes, Mayo-Gamble, & Inniss-Thompson, 2018). In this chapter, we draw on ecological contextually driven theories, as well as strength-based conceptual models, to guide the synthesis of research explaining how settings, in this instance, rural spaces, influence family processes and functioning of African American families. Further, we acknowledge the presence of relative plasticity in humans and that this flexibility may be key to explaining differential responses of families to the challenges of living in and raising children in rural spaces. It is this information that is needed to inform and guide preventive interventions and policies.

We begin by providing a brief rationale for the focus on rural African American families, including historical patterns and current demographic shifts. Next, we summarize theoretical and conceptual models used to frame studies of African American families. Using a critical lens, we identify strengths, effectiveness, and weaknesses of these models and suggest ways to make them more applicable to rural African American families. Following this discussion, we synthesize extant studies of rural African American families. To the extent possible, we identify studies that have examined how family processes are interlocked with contextual processes to explain individual differences in mental, physical, social, and behavioral well-being. Finally, we highlight two studies with rural African American families that integrate strength-based factors and assets, demonstrating ways to translate research on rural African American families into practice.

Why Focus on Rural African American Families?

For African American families in the rural south, everyday life experiences including life opportunities and advancements continue to be affected by the vestiges of slavery, Jim Crow Laws, racism, and discrimination (Murry & Liu, 2014). The everyday life experiences for many African American families who reside in the rural South are more challenging than what is observed in urban areas due to the concentration of poverty (Lichter, Parisi, & Taquino, 2012). Population trend data shows that rural African American families are not only more likely to be poor but are also more likely to be living in situations characterized as persistent "deep poverty." Furthermore, rural environments often lack structural resources that are typically available to families in urban settings (Proctor & Dalaker, 2003). Rural families must deal with a restricted range of employment, long distances to businesses and services, limited public transportation, and lack of recreational facilities for children (Murry, Berkel, Brody, Miller, & Chen, 2009). In addition, families living in rural environments have fewer educational opportunities than do their urban counterparts (Rojewski, 1995; Witherspoon & Ennett, 2011), and most jobs available to rural African Americans are labor intensive and pay low wages (Brody, Kim, Murry, & Brown, 2005). These economic conditions coupled with demographic shifts in rural communities have significance for the current state of African American families living in rural spaces. Yet, research studies of rural African American families describing their unique social location and propose preventions, interventions, and social policies to improve their well-being remain largely invisible.

African American Families in Rural Spaces: Historical Patterns and Current Trends

Reflecting a historical pattern, the majority of African Americans reside in the Southern region of the U.S. (Lichter & Campbell, 2005). Residential concentration in these regions reveals that most African American families are located in the Black Belt, which runs from North and South Carolina through Georgia, Tennessee, Alabama, Mississippi, Arkansas, and Louisiana (Albrecht, Albrecht, & Murguia, 2005). Based on the 2010 Census reports of population growth, while there has been rapid growth in rural communities, African Americans represent the lowest minority group growth (2.9%). Larger growth has occurred among all other groups of color, ranging from 25% to 46% for Latinx, Asian, American Indian, and Native/Pacific Islander (U.S. Census, 2010). This demographic shift may impact dynamics between rural African American families and other groups, particularly in communities that have restricted resources (Lichter, 2012). Furthermore, these demographic patterns and changes may complicate race-related interactions, potentially exacerbating existing economic gaps between high- and low-resource communities and neighborhoods.

Currently, approximately 67% of poor rural blacks live in the South—and primarily in high-poverty counties (Lichter et al., 2012) compared to 38.7% of poor rural Hispanics. While more than half of all poor rural families are European American (Lichter, Qian, & Crowley, 2005), rural minorities are often highly segregated from their White counterparts, regardless of income (Lichter et al., 2012). Changing geographic spatial residence patterns not only decrease opportunities for racial and ethnic mixing, but also increase economic gaps between high resource and low resource communities and neighborhoods. Further, these demographic shifts increase the likelihood that rural African American families will continue to be disproportionately poor (Friedman & Lichter, 1998) and experience restricted opportunities, which will negatively affect their health and well-being in pervasive ways (Murry, Butler-Barnes, et al., 2018). Thus, the changing demographics and neighborhood settlements of families in the U.S. are impacting the life course of all families.

As previously noted, demographic shifts and population growth in rural black communities have been slow. There are some notable shifts though, that may contribute to our understanding of African Americans in rural communities, particularly in reference to their family processes and overall well-being. Over the last 30 years, with greater increases occurring within the last 15 years, a large number of African Americans have begun moving back to the South (Ihrke & Faber, 2012; U.S. Census Bureau, 2016). This demographic shift, termed *reverse migration*, represents an exodus of African Americans from large metropolitan areas to cities in the Southern region of the U.S. For instance, there were dramatic decreases in the African American population of Chicago, New York, and Detroit and an overall 2% population increase for African Americans in the South (U.S. Census, 2010). This demographic trend is noteworthy for a couple of reasons. First, a large number of reverse migrators are composed of African American parents who are returning to the south seeking greater economic opportunities and improved quality of life for their children. Second, a significant number represent older African Americans returning to their homeplaces to retire, which are often located in or near small, rural communities. The long-term implications and impacts of reverse migration for rural African Americans are not immediately clear. However, it may have a direct economic impact as well as influence family processes. For instance, older African Americans who may have been part of the Great Migration, which brought many southern African Americans to the Northeast, Midwest, and Western regions of the U.S., are now returning to the South and bringing with them amassed resources. Additionally, African Americans who return may serve as critical social support, both instrumentally and emotionally, for family members who have maintained residence in these rural communities. Thus, while most of the states where the migration is occurring are those with long-standing poverty, the new or returning residents have the potential to reduce or widen social stratification divides within rural African American families. It is worth noting that there is a dearth of research on reverse migration patterns of African Americans and, given the potential impact that their presence may assuage on economic, political, and social processes in the rural south, future research on this phenomenon is warranted. In sum, efforts to document demographic trends and patterns in rural spaces have primarily sought to describe economic circumstances and shifts in populations migrating into these communities, creating greater ethnic racial diversity. However, there has been limited attention given to understanding how these changes are affecting everyday life experiences of African American families. This lack of knowledge may be attributed to theories commonly used to frame studies of African Americans, in general, and rural families in particular.

In the next section, we provide an overview of theories and models used to study African Americans and consider the applicability to what we know about family relationships and well-being among rural African Americans. We highlight the limitations of what we know about these families including obvious omissions which may be a function of theoretical selection biases. Next, we summarize existing research highlighting family and community assets for rural African Americans. This is followed by an overview of culturally tailored, preventive intervention programs and research designed to enhance protective processes in rural African American families.

Theoretical Frameworks of Rural African American Family Well-Being

In the quest to highlight the lived experiences of rural African American families and the implications for their relationships and well-being, we examine whether studies are framed by contextualized and process-oriented perspectives. Applying these perspectives provides opportunities to more clearly understand the distinct experiences of African Americans (Jarrett, 1998; cf. Wiley, Warren, & Montanelli, 2002). Contextual-focused theories are appropriate to guide studies of African American families in general, and rural families in particular, in order to highlight the impact of historical, economic, social, and political contexts of rural communities. Finally, given the significance of ancestral heritage, religion, and traditions to everyday life experiences of African American families, studies of normative functioning in rural families should include culturally protective and strength-based factors in their theoretical foundations. With this critical lens, we begin by summarizing studies that have applied ecological frameworks in studies of African American families, with specific focus on investigations of families residing in rural spaces.

Ecological and Cultural–Ecological Perspectives

Ecological models posit that individuals' dynamic interactions with their contexts shape development over time (Bronfenbrenner, 2005). Much of the existing research has framed the discussion on rural African American families around macrolevel factors. In particular, research has disentangled, defined, and redefined economic risk to include income, employment opportunities, availability or lack of resources (e.g., health, education), and the intergenerational effects of chronic poverty (Burton, 1996; Wiley et al., 2002). Studies have illuminated the ways in which economic disadvantage influences health care and legal resource availability in rural communities. Prior experiences in the mental health care system, as well as perceptions of stigma held in their communities about mental illness, dissuaded caregivers from seeking care and treatment for their children (Murry, Heflinger, Suiter, & Brody, 2011). Further, while school counselors were the primary source for identifying mental health and behavioral concerns, treatment and care often occurred as a consequence of disciplinary punishment in schools, which then served as a gateway to juvenile justice systems (Murry et al., 2011). This investigation reflects the very real and potentially damaging impact of structural factors in the daily lives of rural Americans, as indicated by the impact on health care seeking, treatment, and utilization of reduced access to quality health care in their communities. Although widespread in rural communities, these issues disproportionately impact African American families, particularly in the rural South.

In addition to restricting opportunity and resources, macrolevel factors may have direct filtrating effects on rural African Americans. We identified three areas for categorizing and assessing how macrolevel factors may have direct filtrating effects, namely (1) influencing parents' well-being; (2) contributing to child well-being; and (3) effecting child well-being via impact on parenting and family processes. Highlighting the link between macrolevel systems and individual micro-level factors, studies have explored how economic context influences *parent* well-being. Investigations examining these associations have centered on an array of outcomes that directly and indirectly relate to parent well-being, including factors such as mental health, stress, coping, and marital/co-partner relationship quality. Among a sample of rural African American mothers, economic strain, and racial discrimination were individually associated with greater depressive symptoms (Murry et al., 2008; Odom, Vernon-Feagans,, & Family Life Project, 2010). These investigations suggest that the combination of economic and race-related stress may adversely influence mothers' mental health through the erosion of self-efficacy and perceptions of diminished control over one's environment. Studies have also indicated that macrolevel processes (e.g., economic stress, racial transgressions, and encounters) can filter through to influence marital and co-partner relationships. For instance, a highly conflicted marital relationship (e.g., less stability, warmth, and stability; greater hostility) was associated with diminished psychological functioning among rural African American women (Murry et al., 2008). However, the potential compromising effects of racial discrimination on rural African American women's psychological well-being were less evident among those in intimate relationships characterized as close, connected, and supportive. Further, examining the buffering effects of supportive spousal relationships in rural African American families is particularly contributory as scholars have asserted that the dual impact of economic conditions and racial discrimination may have long-term implications for the well-being of rural African Americans in general, and marital relationship stability in particular (Murry et al., 2008).

Additionally, ecologically framed studies have examined how macrolevel factors impact micro-level indicators of child well-being. These studies have conceptualized child well-being to include a number of outcomes, including psychological functioning, externalizing behaviors, self-perception, and academic adjustment. Acknowledging the distinct experiences that shape the well-being of African American children, studies have also utilized culturally framed ecological frameworks to further advance understanding of the developmental competencies of ethnic minority youth (Ogbu, 1981; Spencer, Dupree, & Hartmann, 1997). This work has been particularly instrumental in explaining how macrolevel processes shape the academic self-beliefs, expectations, and outcomes of African American youth. Drawing on the social stratification theory, an integrative model for the study of developmental competencies in minority families and children was developed (García Coll et al.'s (1996). The model asserts that there are critical aspects of the youth of color's environments that are profoundly influenced by racism, prejudice, discrimination, oppression, and segregation and are distinct from any comparable influence for white youth. In this regard, studies of the well-being of African American children growing up in rural spaces need to consider ways in which social positions of marginalization and socioeconomic status (SES) contribute to and influence the everyday life experiences and processes in families of children of color. Other macrolevel frameworks include the oppositional cultural identity perspective (Fordham & Ogbu, 1986; Ogbu, 2004), which focuses specifically on explaining variability in academic outcomes of African American children. The perspective contends that the academic achievement of African American children is shaped by the larger social structure and experiences in the social world (Fordham & Ogbu, 1986). This theory was tested by examining the extent to which racial and ethnic socialization buffered rural African American youths from masking their academic abilities to do well in school (Murry et al., 2009). Findings demonstrated that adaptive racial and ethnic socialization did indeed increase academic performance among rural African American children through the enhancement of racial identity and self-esteem. Adolescents who develop positive racial identities are likely to reject stereotypic images of their race and develop high self-esteem. They are less likely to use academic self-presentation strategies as a way to defy oppressions of larger social structures. These studies highlight the importance of rural African American parents teaching their children about racial- and ethnic-related issues, as well as encouraging them to be strong and work hard. The lessons from parents foster a sense of empowerment, confidence, and pride to do well in school.

In fact, research specific to rural African American children has found that race- and economic-related experiences not only shape their interactions but also guide adaptation and response to the social world (Kerpelman, Eryigit, & Stephens, 2008). Based on data from the National Educational Longitudinal Study to examine aspirational differences among rural, urban, and suburban African American male high school students, low-SES and lower achieving African American rural males had lower aspirations in comparison to suburban African American males (Strayhorn, 2009). Findings added further support that ecological contexts influence and shape beliefs about perceived educational opportunity. This investigation highlights ways in social position, in this instance, low SES and low academic performance, interacts with youths' future orientation and in turn influences educational aspirations and academic behaviors.

Other frameworks have connected context to social position and child well-being. The phenomenological variant of ecological systems theory (PVEST; Spencer et al., 1997) demonstrated associations among racial identity, stressful life events, and internalizing problems among rural African American youth. Specifically, a strong sense of racial identity appears to buffer rural African American youth from experiencing depressive symptoms when exposed to multiple negative life events (Mulser, Hucke, Trask-Tate, & Cunningham, 2012). Thus, PVEST and other cultural–ecological frameworks provide an opportunity to not only understand how context shapes developmental processes, risk, and protective factors, but to also understand how individuals, families, and communities make meaning of their own experiences and the process of developing adaptive strategies.

Extending beyond individual (micro) level indicators of child well-being, studies have examined how macrolevel processes have direct filtrating effects on children through their impact on family relationships and parenting. These investigations have incorporated ecological and process models to identify mechanisms and guiding processes (Berkel et al., 2009). Reflecting a Structural Ecosystems approach (Szapocznik & Coatsworth, 1999), Bynum and Brody (2005) sought to identify ways in which maternal education and mother–child relationship quality impacted African American rural youths' externalizing and internalizing behaviors through mother–child relationship quality. Results revealed that mothers with higher levels of education were found to have greater coping resources for navigating their daily experiences. Further, the use of coping resources was associated with more positive mother–child relationships, which in turn decreased children's internalizing and externalizing behaviors through the promotion of self-regulatory skills.

Other parenting behaviors that have influenced rural African American children's well-being are parents' own discrimination experiences that shape family conversations about race and culture. Rural African American mothers who experienced discrimination were more likely to engage in racial-cultural discussions with their children, and the underlying processes of these conversations influenced child outcomes (Berkel et al., 2009). Specifically, conversations about race, often characterized as ethnic and racial socialization messages, are adaptive responses to the social environment of raising a black child in the U.S. These conversations are viewed as adaptive because they are geared toward promoting child resilience through the encouragement of racial pride and positive self-views, balanced with messages to prepare children for encounters with discrimination and racial bias (Murry et al., 2009). The installation of a positive sense of racial self-perception and a sense of group belongingness help youth resist internalizing negative images and stereotypes surrounding African Americans. Collectively, investigations of racial socialization and racial identity demonstrate ways in which African American parents negotiate and navigate macrolevel experiences (e.g., structural and racial inequities) that shape parenting strategies and practices to raise their children and influence well-being and adjustment.

Family Stress and Process Models

Family process and stress coping frameworks (McCubbin et al., 1980; Peters & Massey, 1983) have situated family stress and associated functioning within larger social and economic contexts (Conger et al., 1992). Family stress models, for example, propose that economic disadvantage may lead to greater economic stress, which may adversely influence individual and family well-being (Conger et al., 2002; Dorsey, Forehand, & Brody, 2007; Elder Jr., 1985; McLoyd, 1990). Studies with African American samples have found that economic concerns and adequate housing were prominent stressors for those residing in rural communities (Burton, 1996; Wiley et al., 2002). Moreover, investigations have identified several pathways through which economic stress and strain influence individual and family well-being (Brody & Flor, 1998; Brody, Flor, & Gibson, 1999; Conger et al., 2002; Cutrona et al., 2003; Farmer, Marien, Clark, Sherman, & Selva, 2004; McLoyd, 1998; Murry, Brown, Brody, Cutrona, & Simons, 2001). Using data from the Family and Community Health Study (FACHS), Conger et al. (2002) identified a link between low per capita income and economic stress among two-caregiver rural African American families. Additionally, increased economic stress was associated with depressed mood among both primary and secondary caregivers. Caregivers' depressed mood indirectly impacted their children's adjustment through compromised parenting and a reduction in family relationship quality. Other studies examining family stress processes across the life course also noted direct and indirect spillover effects on child and adolescent adjustment (Taylor, Larsen-Rife, Conger, Widaman, & Cutrona, 2010). Using an adapted version of the original family stress model, the Mundane Extreme Environmental Stress model (Peters & Massey, 1983), researchers demonstrated pathways through which racial discrimination amplified the effects of economic strain and pressure on psychological functioning and marital relationship quality among rural African American women (Murry et al., 2008; Murry, Brown, et al., 2001). Though these models have identified stress-related mechanisms or risk factors, they have not systematically incorporated a strengths-based lens.

Risk and Resilience Frameworks

Although several conceptualizations of risk and resilience have been proposed (Fergus & Zimmerman, 2005; Garmezy, 1996; Masten, 2013; Masten & Coatsworth, 1998), across frameworks there has been broad agreement in two key premises: (1) that adversity or a significant threat exists and (2) there is positive adaptation despite these risks (cf. Luthar, Cicchetti, & Becker, 2000). There has been some debate though about the extent to which positive adaptation is universally defined. Evidence indicates that individual and contextual variation exists in positive development and adaptation. Whether explicitly articulated or implied by the employed methodological approach, a number of studies have sought to identify risks among rural African Americans as well as examine mitigating factors. These studies have revealed that rural African American families and youth are differentially exposed to various social contextual risks (Murry, Bynum, Brody, Willert, & Stephens, 2001; Vazsonyi, Trejos-Castillo, & Young, 2008). Although little variation in risk factors was found between families residing in rural and non-rural spaces, drug use and delinquency were higher for African American rural youth (Vazsonyi et al., 2008). Further, in comparison to non-rural African American youth, the stronger association between family risk factors and rural youth problem behaviors may provide some indication that economic risk factors are mediated by family and neighborhood factors.

Several studies have sought to identify pathways through which families and communities dissuade youth from engaging in risky behaviors. In their efforts to highlight and explain how families overcome adversities, scholars have advocated for the use of resilience frameworks (Murry, Bynum, et al., 2001). Investigations using the resilience framework to study African American families and youth have emphasized that promotive and protective factors are multilevel in nature, encompassing individual, family, cultural, and community domains (Brody, Dorsey, Forehand, & Armistead, 2002; Irvin, Farmer, Leung, Thompson, & Hutchins, 2010). One protective factor that reflects both cultural and community protection is youth's involvement in religious activities (e.g., choir, youth group activities). Involvement in church, after accounting for school activities, promoted higher academic achievement among low-income rural African American adolescents (Irvin et al., 2010). Further, organized classroom environments served a protective function against family difficulties experienced by rural African American elementary and middle school students (Brody et al., 2002). Additionally, in samples with rural and non-rural children, there is some indication of variability in the nature and strength of risk and resilience factors. In comparison to non-rural youth, community risk, and resilience factors were more protective for rural youth (Clark, Nguyen, and Belgrave (2011). Specifically, this investigation noted that family and community factors, in comparison to peer and individual factors, were more strongly associated with reduced substance use risk. Historically, family contexts have been central in the resilience of African Americans. It is likely that the closer proximity of rural youth to extended family members may offer greater opportunities for social interactions and closer monitoring by neighbors, a process characterized as collective socialization. Family- and community-level protection extends adult oversight in monitoring neighborhood children and has implications for encouraging positive developmental pathways for African American youth (Berkel et al., 2009; Burton & Jarrett, 2000; Roche & Leventhal, 2009), thereby serving to protect youth from engagement in risk behaviors.

Research has also explored risk and resilience at the biological level (Evans, 2003). Residing in neighborhoods with increasing poverty was associated with elevated allostatic load among rural African Americans, placing them at risk for early onset of chronic disease, such as hypertension and diabetes, as they transitioned into young adulthood (Brody, Lei, Chen, & Miller, 2014). Additionally, this study demonstrated that emotional support networks, however, mitigated the negative effects of neighborhood poverty on elevated allostatic load and its consequences. Other investigations have alluded to the complexity, and sometimes counterintuitive nature of these relationships. Applying principles of risk and resilience theories and John Henryism (James, 1994), Brody et al. (2013) found that SES-related risk, which included multiple indicators of economic risk (e.g., family poverty level, parental education, employment, family structure, income), moderated the association between self-competence and elevated allostatic load among African American rural youth, such that higher self-competent youth demonstrated greater physiological weathering (i.e., allostatic load) over time compared to lower self-competent youth. This finding offers greater insight on adaptive processes that may be unique among rural African American families and also suggests the need to further contextualize development of African American youth residing in rural spaces.

Integrative Model for the Study of Stress in Black American Families

Aforementioned theoretical frameworks have illuminated the processes that may shape family functioning, health, and well-being in rural African American families. These models have helped to refine existing theories and brought forth new theoretical frameworks that address both the distinctive experiences of this population as well as the inherent within-group variation that exists. Incorporating principles of ecological, family stress, biopsychosocial, and integrative frameworks (García Coll et al., 1996; Myers, 2009; Peters & Massey, 1983), the integrative model for the study of stress in black American families asserts that sociocultural, race-related, and structural stressors are commonplace in the lives of African American families (Murry, Butler-Barnes, et al., 2018). Importantly, the model emphasizes that these stressors, which accumulate and proliferate across the life course, lead to individual-, family-, and community-level vulnerabilities. Responding to their contexts, this model contends that families implement a range of strengths-based assets to mitigate stressors and promote positive development, adjustment, and adaptation. Addressing a need in the theoretical literature, the integrative model for the study of stress in black American families emphasizes the role of cultural strengths-based coping assets, or *ordinary magic* in the lives of African American families (see Fig. 1).

Ordinary magic, emerges as individuals and families' identity opportunities to adapt and respond to their adversity within their social contexts (Masten, 2001; Murry, Butler-Barnes, et al., 2018). A needed focus, this chapter turns attention to *cultural strengths-based coping assets and processes* in the lives of rural African American families. In the following section, we summarize existing studies that have explored ordinary magic through the lens of family and community contexts.

Cultural Strength-Based Coping Assets: Ordinary Magic in Families Theoretical and empirical evidence suggests that macrolevel systems have greatly shaped familial roles and values in rural African American families (Burton et al., 2013), an influence that can be seen within and across generational contexts. These experiences influence African American family's collective responses to their social world as well as individual well-being and family adaptation (Murry, Butler-Barnes, et al., 2018). For instance, support and cohesion among family members has been defined as an important adaptive and coping asset for rural African American families. Considering frequency and quality of contact with family members, investigations have demonstrated that families engaging in consistent and supportive interactions serve a key protective role for rural African American families (Murry et al., 2005).

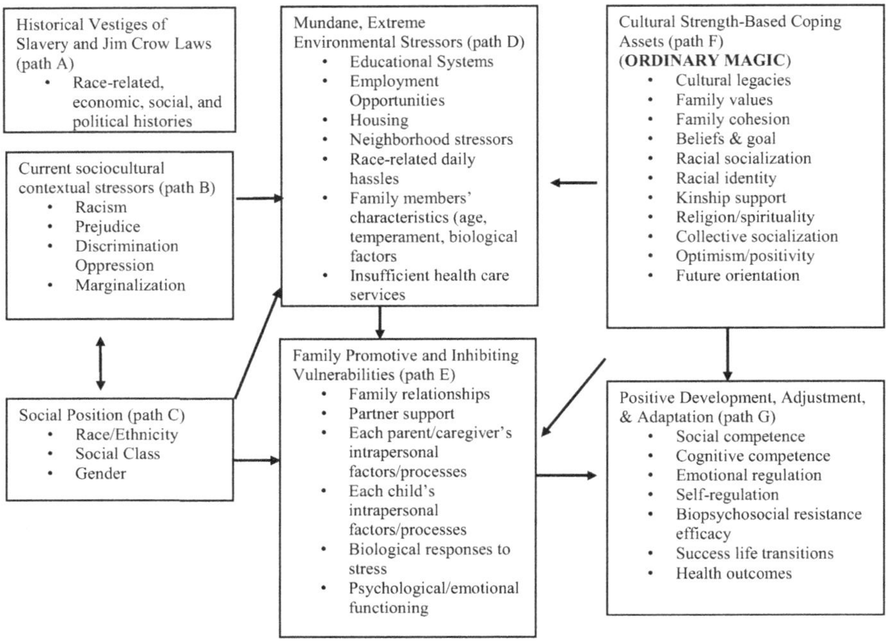

Fig. 1 Integrative model for the study of stress in black American families. Adapted from Murry, Butler-Barnes, et al., 2018

For example, several studies have highlighted how African American families in rural communities contend with racial discrimination and intergenerational economic disenfranchisement. These experiences greatly shape the larger context of parenting and family processes. Racial socialization, which is composed of messages meant to help youth navigate in the face of discrimination and transmit important cultural values is a common strategy for African American parents (Hughes et al., 2006). Research with rural families demonstrate the adaptive nature of cultural socialization, particularly discussions that emphasize group pride and affirmation (Berkel et al., 2009; Murry et al., 2009). Additionally, racial socialization and larger parenting processes have been found to influence a key mechanism for promoting positive child and adolescent outcomes—ethnic-racial identity (Murry et al., 2005; Murry et al., 2009). Thus, these discussions promote positive views about youths' racial or ethnic group and in turn, influence more positive self-beliefs and well-being (Murry et al., 2009).

Also, largely reflecting their awareness of contextual risk, parents are significant socializing agents who transmit attitudes, values, and norms regarding appropriate behavior and consequences for misbehavior (Jaccard & Dittus, 2000; Jaccard, Dittus, & Gordon, 1996; Whitaker & Miller, 2000). Thus, the mechanism through which parents are able to influence their children's behavior is through youths' internalization of parental norms, values, and expectations. Internalization is more likely to occur when youth and parent engage in frequent positive communication behaviors (Brody, Flor, Hollett-Wright, & McCoy, 1998; Whitaker & Miller, 2000). Research has shown that parents' and adolescents' engagement in positive communication can promote positive developmental pathways, including reduced risk behavior engagement. For instance, rural African American parents' articulated expectations regarding sexual activities and substance use significantly influenced their adolescents' decisions about risk engagement (Murry, McNair, Myers, Chen, & Brody, 2014).

In addition to direct associations, evidence has identified indirect pathways through which family relationships in African American rural families influence adolescent outcomes. Open communication between parents and adolescents shape youths' images of risk-taking peers (Williams, 2003), increases self-regulation and self-control, and increases their willingness to avoid risk opportunity situations and resist peer pressure (Berkel et al., 2009; Murry, Simons, Simons, & Gibbons, 2013). Both research and theory support that deviant peer affiliations serve as a proximal link to early sexual debut, onset of alcohol use, and disengagement from conventional activities such as academic achievement (Elliott, Huizinga, & Ageton, 1985; Hawkins, Catalano, & Miller, 1992; Mosbach & Leventhal, 1988; Patterson, DeBaryshe, & Ramsey, 1989). Moreover, previous empirical work contends that positive parent–child communication about risky behaviors moderates the effects of peer pressure on youths' decisions about sexual activity and using alcohol and other substances (Brody et al., 2005; Hill & Craft, 2003; Hill & Tyson, 2009).

Community Context Studies support the influential role of community in rural contexts, for both African American children and families. Community settings where youth and families are presented with opportunities and resources serve to reduce risk and promote adjustment and adaptation. Research has shown that for rural African American mothers living in high-poverty neighborhoods, positive relationships and social support from extended family members becomes an adaptive strategy for positive family functioning (Jarrett, Jefferson, & Kelly, 2010). Kinship support includes both emotional and instrumental support for rural African American parents (Jarrett et al., 2010). Also, living in a neighborhood characterized by high collective socialization positively influences vigilant parenting strategies, a parenting approach known to be protective for rural African American youth (Berkel et al., 2009).

In addition to influencing familial relationships, parenting, and overall functioning (Vazsonyi et al., 2008), community support and connectedness promote positive well-being and reduces risk in adult rural populations (Letvak, 2002). Research has highlighted how community support and cohesion influences family and marital relationships. Connectedness with neighbors moderates the link between partner relationship quality and psychological functioning among rural African American women (Black, Cook, Murry, & Cutrona, 2005). Community connectedness and support have also been linked to positive psychological well-being (Markstrom, Marshall, & Tryon, 2000) and reduced risk behavior engagement among rural African American adolescents (Browning, Burrington, Leventhal, & Brooks-Gunn, 2008; Clark et al., 2011). In comparison to urban youth, community resilience factors (i.e., community cohesion) more strongly predicted delayed onset of alcohol and marijuana use among rural African American adolescents

(Clark et al., 2011). In fact, rural spaces, by nature of reduced mobility and closer proximity, provide increased opportunities for rural youth to interact with members of their community, providing the norms, values, and standards that can guide and inform youth on how to act, including how to avoid risk opportunity situations (Murry, McNair, et al., 2014).

Though studies have linked community contexts to child and adolescent outcomes, the underlying mechanisms illuminating how community contexts or neighborhoods, particularly disadvantaged ones, become linked with adolescents' risky behavior are less clear. A general assumption is that community residents influence youths' behavior by providing the norms, values, and standards that can guide and inform them on how to act. Moreover, growing up in close-knit communities in which adults use strategies to support each other (e.g., monitoring neighborhood children), a process referred to as collective socialization (Burton & Jarrett, 2000), can encourage positive developmental pathways for rural African American adolescents. Community norms and expectations for youth behaviors provide social control, as youth are socialized on behaviors that are sanctioned by the community and protocols and procedures for correcting misbehavior (Simons, Simons, Conger, & Brody, 2004). A benefit of having other adults invest in the well-being of youth is that it provides an additional monitoring system that extends beyond household boundaries. Extant studies of rural communities have shown collective socialization to have long-term protective effects against risk engaging behaviors among rural youth by dissuading them from affiliating with deviant peers (Brody et al., 2001; Murry et al., 2009; Simons et al., 2004).

Historically, the black church has been a support system for African Americans, an institution that still maintains influence within rural communities today. That black churches have a pivotal role in the development of youth is not surprising given that this institution has historically served as a place of refuge and support for African Americans (Chatters, Taylor, Jackson, & Lincoln, 2008; Smith, Faris, Denton, & Regnerus, 2003). Asset-based studies have shown that church involvement facilitates moral development, racial pride, healthy self-esteem, and self-efficacy, and in turn, increased prosocial competence including academic success and civic engagement among both rural and non-rural African American youth (Brody, Stoneman, Flor, & McCrary, 1994; Lincoln & Mamiya, 1990; Williams, 2000). For African American youth, the church also increases their connections to other adults with whom they can build supportive relationships. The black church is characterized as "a village opportunity to provide positive experiences for youth" (Williams, 2003, p. 27) and exemplifies the collective socialization found in many rural African American communities (Berkel et al., 2009). The benefits of "the village" have been found to impact adolescents directly. For instance, a number of studies have indicated that church involvement reduces adolescents' likelihood of risk behavior engagement in rural communities (Nasim, Fernander, Townsend, Corona, & Belgrave, 2011; Piko, Kovacs, Kriston, & Fitzpatrick, 2012). Moreover, church involvement may influence children's outcomes indirectly through the support that their parents' gain from church members and neighbors (Black et al., 2005).

Taken together, these studies emphasize the role of family- and community-specific strengths-based assets in adjustment and adaptation. While previous theories have typically focused on the role of macrolevel influences, they have not fully acknowledged the ordinary magic that exists within rural African American families through inclusion or integration in study frameworks and designs. Building upon this work and applying the integrative model for the study of stress in black American families, the following section discusses two critical areas of focus in the continued study of rural African American families: (1) the role of preventive interventions in bolstering protective processes among rural African American families and (2) a need to examine the roles, experiences, and contributions of African American rural fathers.

Harnessing Strengths-Based Assets Through Preventive Interventions

Powerful factors that protect African American youth from high-risk behaviors originate in the family environment, particularly in parents' caregiving practices (Murry et al., 2005) which have been shown to buffer their children from engaging in numerous risky behaviors. An ongoing challenge for prevention scientists, however, has been how to effectively harness African American families' protective capacities as malleable targets in preventive intervention programs and identify ways to increase access to such programs. Prevention research is not only a means of testing an intervention's effectiveness; it can also be used to test the theory on which the intervention is based (Cicchetti & Toth, 1992; Dishion & Patterson, 1999). In this section, we summarize two programs that have integrated a strengths-based approach in the design, development, and implementation of family-based preventive intervention programs targeting rural African Americans: Strong African American Families Program (SAAF), Pathways for African American Success (PAAS). Also, highlighting African American fathers, the Fathers and Mothers in the Lives of Youth (F.A.M.I.L.Y) study emphasizes the roles, experiences, and contributions of fathers as an important context for understanding prevention in African American rural families. Most notable about this collective work is the inclusion of both universal and culturally specific strength-based assets of African American families as intervention targets. These programs are designed to enhance parenting and family relationships, and in turn promote health and well-being, as evidenced by positive development and adjustment among parents and their children.

Culturally Tailored Family-Based Preventive Interventions

We begin with an overview of Strong African American Families (SAAF) and Pathways for African American Success (PAAS) Programs. Both programs are universal preventive interventions designed to deter HIV risk vulnerability among rural African American youth. They differ in testing sites of rural spaces, randomization sequences, and in the delivery platform of the experimental conditions.

SAAF is a two-arm randomized control trial (RCT) tested on 677 families with a child who was 11-years old at recruitment from nine rural counties in Georgia. In constructing the randomization sequence of the nine counties, two were small and contiguous and were combined into a single population unit, yielding eight county units. These eight county units were randomly assigned to either the control or the intervention condition, resulting in four county units in each condition. Families and youths were pretested before the intervention, post-tested 3 months after the intervention, and given a long-term follow-up assessment 24 months post-intervention when the target youths were 13.5 years old, with additional follow-ups as youth transitioned into young adulthood.

The PAAS program is a 3-arm RCT tested on 421 African American families recruited from five rural counties in Tennessee. At the county level, families were randomized into the following conditions: (1) self-directed, technology-based ($N = 141$); (2) in-person, small group led by facilitators ($N = 141$); and (3) noninteractive literature control with home-mailed educational materials ($N = 141$). Criteria for county selection was based on rurality, proportion of African American residents, evidence of high rates of teen pregnancy, and negative overall health indicators. Specifically, counties were selected based on the following characteristics: (1) rurality index scores greater than 11 (scale of 0 = least rural to 16 or greater = most rural), (2) over 30% African American residents, (3) over 600 African American teens in the targeted age range, (4) teen pregnancy rates of 69% (which is 13% higher than the average for TN), and (5) TN state health indicators reflect poor health determinant outcomes including health care, health behaviors, socioeconomic factors related to health, and physical environment (U.S. Census Bureau, 2010). Families and youths were pretested before the intervention, reinterviewed at post-test (on average, 4.4 months post-intervention), when youth were on average 14.5 years old, and again at long-term follow-up approximately 4 months after post-test when youth were transitioning from junior high to high school.

Theoretical Underpinnings of SAAF and PAAS Both SAAS and PAAS were informed by findings from Murry and colleagues' longitudinal developmental research program with rural African American youths and their families. SAAF and PAAS's causative model, illustrated in Figure 2, includes factors and processes

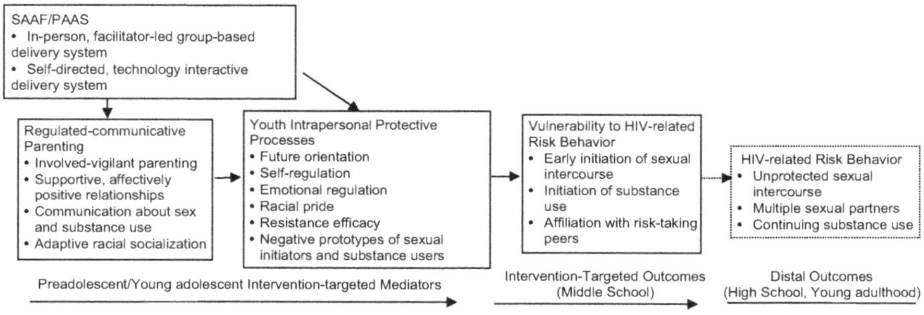

Fig. 2 SAAF/PAAS causative model

designed to change parenting and youth behaviors, and in turn, dissuade youth from engaging in risky behaviors. Results demonstrate that powerful protective factors for child and adolescent problem behaviors originate in the family, particularly in parents' caregiving practices (Murry & Brody, 1999). Caregiving practices play a pivotal role in children's and adolescents' positive development. Effective caregiver–youth relationships foster self-regulation, academic competence, psychological adjustment, and avoidance of alcohol and other substance use (e.g., Wills et al., 2007). Based on this research program, feedback from focus groups with rural African American parents and youths, and the research literature, Murry and associates defined proximal, malleable strengths-based factors and protective assets for primary caregivers and youths. That information was used to design, development, and implemented these curricula.

Recent advances in computer-based interactive technology offer a potentially cost-effective means to increase rural African American families' access to evidence-based prevention programming. The impetus for developing the technology arm of PAAS was in response to the need for increased access. In so doing, theories that inform which program delivery modalities would facilitate programmatic effects on participants' behavioral outcomes were selected. In this regard, traditional learning theories including cognitionism, constructionism, and behaviorism were used to explain linkages among program content, graphics, and computer-driven interactive activities. Traditional learning theories were also used to explain linkages among intervention-induced changes in knowledge, attitudes, decision-making, and skill development that were conferred to be manifested through changes in parent and youth intervention-targeted behaviors.

Family-Based Efficacy and Effectiveness Trials

SAAF Effects on Parent-Level Processes SAAF facilitated intervention-induced changes in strength-based factors and assets in parents, including involved-vigilant parenting, adaptive racial socialization, open, clear, supportive communication in families, and supportive family relationships. Changes in strength-based factors, in turn, fostered increases in youths' protective factors (e.g., positive racial identity, future orientation, internalization of parental norms, and values regarding risk avoidance behaviors). Increases in youth's protective factors were associated with avoidance of deviant peer affiliation, delayed sexual onset and initiation of substance use and changes in alcohol use over time. Increases in rural African American adolescents' future orientations, negative attitudes toward alcohol, negative images of drinkers, and resistance efficacy, promoted greater alcohol avoidance self-efficacy. This in turn reduced youths' vulnerability to HIV-related risk behavior (e.g., delayed sexual onset and the initiation/escalation of alcohol and other drugs) 2 years post-intervention.

SAAF Effects on Youth-Level Processes SAAF participants increased their alcohol use at a slower rate than did adolescents in the control condition across the follow-up assessments. At the 65-month assessment, SAAF participants' reported having drunk alcohol half as often as did youth in the control group. SAAF's effects on deterring initiation carried forward to account for its effects on alcohol use across time as youth transitioned into late adolescence. These findings suggest that offering psychoeducational programs to rural African American families on protective parenting processes and self-regulatory skills during preadolescence may contribute to a self-sustaining trajectory of disinterest in, and avoidance of, alcohol use during adolescence when peers begin to model and sanction it. Results from another examination of long-term follow-up assessments when youth were 17 years old revealed that intervention-induced changes in parenting practices mediated the effect of intervention-group influences on changes in the onset and escalation of risky sexual behaviors over 65 months through its positive influence on adolescents' self-pride and their sexual norms. Results underscore the powerful effects of parenting practices among rural African American families. Over time, the parenting practices serve a protective role in reducing youth's risk behavior including HIV vulnerable behaviors (Murry et al., 2011).

Finally, some consideration has been given to the potential spillover effect of SAAF on non-targeted outcomes for both parents and youth. For example, the effect of SAAF on primary caregivers' depressive symptoms was examined by selecting 167 caregivers with elevated scores on the Center for Epidemiologic Studies-Depression Scale. Results revealed that SAAF participation was associated with reduced depressive symptoms, enhanced parenting, and perceived improvements in youth behavior (Beach et al., 2008). Results support the link between reduced depressive symptoms and stronger family relationships, in particular, the importance of enhanced parenting efficacy in alleviating depressive symptoms among rural African American parents.

While SAAF was not specifically designed to reduce conduct problems among youth, results revealed that SAAF youth were less involved than control-group youth in aggressive and rule-breaking behaviors across time (Brody et al., 2008; Murry et al., 2014). Moreover, SAAF effects were stronger for youth at greater risk of developing conduct problems. Youth assigned to the SAAF program demonstrated increases in self-control that in turn was associated with avoidance of affiliating with deviance-prone peers.

PAAS Intervention Induced Changes in Parenting Protective Processes Concern for the acceptability of a computer-based intervention for rural African American families was allayed in that more families attended the technology condition than the small group condition, irrespective of parent's age, education, or SES (Murry, Berkel, & Liu, 2018). In another study, differential responsiveness of parents to PAAS was based on the assigned delivery platform, with both experimental groups outperforming families assigned to the literature-based control arm (Murry, Berkel, Inniss-Thompson, & Debreaux, 2019). Further, rural African American parents assigned to the small group facilitator-led condition, compared to those assigned to the technology arm, demonstrated greater improvements in intervention targeted, universal parenting processes, including more frequent and in-depth discussions about sensitive topics related to pubertal development, sexual-related issues, and clarification of rules, norms, and expectations about alcohol and substance use (β = 0.31; p = 0.03). Finally, Murry and colleagues (Murry, 2019) conducted a comparative effectiveness evaluation of PAAS to determine the potential promise of the technology arm as an effective delivery platform for increasing access to evidence-based youth risk prevention programs among those in greatest need. Results revealed that compared to families in the literature control condition, families assigned to the PAAS self-directed technology or small group facilitator-led conditions reported significantly stronger positive changes in parenting processes, reflective of both universal and culturally specific strengths-based assets (e.g., enhanced discussion quality, clearly articulated norms, and parental expectations about risk engagement).

PAAS Intervention Induced Changes on Youth Protective Processes Results from mediational test of PAAS' effect on youth risk engaging behaviors revealed that youth assigned to the PAAS technology condition experienced a significant decline in behavioral intent to engage in risk behaviors from baseline to post-test (β = −0.12; p = 0.04). On the other hand, youth in the small group facilitator-led condition experienced a significant increase in affiliation with deviant peers (β = 0.16; p = 0.002). Further, examining the influence of condition on sexual risk behavior and substance use from pretest to long-term follow-up, revealed that random assignment to receive PAAS via the technology platform was associated with a significant decrease in risk behavior over time (β = −0.17; p = 0.04) among youth. No significant change in risk protection via PAAS was observed for youth assigned to the small group facilitator-led condition (β = −0.05; p = 0.58). Based on these findings, the PAAS technology arm demonstrated greater changes in intervention targeted behaviors than either of the other two platforms, with notable changes in family processes that in turn fostered positive adjustment and well-being among youth (Murry, Kettrey, Berkel, & Inniss-Thompson, 2019).

Taken together, results from SAAF and PAAS hold promise for addressing numerous disparities confronting African American families residing in rural spaces. The enhancement of culturally specific strengths-based processes increased parents' capacity and ability to perform their roles as supportive, involved, nurturant, and vigilant parents. That, in turn, fostered positive developmental outcomes and well-being in their children.

The F.A.M.I.L.Y Study

As studies have indicated higher unemployment rates for men in rural communities, particularly among African American men (Burton et al., 2013), there has been discussion on how this economic context shapes fathers' roles, parenting practices, and family processes. Though a large focus of the existing literature on rural African American families has been centered on how economic stress influences individual functioning and parenting among African American single mothers (Murry, Bynum, et al., 2001), studies have shown that fathers' experiences, regardless of their residential status, influence larger family processes and child outcomes (Jarrett, Roy, & Burton, 2002; Roy, 2006). Building on and extending this work, the Fathers and Mothers in the Lives of Youth (F.A.M.I.L.Y) study was born and includes a subsample of rural families (Cooper, Smalls-Glover, Metzger, & Griffin, 2015; Cooper, Smalls-Glover, Neblett, & Banks, 2014). F.A.M.I.L.Y examines determinants of fathers' parenting practices (e.g., ideologies, intergeneration relationships) as well as contributions to African American adolescents' developmental and social adjustment. This study highlights a needed focus on the roles, experiences, and contributions of African American fathers.

African American fathers were shown to have a diverse strategy for discussing issues of race with their children, emphasizing the larger racial context of parenting for many African American families residing in small and rural communities (Cooper et al., 2015; Cooper et al., 2019). Moreover, there was some indication that fathers' discrimination experiences and awareness of others' views of African Americans profoundly influenced discussions about race and inequities with their children. Overall, this study supports the race-related context often experienced by many rural African American men, including direct experiences with racial discrimination and awareness of others' negative views about their racial group. Additional research with this sample has found that African American fathers' experiences with racial discrimination and racial identity beliefs were related to dyadic congruence in mothers' and fathers' ethnic–racial socialization practices. These findings are particularly notable as they suggest that African American fathers' discrimination experiences and race-relations beliefs extend beyond an individual impact to also shape dyadic interactions and family processes.

Studies have noted that Southern African American men, in comparison to their counterparts in other geographic regions, hold more traditionally masculine ideologies (Levant, Majors, & Kelley, 1998). Given larger discussions about the impacts of poverty and economic disenfranchisement on the father's presence in many rural households, understanding determinants of fathering role ideologies may be particularly relevant for rural African American men. Existing economic and employment conditions exacerbated by race-related barriers within rural communities can have widespread impacts on African American fathers' parenting efficacy as well as engagement in the parenting and co-parenting process. Research suggests these impacts are best understood within a multigenerational context and are critical to the understanding of African American fathers' paternal identities, as they are shaped by the larger social environment (Cooper, Ross, Dues, Golden, & Burnett, 2019; Hunter et al., 2006; Roy, 2004; Shears, Robinson, & Emde, 2002). Further, studies have revealed both proximal and distal impacts of African American fathers' intergenerational influences on their involvement with their children and larger family processes (Allen & Doherty, 1996; Brown, Kogan, & Kim, 2018; Fagan, 1998; Hunter et al., 2006; Roy, 2006).

For African American fathers, role ideologies and beliefs may serve as an impetus for parental engagement or disengagement (Smetana & Daddis, 2002). Findings from the F.A.M.I.L.Y study support that African American fathers' parenting role ideologies are an important mechanism for understanding the relationship between intergenerational experiences and involvement with their adolescent children (Cooper, Banerjee, et al., 2019). Further, building off of the contributions of existing work, this study indicates that African American fathers' role ideologies are shaped by a number of factors, including individual (perceived parenting competence), contextual (residential status), and child characteristics (gender). These findings suggest that the larger social context, reflecting the collective impacts of economic- and race-related factors, has complex implications for the development of African American rural fathers' parenting identities and perceived roles as well as how they contribute to family processes.

Highlighting the ecologically embedded context of fathering for rural African American men, the F.A.M.I.L.Y study suggests important areas of focus in the development of father-focused preventive interventions with this population. Undoubtedly, the race-related experiences of African American men, including person-level transgressions, pervasive negative stereotypes, and structural inequities have multilayered impacts on their health and well-being. Masculinity ideologies and awareness of negative views about African American fathers can further complicate coping processes (Hammond, Banks, & Mattis, 2006). However, these effects can extend far beyond the individual to influence larger family systems. Preventive interventions with rural fathers should openly address the multiple intersections and contexts of African American fatherhood. Additionally, buttressed by research indicating that family relationships are especially important in the lives of rural African Americans (Clark et al., 2011), intergenerational factors and influences continue to impact fathers' parenting identities and related behaviors across the life span. Resources and opportunities for rural African American fathers to enhance social relationships with their fathers and father-figures are key components for preventive interventions targeting this population. Further, opportunities to enhance and support these relationships, especially within the context of high poverty, economic disenfranchisement, and racial inequity, have the potential to serve as critical sources of coping and support as well as positively impact family processes (Young, 2016).

Conclusions and Recommendations

This narrative review of extant studies of rural African American families was conducted to inform the fields of social, behavioral, and health sciences, as well as economics, demography, and social policy on what is known about factors, processes, and context that impact and influence what goes on inside African American families residing in and raising children in rural spaces. Further, we acknowledge the presence of relative plasticity in humans and that this flexibility may be key in explaining differential responses of families to socio-eco-political and environmental challenges associated with living in and raising children in rural spaces. In this regard, our review includes studies that have examined the processes through which strengths-based cultural assets serve protective functions that in turn explain how these families negotiate and navigate life challenges to be healthy and raise healthy children (Murry, 2019). To set the stage for our chapter, we posed a question—*Why focus on rural African American families*? Our rationale was embedded in three reasons: (1) that, while historically, the majority of African Americans in the southern region of the U.S. resided in rural communities (Lichter & Campbell, 2005), in recent years African Americans families are the smallest minority group in rural spaces as migration of Latinx, Asian, American Indian, and Native/Pacific Islander to rural spaces have created a demographic shift; (2) the extent to which this demographic shift has impacted dynamics between rural African American families and other groups, particularly in communities, needs to be examined and understood; and (3) what we know about the everyday life experiences of rural African American families can provide us with greater insights on how they negotiate and navigate their environment. Concluding remarks reflect the extent to which our systematic review was useful in addressing these questions and issues and encourage the expansion of our review in light of the population shifts occurring in rural communities in the U.S.

Population Shifts

Notable changes in the populations' shifts in rural spaces include complicated race-related interactions and potentially exacerbate economic gaps between high- and low-resource communities and neighborhoods. These shifting dynamic processes have implications for adding to the existing struggles and life challenges that rural African Americans have experienced. Historically, restricted life opportunities and economic fragility experienced by African American families were associated with racial segregation and the consequences of Jim Crow Laws. Many African American families in the rural South are more likely to be living in situations characterized as persistent deep poverty. Further, while historically, the land was used for livelihood, farming and gardening, rural farmland has been identified as a place for toxic waste dumping and prisons (Burton et al., 2013). This shift in the nature, functionality, and landscape of rural spaces created communities that are now classified as "food deserts." Further, many rural communities are witnessing an age drain, such that young families are relocating to urban settings, often to seek employment and greater access to resources and services, leaving behind relatives who are older, less educated, and poor (Morton & Blanchard, 2007). These circumstances may explain the decline in land ownership among rural southern African Americans, as those left behind are unable to meet the financial demands associated with maintaining the property (Gilbert, Sharp, & FeZin, 2002). The connections among demographic shifts, economic fragility, social isolation, and family process and health outcomes of rural African American families have not been examined in extant studies. Thus, insights about ways in which various population shifts have implications for and explain everyday life experiences, relationships, and well-being of rural African American families remain unexplored. Given that, we turn to some concluding statements about what is known about the everyday life experiences of rural African American families and how they negotiate and navigate their environment. Consideration is given to highlighting unexpected findings and also obvious omissions.

First, the majority of studies focus on macrolevel systems to frame investigations of rural settings, demonstrating ways in which economic stress and chronic persistent poverty are linked with unemployment, population decline, resource scarcity, including substandard housing, underperforming educational systems, and low quality or no health care due to hospital closings. Further, the economic fragility of these communities has been associated with rising crime and drug use. For example, drug use and delinquency were found to be higher for African American rural youth in comparison to non-rural African American youth (Vazsonyi et al., 2008). In addition, poverty has been linked to long-term health decline among African Americans. Increases in allostatic load as rural African American youth age is associated with elevating the risk for early aging with regard to chronic disease (Brody et al., 2014). Several questions remain in terms of identifying the mechanisms through which poverty affects families, as poverty, while measured as a static state, is often conceptualized as process.

This macrosystem approach has also been used by a few studies that sought to explain how economic stress impacts and influences what goes on inside rural African American families. Emerging from these studies is the conclusion that not having enough income to meet family needs adversely influences individual and family well-being (Conger et al., 2002; Dorsey et al., 2007; Elder Jr., 1985; McCubbin et al., 1980; McLoyd, 1990). This pathway is thought to result from the toll that economic stress has on parents' psychological functioning. Increased economic stress elevates parental depressive mood, which in turn compromises positive interactions, which negatively influences marital relationships (Kerpelman et al., 2008). Unhappy couples often are unable to muster energy to be actively engaged in parenting, and disrupted parenting, in turn, adversely impacts children's adjustment. While economic stress can compromise family functioning, adjustment, and development regardless of race/ethnicity or geographic residence, studies have demonstrated that racial discrimination amplifies and elevates stress in rural African Americans (Murry, Brown, et al., 2001).

A paucity of studies has shown that racial discrimination is closely linked to persistent poverty and intergenerational economic disenfranchisement (Lichter et al., 2012). For many rural families, racial discrimination greatly shapes the larger context of parenting and family processes. Aware of the increased likelihood that their children will be exposed to racial discrimination, many African American parents use practices and approaches to protect their children from the environmental circumstances and situations that may impede their development. For example, to help their children navigate growing up in a racially oppressed environment, parents integrate racial socialization with universal parenting strategies, overlaying cultural values and racial pride and affirmation (Berkel et al., 2009; Murry et al., 2009). Further, because of their awareness of detrimental consequences of contextual risk, rural African Americans parents have open dialogues with their children to ensure that they clearly articulate attitudes, values, and norms of appropriate behavior and consequences of misbehavior to their children (Murry, McNair, et al., 2014). The combination of these race-specific parenting processes increases youths' self-regulation and self-control, encouraging them to avoid risk opportunity situations and resist peer pressure (Berkel et al., 2009; Murry, McNair, et al., 2014).

Based on our review, we conclude that most studies of rural African American families, while framed using traditional models, are done so from a social and cultural deficit perspective, perpetuating the notion that these families are deficient when compared with their urban counterparts. Also implied is that they are different from rural white families. This difference or deficit is often attributed to their residential context and its consequences, including economic, social, political, educational, and other disparities which spillover to influence internal family interactions (Kerpelman et al., 2008; Stewart, Simons, & Conger, 2002). The toll that these challenging circumstances take in rural African American families has been associated with maladaptive behaviors such as drug use (Vazsonyi et al., 2008), psychological and physical health decline, and compromised marital relations and parenting in these families (Brody et al., 2014; Murry et al., 2008).

A few scholars recognize the need to acknowledge the presence of relative plasticity and flexibility of African American families, as some families are able to overcome the challenges associated with living in and raising children in rural spaces. Emphasized in those studies are protective processes that have been characterized as strengths-based cultural assets. These assets can be traced back to patterns of family life established in African societies and modified in response to enslavement in America (Sudarkasa, 1988). A model to explain the linkages among racial oppression, race-related stress, and resources that enhance adaptive coping—particularly important and protective for black families—has been developed by Murry, Butler-Barnes, et al. (2018).

Despite exposure to multiple stressors, rural African American families, including economically stressed families, may function well due to access to kinship support, which may compensate for the negative impact of poverty on family functioning. While there is a paucity of strengths-based studies of rural African American families, those studies have informed and guided the development of preventive interventions shown to enhance protective processes in families that lead to higher functioning (Cooper et al., 2014, 2015; Murry et al., 2008, 2011; Murry, Kettrey, et al., 2019).

Call for Action

There is an urgent need for more culturally tailored programs targeting rural African American families, including programs that span the life course. Further, there is a need for more research and for systematic reviews of rural African Americans to facilitate a greater understanding of normative family developmental processes and strength-based asset perspectives. Greater emphasis needs to be given to how rural African American families muster the energy and the capacity to adapt, cope, overcome, and then achieve healthy relationships and healthy members. Murry, Butler-Barnes, et al. (2018) provide an integrative approach to guide and advance this research charge. Finally, because families do not function in a vacuum, there is a need to consider how structurally and functionally integrated systems, including public policy, governmental, economical, employment, educational, and health care, affect the everyday life experiences of African American families residing in rural spaces.

Acknowledgments This research was supported by the National Institute of Mental Health Grant MH063043 awarded through funding to Peabody College, Vanderbilt University. Velma McBride Murry's involvement was also supported by funding from the Lois Autrey Betts Chair in Education and Human Development.

References

Albrecht, D. E., Albrecht, C. M., & Murguia, E. (2005). Minority concentration, disadvantage, and inequality in the nonmetropolitan United States. *The Sociological Quarterly, 46*(3), 503–523. https://doi.org/10.1111/j.1533-8525.2005.00024.x

Allen, W., & Doherty, W. (1996). The responsibilities of fatherhood as perceived by African American teenage fathers. *Families in Society: The Journal of Contemporary Social Services, 77*(3), 142–155.

Beach, S. R., Kogan, S. M., Brody, G. H., Chen, Y. F., Lei, M. K., & Murry, V. M. (2008). Change in caregiver depression as a function of the Strong African American Families Program. *Journal of Family Psychology, 22*(2), 241–252.

Berkel, C., Murry, V. M., Hurt, T. R., Chen, Y. F., Brody, G. H., Simons, R. L., … Gibbons, F. X. (2009). It takes a village: Protecting rural African American youth in the context of racism. *Journal of Youth and Adolescence, 38*(2), 175–188. https://doi.org/10.1007/s10964-008-9346-z

Black, A. R., Cook, J. L., Murry, V. M., & Cutrona, C. E. (2005). Ties that bind: Implications of social support for rural, partnered African American women's health functioning. *Women's Health Issues, 15*(5), 216–223. https://doi.org/10.1016/j.whi.2005.05.003

Brody, G. H., Conger, R., Gibbons, F. X., Ge, X., Murry, V. M., Gerrard, M., & Simons, R. L. (2001). The influence of neighborhood disadvantage, collective socialization, and parenting on African American children's affiliation with deviant peers. *Child Development, 72*(4), 1231–1246. https://doi.org/10.1111/1467-8624.00344

Brody, G. H., Dorsey, S., Forehand, R., & Armistead, L. (2002). Unique and protective contributions of parenting and classroom processes to the adjustment of African American children living in single-parent families. *Child Development, 73*(1), 274–286.

Brody, G. H., & Flor, D. L. (1998). Maternal resources, parenting practices, and child competence in rural, single-parent African American families. *Child Development, 69*(3), 803–816. https://doi.org/10.1111/j.1467-8624.1998.tb06244.x
Brody, G. H., Flor, D. L., & Gibson, N. M. (1999). Linking maternal efficacy beliefs, developmental goals, parenting practices, and child competence in rural single-parent African American families. *Child Development, 70*(5), 1197–1208. https://doi.org/10.1111/1467-8624.00087
Brody, G. H., Flor, D. L., Hollett-Wright, N., & McCoy, J. K. (1998). Children's development of alcohol use norms: Contributions of parent and sibling norms, children's temperaments, and parent–child discussions. *Journal of Family Psychology, 12*(2), 209–219.
Brody, G. H., Kim, S., Murry, V. M., & Brown, A. C. (2005). Longitudinal links among parenting, self-presentations to peers, and the development of externalizing and internalizing symptoms in African American siblings. *Development and Psychopathology, 17*(1), 185–205. https://doi.org/10.1017/S0954579405050108
Brody, G. H., Kogan, S. M., Chen, Y. F., & Murry, V. M. (2008). Long-term effects of the strong African American families program on youths' conduct problems. *Journal of Adolescent Health, 43*(5), 474–481.
Brody, G. H., Lei, M. K., Chen, E., & Miller, G. E. (2014). Neighborhood poverty and allostatic load in African American youth. *Pediatrics, 134*(5), 1362–1368.
Brody, G. H., Stoneman, Z., Flor, D., & McCrary, C. (1994). Religion's role in organizing family relationships: Family process in rural, two-parent African American families. *Journal of Marriage and the Family, 56*(4), 878–888. https://doi.org/10.2307/353600
Brody, G. H., Yu, T., Chen, E., Miller, G. E., Kogan, S. M., & Beach, S. R. (2013). Is resilience only skin deep? Rural African Americans' socioeconomic status–related risk and competence in preadolescence and psychological adjustment and allostatic load at age 19. *Psychological Science, 24*(7), 1285–1293. https://doi.org/10.1177/0956797612471954
Bronfenbrenner, U. (Ed.). (2005). *Making human beings human: Bioecological perspectives on human development*. Thousand Oaks, CA: Sage.
Brown, G. L., Kogan, S. M., & Kim, J. (2018). From fathers to sons: The intergenerational transmission of parenting behavior among African American young men. *Family Process, 57*(1), 165–180.
Browning, C. R., Burrington, L. A., Leventhal, T., & Brooks-Gunn, J. (2008). Neighborhood structural inequality, collective efficacy, and sexual risk behavior among urban youth. *Journal of Health and Social Behavior, 49*(3), 269–285. https://doi.org/10.1177/002214650804900303
Burton, L. M. (1996). Age norms, the timing of family role transitions, and intergenerational caregiving among aging African American women. *The Gerontologist, 36*(2), 199–208. https://doi.org/10.1093/geront/36.2.199
Burton, L. M., & Jarrett, R. L. (2000). In the mix, yet on the margins: The place of families in urban neighborhood and child development research. *Journal of Marriage and Family, 62*(4), 1114–1135. https://doi.org/10.1111/j.1741-3737.2000.01114.x
Burton, L. M., Lichter, D. T., Baker, R. S., & Eason, J. M. (2013). Inequality, family processes, and health in the "new" rural America. *American Behavioral Scientist, 57*(8), 1128–1151. https://doi.org/10.1177/0002764213487348
Bynum, M. S., & Brody, G. H. (2005). Coping behaviors, parenting, and perceptions of children's internalizing and externalizing problems in rural African American mothers. *Family Relations, 54*(1), 58–71. https://doi.org/10.1111/j.0197-6664.2005.00006.x
Chatters, L. M., Taylor, R. J., Jackson, J. S., & Lincoln, K. D. (2008). Religious coping among African Americans, Caribbean blacks and non-Hispanic whites. *Journal of Community Psychology, 36*(3), 371–386. https://doi.org/10.1002/jcop.20202
Cicchetti, D., & Toth, S. L. (1992). The role of developmental theory in prevention and intervention. *Development and Psychopathology, 4*(4), 489–493.
Clark, T. T., Nguyen, A. B., & Belgrave, F. Z. (2011). Risk and protective factors for alcohol and marijuana use among African-American rural and urban adolescents. *Journal of Child & Adolescent Substance Abuse, 20*(3), 205–220.

Conger, R. D., Conger, K. J., Elder, G. H., Jr., Lorenz, F. O., Simons, R. L., & Whitbeck, L. B. (1992). A family process model of economic hardship and adjustment of early adolescent boys. *Child Development, 63*(3), 526–541. https://doi.org/10.1111/j.1467-8624.1992.tb01644.x

Conger, R. D., Wallace, L. E., Sun, Y., Simons, R. L., McLoyd, V. C., & Brody, G. H. (2002). Economic pressure in African American families: A replication and extension of the family stress model. *Developmental Psychology, 38*(2), 179–193. https://doi.org/10.1037/0012-1649.38.2.179

Cooper, S. M., Banerjee, M., Griffin, C., Glover, C., Shaheed, J., McBride, M., & Burnett, M. (2019). African American fathers' race-related discussions with their children: Associations with racial identity beliefs and sociodemographic factors. *Journal of Child and Family Studies*, 1–13.

Cooper, S. M., Ross, L., Dues, A., Golden, A., & Burnett, M. (2019). Intergenerational experiences and involvement among African American fathers: Building the case for a mediated pathway. *Journal of Family Issues, 40*(15), 0192513X1984962.

Cooper, S. M., Smalls-Glover, C., Metzger, I., & Griffin, C. (2015). African American fathers' racial socialization patterns: Associations with racial identity beliefs and discrimination experiences. *Family Relations, 64*(2), 278–290.

Cooper, S. M., Smalls-Glover, C., Neblett, E. W., & Banks, K. H. (2014). Racial socialization practices among African American fathers: A profile-oriented approach. *Psychology of Men & Masculinity, 16*(1), 11–22.

Cutrona, C. E., Russell, D. W., Abraham, W. T., Gardner, K. A., Melby, J. N., Bryant, C., & Conger, R. D. (2003). Neighborhood context and financial strain as predictors of marital interaction and marital quality in African American couples. *Personal Relationships, 10*(3), 389–409. https://doi.org/10.1111/1475-6811.00056

Dishion, T. J., & Patterson, G. R. (1999). Model building in developmental psychopathology: A pragmatic approach to understanding and intervention. *Journal of Clinical Child Psychology, 28*(4), 502–512.

Dorsey, S., Forehand, R., & Brody, G. (2007). Coparenting conflict and parenting behavior in economically disadvantaged single parent African American families: The role of maternal psychological distress. *Journal of Family Violence, 22*(7), 621–630. https://doi.org/10.1007/s10896-007-9114-y

Elder, G. H., Jr. (1985). *Life course dynamics: Trajectories and transitions 1968–1980*. Ithaca, NY: Cornell University Press.

Elliott, D. S., Huizinga, D., & Ageton, S. S. (1985). *Explaining delinquency and drug use*. Thousand Oaks, CA: Sage.

Evans, G. W. (2003). A multimethodological analysis of cumulative risk and allostatic load among rural children. *Developmental Psychology, 39*(5), 924–933. https://doi.org/10.1037/0012-1649.39.5.924

Fagan, J. (1998). Correlates of low-income African American and Puerto Rican fathers' involvement with their children. *Journal of Black Psychology, 24*(3), 351–367.

Farmer, J. E., Marien, W. E., Clark, M. J., Sherman, A., & Selva, T. J. (2004). Primary care supports for children with chronic health conditions: Identifying and predicting unmet family needs. *Journal of Pediatric Psychology, 29*(5), 355–367. https://doi.org/10.1093/jpepsy/jsh039

Fergus, S., & Zimmerman, M. A. (2005). Adolescent resilience: A framework for understanding healthy development in the face of risk. *Annual Review of Public Health, 26*, 399–419. https://doi.org/10.1146/annurev.publhealth.26.021304.144357

Fordham, S., & Ogbu, J. U. (1986). Black students' school success: Coping with the "burden of 'acting white'". *The Urban Review, 18*(3), 176–206. https://doi.org/10.1007/BF01112192

Friedman, S., & Lichter, D. T. (1998). Spatial inequality and poverty among American children. *Population Research and Policy Review, 17*(2), 91–109. https://doi.org/10.1023/A:1005740205017

García Coll, C., Lamberty, G., Jenkins, R., McAdoo, H. P., Crnic, K., Wasik, B. H., & Vázquez García, H. (1996). An integrative model for the study of developmental competencies in minority children. *Child Development, 67*(5), 1891–1914.

Garmezy, N. (1996). Reflections and commentary on risk, resilience, and development. In R. J. Haggerty, L. R. Sherrod, N. Garmezy, & M. Rutter (Eds.), *Stress, risk, and resilience in children and adolescents: Processes, mechanisms, and interventions* (pp. 1–18). Cambridge: Cambridge University Press.

Gilbert, J., Sharp, G., & FeZin, M. S. (2002). The loss and persistence of black-owned farms and farmland: A review of the research literature and its implications. *Southern Rural Sociology, 18*(2), 1–30.

Hammond, W. P., Banks, K. H., & Mattis, J. S. (2006). Masculinity ideology and forgiveness of racial discrimination among African American men: Direct and interactive relationships. *Sex Roles, 55*(9–10), 679–692.

Hawkins, J. D., Catalano, R. F., & Miller, J. Y. (1992). Risk and protective factors for alcohol and other drug problems in adolescence and early adulthood: Implications for substance abuse prevention. *Psychological Bulletin, 112*(1), 64–105.

Hill, N. E., & Craft, S. A. (2003). Parent-school involvement and school performance: Mediated pathways among socioeconomically comparable African American and euro-American families. *Journal of Educational Psychology, 95*(1), 74–81. https://doi.org/10.1037/0022-0663.95.1.74

Hill, N. E., & Tyson, D. F. (2009). Parental involvement in middle school: A meta-analytic assessment of the strategies that promote achievement. *Developmental Psychology, 45*(3), 740–763. https://doi.org/10.1037/a0015362

Hughes, D., Rodriguez, J., Smith, E. P., Johnson, D. J., Stevenson, H. C., & Spicer, P. (2006). Parents' ethnic and racial socialization practices: A review of research and directions for future study. *Developmental Psychology, 42*(5), 747–770. https://doi.org/10.1037/0012-1649.42.5.747

Hunter, A. G., Friend, C. A., Murphy, S. Y., Rollins, A., Williams-Wheeler, M., & Laughinghouse, J. (2006). Loss, survival, and redemption: African American male youths' reflections on life without fathers, manhood, and coming of age. *Youth & Society, 37*(4), 423–452.

Ihrke, D. K., & Faber, C. (2012, December). *Geographical mobility: 2005 to 2010.* (Report No. P20–567). Washington, DC: U.S. Census Bureau. Retrieved from https://www.census.gov/library/publications/2012/demo/p20-567.html

Irvin, M. J., Farmer, T. W., Leung, M.-C., Thompson, J. H., & Hutchins, B. C. (2010). School, community, and church activities: Relationship to academic achievement of low-income African American early adolescents in the rural deep south. *Journal of Research in Rural Education, 25*(4), 1–21.

Jaccard, J., & Dittus, P. J. (2000). Adolescent perceptions of maternal approval of birth control and sexual risk behavior. *American Journal of Public Health, 90*(9), 1426–1430.

Jaccard, J., Dittus, P. J., & Gordon, V. V. (1996). Maternal correlates of adolescent sexual and contraceptive behavior. *Family Planning Perspectives, 28*(4), 159–165+185. https://doi.org/10.2307/2136192

James, S. A. (1994). John Henryism and the health of African-Americans. *Culture, Medicine and Psychiatry, 18*(2), 163–182. https://doi.org/10.1007/BF01379448

Jarrett, R. L. (1998). African American mothers and grandmothers in poverty: An adaptational perspective. *Journal of Comparative Family Studies, 29*(2), 387–396.

Jarrett, R. L., Jefferson, S. R., & Kelly, J. N. (2010). Finding community in family: Neighborhood effects and African American kin networks. *Journal of Comparative Family Studies, 41*(3), 299–328.

Jarrett, R. L., Roy, K. M., & Burton, L. M. (2002). Fathers in the "hood": Insights from qualitative research on low income African American men. In N. J. Cabrera & C. S. Tamis-LeMonda (Eds.), *Handbook of father involvement: Multidisciplinary perspectives* (pp. 211–248). Mahwah, NJ: Earlbaum.

Kerpelman, J. L., Eryigit, S., & Stephens, C. J. (2008). African American adolescents' future education orientation: Associations with self-efficacy, ethnic identity, and perceived parental support. *Journal of Youth and Adolescence, 37*(8), 997–1008. https://doi.org/10.1007/s10964-007-9201-7

Lee, M. A., & Singelmann, J. (2006). Welfare reform amidst chronic poverty in the Mississippi Delta. In W. A. Kandel & D. L. Brown (Eds.), *Population change and rural society* (pp. 381–403). Dordrecht: Springer.

Letvak, S. (2002). The importance of social support for rural mental health. *Issues in Mental Health Nursing, 23*(3), 249–261.

Levant, R. F., Majors, R. G., & Kelley, M. L. (1998). Masculinity ideology among young African American and European American women and men in different regions of the United States. *Cultural Diversity and Mental Health, 4*(3), 227–236.

Lichter, D. T. (2012). Immigration and the new racial diversity in rural America. *Rural Sociology, 77*(1), 3–35. https://doi.org/10.1111/j.1549-0831.2012.00070.x

Lichter, D. T., & Campbell, L. A. (2005). *Changing patterns of poverty and spatial inequality in Appalachia.* Washington, DC: Appalachian Regional Commission. Retrieved from https://www.prb.org/changingpatternsofpovertyandspatialinequalityinappalachiapdf676kb/

Lichter, D. T., Parisi, D., & Taquino, M. C. (2012). The geography of exclusion: Race, segregation, and concentrated poverty. *Social Problems, 59*(3), 364–388. https://doi.org/10.1525/sp.2012.59.3.364

Lichter, D. T., Qian, Z., & Crowley, M. L. (2005). Child poverty among racial minorities and immigrants: Explaining trends and differentials. *Social Science Quarterly, 86*(s1), 1037–1059.

Lincoln, C. E., & Mamiya, L. H. (1990). *The black church in the African American experience.* Durham, NC: Duke University Press.

Luthar, S. S., Cicchetti, D., & Becker, B. (2000). The construct of resilience: A critical evaluation and guidelines for future work. *Child Development, 71*(3), 543–562.

Markstrom, C. A., Marshall, S. K., & Tryon, R. J. (2000). Resiliency, social support, and coping in rural low-income Appalachian adolescents from two racial groups. *Journal of Adolescence, 23*(6), 693–703. https://doi.org/10.1006/jado.2000.0353

Masten, A. S. (2001). Ordinary magic: Resilience processes in development. *American Psychologist, 56*(3), 227–238.

Masten, A. S. (2013). Risk and resilience in development. In P. D. Zelazo (Ed.), *Oxford library of psychology. The Oxford handbook of developmental psychology, Vol. 2: Self and other* (pp. 579–607). New York, NY: Oxford University Press.

Masten, A. S., & Coatsworth, J. D. (1998). The development of competence in favorable and unfavorable environments: Lessons from research on successful children. *American Psychologist, 53*(2), 205–220. https://doi.org/10.1037/0003-066X.53.2.205

McCubbin, H. I., Joy, C. B., Cauble, A. E., Comeau, J. K., Patterson, J. M., & Needle, R. H. (1980). Family stress and coping: A decade review. *Journal of Marriage and the Family, 42*(4), 855–871. https://doi.org/10.2307/351829

McLoyd, V. C. (1990). The impact of economic hardship on black families and children: Psychological distress, parenting, and socioemotional development. *Child Development, 61*(2), 311–346. https://doi.org/10.1111/j.1467-8624.1990.tb02781.x

McLoyd, V. C. (1998). Socioeconomic disadvantage and child development. *American Psychologist, 53*(2), 185–204.

Morton, L. W., & Blanchard, T. C. (2007). Starved for access: Life in rural America's food deserts. *Rural Realities, 1*(4), 1–10. Retrieved from https://www.ruralsociology.org/assets/docs/rural-realities/rural-realities-1-4.pdf

Mosbach, P., & Leventhal, H. (1988). Peer group identification and smoking: Implications for intervention. *Journal of Abnormal Psychology, 97*(2), 238–245.

Mulser, R. M., Hucke, K., Trask-Tate, A., & Cunningham, M. (2012). When racial identity matters: Stressful events and mental health in rural African American adolescents. In J. M. Sullivan & A. M. Esmail (Eds.), *African American identity: Racial and cultural dimensions of the black experience* (pp. 171–187). Lanham, MD: Lexington Books.

Murry, V. M. (2019). Healthy African American families in the 21st Century: Navigating opportunities and transcending adversities. *Journal of Family Relations, 68*(3), 342–357. https://doi.org/10.1111/fare.12363

Murry, V. M., Berkel, C., Brody, G. H., Miller, S. J., & Chen, Y. F. (2009). Linking parental socialization to interpersonal protective processes, academic self-presentation, and expectations among rural African American youth. *Cultural Diversity and Ethnic Minority Psychology, 15*(1), 1–10. https://doi.org/10.1037/a0013180

Murry, V. M., Berkel, C., Inniss-Thompson, M. N., & Debreaux, M. L. (2019). Pathways for African American success: Results of three-arm randomized trial to test the effects of technology-based delivery for rural African American families. *Journal of Pediatric Psychology, 44*(3), 375–387.

Murry, V. M., Berkel, C., & Liu, N. (2018). The closing digital divide: Delivery modality and family attendance in the pathways for African American success (PAAS) program. *Prevention Science, 19*(5), 1–10.

Murry, V. M., Berkel, C., Simons, R. L., Simons, L. G., & Gibbons, F. X. (2014). A twelve-year longitudinal analysis of positive youth development among rural African American males. *Journal of Research on Adolescence, 24*(3), 512–525.

Murry, V. M., & Brody, G. H. (1999). Self-regulation and self-worth of Black children reared in economically stressed, rural, single mother-headed families: The contribution of risk and protective factors. *Journal of Family Issues, 20*(4), 458–484.

Murry, V. M., Brody, G. H., McNair, L. D., Luo, Z., Gibbons, F. X., Gerrard, M., & Wills, T. A. (2005). Parental involvement promotes rural African American youths' self-pride and sexual self-concepts. *Journal of Marriage and Family, 67*(3), 627–642.

Murry, V. M., Brown, P. A., Brody, G. H., Cutrona, C. E., & Simons, R. L. (2001). Racial discrimination as a moderator of the links among stress, maternal psychological functioning, and family relationships. *Journal of Marriage and Family, 63*(4), 915–926.

Murry, V. M., Butler-Barnes, S. T., Mayo-Gamble, T. L., & Inniss-Thompson, M. N. (2018). Excavating new constructs for family stress theories in the context of everyday life experiences of black American families. *Journal of Family Theory & Review, 10*(2), 384–405.

Murry, V. M., Bynum, M. S., Brody, G. H., Willert, A., & Stephens, D. (2001). African American single mothers and children in context: A review of studies on risk and resilience. *Clinical Child and Family Psychology Review, 4*(2), 133–155. https://doi.org/10.1023/A:1011381114782

Murry, V. M., Harrell, A. W., Brody, G. H., Chen, Y. F., Simons, R. L., Black, A. R., ... Gibbons, F. X. (2008). Long-term effects of stressors on relationship well-being and parenting among rural African American women. *Family Relations, 57*(2), 117–127. https://doi.org/10.1111/j.1741-3729.2008.00488.x

Murry, V. M., Heflinger, C. A., Suiter, S. V., & Brody, G. H. (2011). Examining perceptions about mental health care and help-seeking among rural African American families of adolescents. *Journal of Youth and Adolescence, 40*(9), 1118–1131. https://doi.org/10.1007/s10964-010-9627-1

Murry, V. M., Kettrey, H. H., Berkel, C., & Inniss-Thompson, M. N. (2019). The Pathways for African American Success (PAAS): Does delivery platform matter in the prevention of youth risk engagement? *Journal of Adolescent Health, 65*(2), 255–261. https://doi.org/10.1016/j.jadohealth.2019.02.013

Murry, V. M., & Liu, N. (2014, February). *Are African Americans living the dream 50 years after passage of the civil rights act*? Council on Contemporary Families Civil Rights Symposium. Retrieved from https://contemporaryfamilies.org/are-african-americans-living-the-dream/

Murry, V. M., McNair, L. D., Myers, S. S., Chen, Y. F., & Brody, G. H. (2014). Intervention induced changes in perceptions of parenting and risk opportunities among rural African American. *Journal of Child and Family Studies, 23*(2), 422–436.

Murry, V. M., Simons, R. L., Simons, L. G., & Gibbons, F. X. (2013). Contributions of family environment and parenting processes to sexual risk and substance use of rural African American males: A 4-year longitudinal analysis. *American Journal of Orthopsychiatry, 83*(2 Pt 3), 299–309.

Myers, H. F. (2009). Ethnicity-and socio-economic status-related stresses in context: An integrative review and conceptual model. *Journal of Behavioral Medicine, 32*(1), 9–19. https://doi.org/10.1007/s10865-008-9181-4

Nasim, A., Fernander, A., Townsend, T. G., Corona, R., & Belgrave, F. Z. (2011). Cultural protective factors for community risks and substance use among rural African American adolescents. *Journal of Ethnicity in Substance Abuse, 10*(4), 316–336. https://doi.org/10.1080/15332640.2011.623510

Odom, E. C., Vernon-Feagans, L., & Family Life Project Key Investigators. (2010). Buffers of racial discrimination: Links with depression among rural African American mothers. *Journal of Marriage and Family, 72*(2), 346–359. https://doi.org/10.1111/j.1741-3737.2010.00704.x

Ogbu, J. U. (1981). Origins of human competence: A cultural-ecological perspective. *Child Development, 52*(2), 413–429.

Ogbu, J. U. (2004). Collective identity and the burden of "acting White" in Black history, community, and education. *The Urban Review, 36*(1), 1–35.

Parisi, D., Grice, S. M., Taquino, M., & Gill, D. A. (2005). Community concentration of poverty and its consequences on nonmetro county persistence of poverty in Mississippi. *Sociological Spectrum, 25*(4), 469–483. https://doi.org/10.1080/027321790947234

Patterson, G. R., DeBaryshe, B., & Ramsey, E. (1989). A developmental perspective on antisocial behavior. *American Psychologist, 44*(2), 329–335.

Peters, M. F., & Massey, G. (1983). Mundane extreme environmental stress in family stress theories: The case of black families in white America. *Marriage & Family Review, 6*(1–2), 193–218. https://doi.org/10.1300/J002v06n01_10

Piko, B. F., Kovacs, E., Kriston, P., & Fitzpatrick, K. M. (2012). "To believe or not to believe?" religiosity, spirituality, and alcohol use among Hungarian adolescents. *Journal of Studies on Alcohol and Drugs, 73*(4), 666–674. https://doi.org/10.15288/jsad.2012.73.666

Proctor, B. D., & Dalaker, J. (2003). *Poverty in the United States: 2002* (Report No. P60-222) Washington, DC: U.S. Census Bureau, Current Population Reports. Retrieved from https://www.census.gov/library/publications/2003/demo/p60-222.html

Ricketts, T. C. (2000). The changing nature of rural health care. *Annual Review of Public Health, 21*(1), 639–657.

Roche, K. M., & Leventhal, T. (2009). Beyond neighborhood poverty: Family management, neighborhood disorder, and adolescents' early sexual onset. *Journal of Family Psychology, 23*(6), 819–827.

Rojewski, J. W. (1995). Impact of at-risk behavior on the occupational aspirations and expectations of male and female adolescents in rural settings. *Journal of Career Development, 22*(1), 33–48. https://doi.org/10.1177/089484539502200103

Roy, K. M. (2004). You can't eat love: Constructing provider role expectations for low-income and working-class fathers. *Fathering, 2*(3), 253–277.

Roy, K. M. (2006). Father stories: A life course examination of paternal identity among low-income African American men. *Journal of Family Issues, 27*(1), 31–54.

Shears, J., Robinson, J., & Emde, R. N. (2002). Fathering relationships and their associations with juvenile delinquency. *Infant Mental Health Journal, 23*(1–2), 79–87.

Simons, L. G., Simons, R. L., Conger, R. D., & Brody, G. H. (2004). Collective socialization and child conduct problems: A multilevel analysis with an African American sample. *Youth & Society, 35*(3), 267–292. https://doi.org/10.1177/0044118X03255005

Smetana, J. G., & Daddis, C. (2002). Domain-specific antecedents of parental psychological control and monitoring: The role of parenting beliefs and practices. *Child Development, 73*(2), 563–580.

Smith, C., Faris, R., Denton, M. L., & Regnerus, M. (2003). Mapping American adolescent subjective religiosity and attitudes of alienation toward religion: A research report. *Sociology of Religion, 64*(1), 111–133. https://doi.org/10.2307/3712271

Spencer, M. B., Dupree, D., & Hartmann, T. (1997). A phenomenological variant of ecological systems theory (PVEST): A self-organization perspective in context. *Development and Psychopathology, 9*(4), 817–833.

Stewart, E. A., Simons, R. L., & Conger, R. D. (2002). Assessing neighborhood and social psychological influences on childhood violence in an African American sample. *Criminology, 40*(4), 801–830.

Strayhorn, T. L. (2009). Different folks, different hopes: The educational aspirations of black males in urban, suburban, and rural high schools. *Urban Education, 44*(6), 710–731. https://doi.org/10.1177/0042085908322705
Sudarkasa, N. (1988). Reassessing the black family: Dispelling the myths, reaffirming the values. *Sisters, 1*(1), 22–23.
Szapocznik, J., & Coatsworth, J. D. (1999). An ecodevelopmental framework for organizing the influences on drug abuse: A developmental model of risk and protection. In M. D. Glantz & C. R. Hartel (Eds.), *Drug abuse: Origins & interventions* (pp. 331–366). Washington, DC: American Psychological Association. https://doi.org/10.1037/10341-014
Taylor, Z. E., Larsen-Rife, D., Conger, R. D., Widaman, K. F., & Cutrona, C. E. (2010). Life stress, maternal optimism, and adolescent competence in single mother, African American families. *Journal of Family Psychology, 24*(4), 468–477. https://doi.org/10.1037/a0019870
U.S. Census Bureau. (2010). *Profile of general population and housing characteristics: 2010 Demographic profile data*. Retrieved from https://factfinder.census.gov/faces/tableservices/jsf/pages/productview.xhtml?pid=DEC_10_DP_DPDP1&src=pt
U.S. Census Bureau. (2016) *Current Population Survey: Annual Social and Economic Supplement*. Retrieved from https://www.census.gov/data/tables/2016/demo/geographic-mobility/cps-2016.html
Vazsonyi, A. T., Trejos-Castillo, E., & Young, M. A. (2008). Rural and non-rural African American youth: Does context matter in the etiology of problem behaviors? *Journal of Youth and Adolescence, 37*(7), 798–811. https://doi.org/10.1007/s10964-007-9239-6
Whitaker, D. J., & Miller, K. S. (2000). Parent-adolescent discussions about sex and condoms: Impact on peer influences of sexual risk behavior. *Journal of Adolescent Research, 15*(2), 251–273. https://doi.org/10.1177/0743558400152004
Wiley, A. R., Warren, H. B., & Montanelli, D. S. (2002). Shelter in a time of storm: Parenting in poor rural African American communities. *Family Relations, 51*(3), 265–273. https://doi.org/10.1111/j.1741-3729.2002.00265.x
Williams, O. (2000). *An examination of the influence that community assets have on the positive development of African American adolescent females from Michigan* (Unpublished doctoral dissertation). Michigan State University, East Lansing.
Williams, O. A. (2003). Effects of faith & church involvement on African American female adolescents. *Michigan Family Review, 8*(1), 19–27.
Wills, T. A., Murry, V. M., Brody, G. H., Gibbons, F. X., Gerrard, M., Walker, C., & Ainette, M. G. (2007). Ethnic pride and self-control related to protective and risk factors: Test of the theoretical model for the Strong African American Families Program. *Health Psychology, 26*(1), 50–59.
Wilson, W. J. (1987). *The truly disadvantaged: The inner city, the underclass, and social policy*. Chicago, IL: University of Chicago.
Witherspoon, D., & Ennett, S. (2011). Stability and change in rural youths' educational outcomes through the middle and high school years. *Journal of Youth and Adolescence, 40*(9), 1077–1090.
Young, A. (2016). Safe spaces for vulnerability: New perspectives on African Americans who struggle to be good fathers. In L. Burton, D. Burton, S. M. McHale, V. King, & J. Van Hook (Eds.), *Boys and Men in African American Families* (pp. 173–183). New York: Springer.

Early Development and Family Life in Rural America

Lynne Vernon-Feagans and Margaret M. Swingler

Life in Rural America

What does growing up in low wealth rural America really look like in the twenty-first century, and how have the dramatic shifts over the last 50 years impacted young rural families and their children? This chapter will try to briefly answer that question by synthesizing the limited, but important, previous research on families and young children living in rural areas. In particular, we describe how large changes in rural communities have impacted family work, childcare, parenting, and schooling for young rural children. We describe some of the impacts these changes have had on child cognitive, emotional, and physiological well-being and outcomes. To illustrate these points, we will use data from the Family Life Project (FLP). This 15-year NICHD-funded project has followed a representative sample of every baby born between 2003 and 2004 to a mother who resided in one of six rural poor counties in Pennsylvania and North Carolina, oversampling for African American families in North Carolina and families living in poverty in both states. The 1292 children in this project have been followed from birth and have received many home, childcare, and school visits. Thus, data from this project can help us understand rural families and their lives today in this country.

Although geographic isolation related to the history of farming in rural areas may be the most salient marker that differentiates urban and rural life, family farming with its vast and rich landscapes has historically been the idealized image of rural family life compared to more urban life. Yet, over the last 50 years, dramatic changes in rural life have greatly altered this idealized picture and had ripple effects across poor rural communities as family farms and small businesses have almost disappeared and talented young adults with higher education and skill levels have

L. Vernon-Feagans · M. M. Swingler (✉)
University of North Carolina at Chapel Hill, Chapel Hill, NC, USA
e-mail: lynnevf@email.unc.edu; mmswing@email.unc.edu

J. E. Glick et al. (eds.), *Rural Families and Communities in the United States*,
National Symposium on Family Issues 10, https://doi.org/10.1007/978-3-030-37689-5_8

left to find better economic futures in urban areas. These changes have left behind less-educated adults who struggle to raise their children with less income and resources than were available in the past. However, many families are committed to their rural roots and remain in their rural communities because of the presence of extended family and friends as sources of support, as well as the availability of affordable single-family homes (vs. high-density housing common in urban areas) and safe neighborhoods (Duncan, 1999; O'Hare, 2009).

Defining Rural

Understanding rural life and the ways in which it differs from life in urban settings is complicated by different definitions of rural. Indeed, a report by Mathematica on the needs of rural areas described six definitions of rural that have been used by U.S. Federal Agencies (Strong, Del Grosso, Burwick, Jethwani, & Ponza, 2005). Two key agencies, the U.S. Census Bureau in conjunction with the Office of Management and Budget (OMB) and the Department of Education, have used these definitions to better define and help clarify what is meant by *rural* (Vernon-Feagans, Garrett-Peters, DeMarco & Bratsch-Hines, 2012). The first definition of urban/rural used by the U.S. Census Bureau and OMB, has provided a rural/urban continuum code to categorize counties as either metro (urban) or nonmetro (rural). Under this definition, there are three categories of population size for metro counties that range from very large (millions of people) to rather small urban areas of up to 50,000 people (Vernon-Feagans, Gallagher & Kainz, 2010). Nonmetro counties, on the other hand, are classified into six categories by population size and adjacency to metro areas beginning with populations of less than 50,000 people.

The second commonly used definition comes from the U.S. Department of Education, which has developed more detailed guidelines for urban/rural that reflect advances in technology and research, to better classify schools as located in an urban or rural setting (National Center for Educational Statistics, 2006). This 12-locale code system includes four major categories: city, suburban, town, and rural. The first three codes are for places with populations above 50,000. Locations categorized as rural may be coded as fringe, distant, or remote, depending on the distance from an urbanized area of greater than 50,000 people or an urban cluster of between 25,000 and 50,000 people. Even though the definition of rural used by these two key agencies differ, there are two central constructs that they both endorse. First, both definitions capture areas of the countryside that are geographically far from large urban areas and their suburbs, so it is less likely that families would commute for work into these large populated areas. Second, the definition of rural generally includes only areas/counties that have towns or areas with fewer than 50,000 people. Data and studies presented in this chapter include reports and research that use a range of definitions for rural but generally fall within the scope of these two key criteria: (1) places far from an urban center and (2) places with populations under 50,000 people.

Rural Life in Twenty-First Century U.S.

The twentieth century, and especially the last half of the twentieth century, saw major changes in the lives of many families living in rural areas. Early twentieth century agriculture was an intensive family affair with over half the population living and working on small family farms. This bucolic view of happy rural family life focused mostly on white families and their children and was depicted in fictional books such as *Little House on the Prairie.* Many in the U.S. saw this idealized description of rural as characterizing typical rural family life. Clearly, these fictional depictions were exaggerated and did not detail the hardships that many families endured, especially during the early twentieth century droughts, dust bowls, and the Great Depression. Especially lacking in the popular literature was a description of the lives of minority families in rural America, particularly African American families. There were some good ethnographic descriptions of rural family life in academic books such as *Ways with Words* (Heath, 1983), *Call to Home* (Stack, 1996), and *Children's Talk in Communities and Classrooms* (Vernon-Feagans, 1996). These books detailed the challenges of rural life for African American and non-African American children and families. They also highlighted, the many advantages of living and working in small towns and communities where extended family, friends, and religious institutions often provided emotional and resource support that resulted in a real sense of belonging and a commitment to "place." Unfortunately, in the twenty-first century many of these advantages of rural life have been dwindling.

Farming in the twenty-first century is concentrated on a smaller number of large corporate farms in rural areas where now less than a fourth of the U.S. population live; half of what the rural population was a century ago. By 1970, more than half of family farms had income from other sources of work; this number increased to 93% of farms by the year 2000 (Dimitri, Effland, & Conklin, 2005). Today's average corporate farmer provides six times as much food compared to the average family farm's yield in 1960. The increased output by farms is impressive nationally, but this productivity has reduced the number of jobs available in farming communities so that farming supports only about 6% of rural jobs (USDA ERS, 2017).

In addition to the disappearance of small family farming as it used to be, there has been a marked disappearance of key industries, such as furniture, textile, steel, mining, and railroad in rural areas (Smith & Tickamyer, 2011; Vernon-Feagans, Burchinal, & Mokrova, 2015). These industries provided important additional employment for rural families 50 years ago, but have now almost completely disappeared or been outsourced to other countries. Unfortunately, jobs in these industries have been replaced by jobs in the service industry (gas stations, grocery stores, and large retail chains) which are usually less desirable because of lower wages, poorer benefits, and nonstandard work hours (Smith & Tickamyer, 2011).

These economic changes in rural areas of the U.S. have been accompanied by a large outmigration of talented young adults from rural areas to more urban areas, leaving behind an older and less-educated population (Vernon-Feagans et al., 2015).

As a result of this outmigration, as well as less access to higher education in rural America, there are now dramatic differences in the college graduation rates between urban and rural adults. Thirty percent of urban adults have a college degree, while only 17.5% of rural adults have a college degree (USDA ERS, 2018). In addition, while 42% of people aged 18 to 24 years are enrolled in some form of higher education, only 29% come from rural areas, compared to nearly 48%from cities or urban areas (NCES, 2017).

These differences in education levels and the pursuit of higher education have more dire consequences in rural areas now than they did in the twentieth century. For instance, in 1970, almost half of adults without a high school degree and 60% of adults with a high school degree were in the middle class, but by 2007, that proportion had fallen to 33% and 45%, respectively. Since 1970, people with a college degree or higher have greatly benefitted economically, compared to those with only a high school degree who have lost ground economically since 1970 and experienced much lower increases in income over the years (Carnevale, Smith, & Strohl, 2010). Nationally, more than half (51%) of rural families with children have incomes below 200% of the federal poverty line compared to only 37% of urban families. This high rural poverty rate occurs despite the fact that 80% of all rural families have a family member working full time; in fact, one-quarter of poor rural families with two or more employed household members are still living in poverty (Rivers, 2005).

The much lower proportion of college-educated adults in rural areas in the U.S. has created even greater disparities between these college-educated adults and their less-educated neighbors. Thus, adults with less than a high school education and those with a high school education are now more alike compared to the more advantaged college-educated adults living in rural areas today. In addition, jobs that may have been relegated previously to the least-educated (adults without a high school degree) are now being filled by adults with a high school degree or some college, but without a college degree. This downward trend for high school graduates to be employed in lower paying jobs that once were mostly filled by non-high school graduates may be one of the reasons for the rising income gap between college-educated and non-college-educated groups, especially in rural areas (Presser, 2003).

Despite the many challenges of living in low wealth rural America, there are also some real strengths of living in rural communities. Rural families still have more connections to extended family and social networks in the community and a greater commitment to the place where they live (Vernon-Feagans et al., 2010). The lower population density, accompanied by more families living in single-family homes and owning their homes compared to urban families, may mean that rural children have greater access to nature and larger play areas around homes (Jaure, Rapoza & Swesnik, 2000; Kannapel & DeYoung, 1999). In addition, people living in rural places are exposed to almost four times less violent crime compared to those living in urban places (Donnermeyer, 1994). Thus, neighborhoods for children are likely to be quieter, safer, and more secure in rural areas and small towns than in urban areas. Schools are also rated more favorably by rural adults; teachers in rural America have more experience and often live in the small community where they teach unlike their urban counterparts (Provasnik et al., 2007).

Child Poverty in Rural Communities

The economic and demographic shifts in rural life just described (fewer college-educated adults, the outmigration of talented young adults, the loss of good jobs, and lower wages) have resulted in higher child poverty rates in rural areas. Child poverty rates have been as high as 29% for young children (Mattingly & Stransky, 2010), compared to about 23% for young children in urban areas. These rates have decreased over the last few years but still, remain greater in rural areas as can be seen in Fig. 1. There remains a five-point percentage difference in poverty rates between rural and urban young children. Children under 6 years living in rural areas have a poverty rate of 27.6% which is more than one in four children, compared to the poverty rate of 22. 5% for similar age children living in more urban areas. These high poverty rates are likely due to the combination of rural adults having fewer college degrees and lack of jobs that pay well.

Despite the relative prevalence of children living in poverty in nonurban rural areas, there have been very few developmental studies of young rural children living in low-wealth communities and especially few that have included large minority populations. The FLP recruited a diverse, representative sample of children born between 2003 and 2004 in rural areas in North Carolina and Pennsylvania (see Vernon-Feagans & Cox, 2013 for more details). The study aimed at examining the lives of these rural children as they developed within the context of their families, schools, and communities, with the hope of better understanding the risk and resilience factors related to

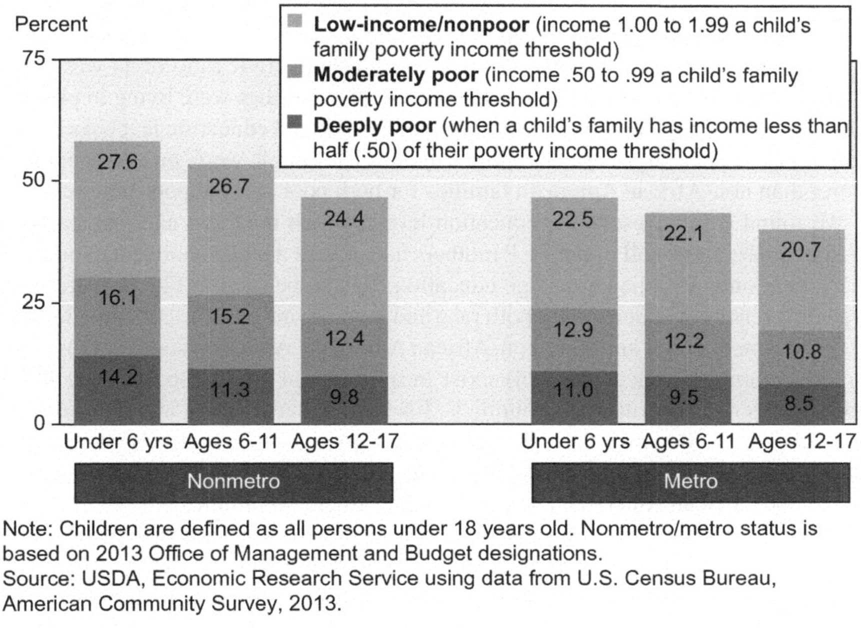

Fig. 1 Children by age, poverty status, and metro/nonmetro residence, 2013

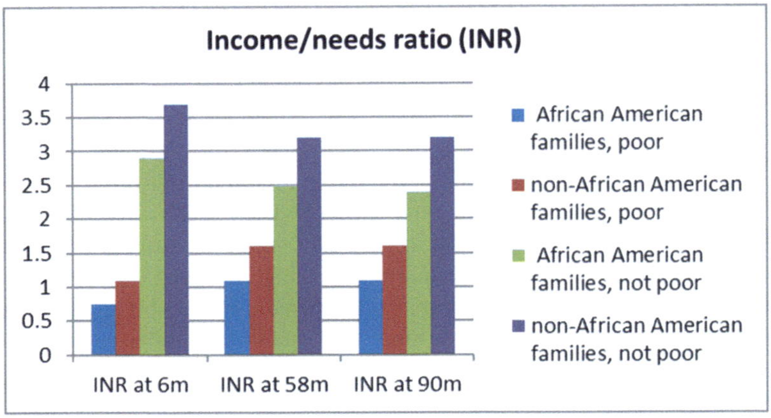

Fig. 2 Income/needs ratio (INR). Source: Vernon-Feagans et al., 2015

developmental outcomes throughout childhood, in the face of the potential challenges and rewards of living in these low wealth communities.

Importantly, this study was one of the few undertaken in the context of the rural U.S. in the twenty-first century with all the recent changes in rural communities just described in the preceding paragraphs. In addition, a focus on African American families has helped to describe the even greater challenges experienced by these families in the current context of rural America. We asked parents to tell us all sources of income from anyone living in their household and then calculated an income to needs ratio (INR) based on the total income for the number of people in their household as our measure of poverty. In 2005, the poverty threshold (INR ratio of 1) was about $20,000 a year for a family of four. Many of the FLP families were living in poverty, and there were fairly large income differences by race and education level. As can be seen in Fig. 2, African American families in our FLP sample were, on average, much poorer than non-African American families for both poor and nonpoor families.

We found similar results for education levels, which mirrored national statistics on rural areas; almost all of our FLP mothers had at least a high school education, but on average only 15% had a college education. As can be seen in Fig. 3, there were large differences in education by both race and income; most of the college-educated mothers were not poor and were non-African American. Although some of these race and education differences probably exist in more urban areas also, they are likely more exaggerated in rural communities. Taken together, Figs. 2 and 3 mirror the national data of a downward trend in income and good jobs for high school-educated parents compared to college-educated parents, and replicate this trend in a rural sample for both African American and non-African American families.

Previous research suggests that early child poverty may be one of the most powerful predictors of child achievement and adult competence; greater than single motherhood, maternal education, and other traditional risk factors (Brooks-Gunn & Duncan, 1997; McLoyd, 1998; Duncan, Ziol-Guest, & Kalil, 2010).

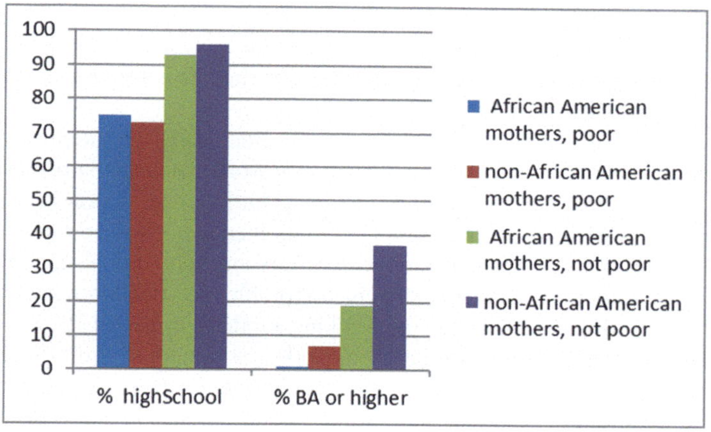

Fig. 3 Education by both race and income

Early childhood poverty probably exerts its influence indirectly through other pathways such as lack of parental education opportunities, workplace conditions, and parenting time and quality (Reardon, 2011; Duncan & Murnane, 2011).

Parenting and Work Schedules in Low Wealth Rural Communities

For both urban and rural families, there has been a dramatic shift in work life for less-educated adults, termed the *24-hour economy* (Presser, 2004). Jobs for adults with less than a college degree are increasingly less desirable in terms of pay, benefits, and work hours, which often interfere with family life. A number of studies have shown that low-income families earning below 200% of the federal poverty level are much more likely to work nonstandard work hours, have jobs with few benefits, and have seasonal or unpredictable work schedules (Joshi & Bogen, 2007). Rural adults are more commonly starting work either late in the evening or the middle of the night compared to urban adults who are more likely to start work in the morning around 8:30 am (Saenz, 2009).

Nonstandard and unpredictable parental work schedules have created real changes in children's lives by decreasing the number of waking hours parents have with their children and impacting the type and timing of childcare families need for their young children, often resulting in very limited options for working parents. A recent study examined diary entries recording the amount of time parents spent with their children as a function of whether they had a standard or nonstandard work schedule (Enchautegui, 2013). Mothers and fathers who worked nonstandard work schedules spent less time with their children from infancy to age 18 years. Similarly, parents who worked night shifts spent many fewer nights having dinner with their children (Presser, 2004). Sixty-four percent of single working mothers who worked nights missed about half the dinners with their children each week, compared to only 23% of single mothers who work during the day. This trend was similar for both mothers and fathers in dual-earner families.

Nonstandard work hours have consequences for the quality of parenting and subsequent child outcomes. For instance, mothers who worked nonstandard hours during the early years of their child's life tended to have children with poorer language and cognitive skills in early childhood compared to mothers who worked standard hours (Han, 2005). This pattern was evident in elementary aged children also; nonstandard work hours have been linked to greater behavior problems for children in elementary school (Joshi & Bogen, 2007). Of the working mothers in the FLP, 38% of poor mothers and about 25% of not poor mothers worked nonstandard shifts. We also saw a marked difference in standard vs. nonstandard work hours if we examined the FLP mothers by the level of education. There was a stark difference in the work schedules experienced by our college-educated versus non-college educated mothers (Fig. 4).

We examined the role of nonstandard work hours among the African American families only in the FLP and found, consistent with previous work, that nonstandard work schedules were associated with detrimental effects on children's early expressive language. However, we also uniquely identified maternal positive engagement and negative work–family spillover as partial mediators of this effect (Odom, Vernon-Feagans, & Crouter, 2013).

In addition to impacts on child outcomes, nonstandard work hours have been related to higher stress levels, more marital problems, and less general satisfaction with family relationships (Presser, 2003; Grosswald, 2004). Although there is also evidence that nonstandard work hours often increase father–child interactions among dual-earner couples compared to couples working day shifts. (A discussion of the role of fathers appears later in this chapter.) Sharing of childcare because of alternating work schedules may be viewed by parents as financially and emotionally

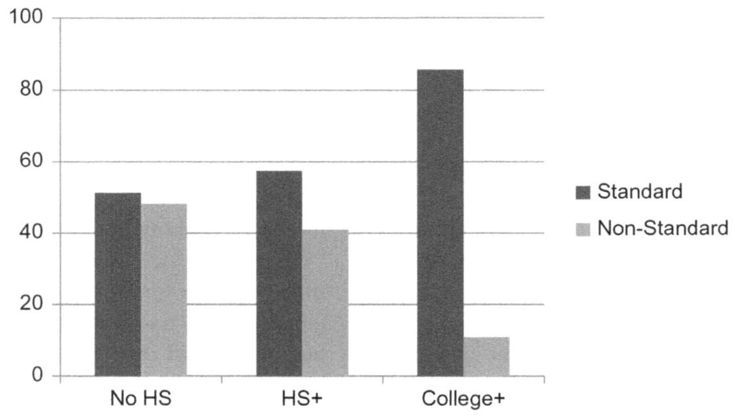

Fig. 4 Proportion of FLP working mothers who reported standard versus nonstandard work hours when their child was 36 months old. Source: Vernon-Feagans et al., 2015

advantageous over other childcare arrangements. Although, the stress (including lack of sleep and not seeing your partner often) of these arrangements may also have negative impacts on well-being. Indeed, overall, evening and rotating shifts have been found to have a negative effect on the quality of time spouses spend with each other, relative to those on day shifts (Presser, 2007). Clearly, adults living in rural areas may struggle with time for family and children because of challenges in work schedules. These struggles are often exacerbated because of the lack of public transportation and longer distances to work than urban families experience. Among the six rural counties in which our FLP study families lived, there was almost no public transportation that could help families navigate their way to work or childcare.

Work, Childcare, and Children's Development

One of the major challenges for families in which one or two parents work is childcare, especially when the work requires nonstandard work hours. Families in rural areas are farther away from childcare centers and other sources of care for their children (Vernon-Feagans et al., 2010). This challenge is further complicated by the relative lack of availability of childcare during nonstandard work hours. Although this is likely also an issue in more urban areas, the geographic isolation of many rural families makes childcare challenges particularly problematic. Families must cobble together care from a variety of sources, including relatives, babysitters, family childcare homes, and childcare centers. Examination of childcare practices in the FLP revealed that parents used many different forms of care, and children were often in a number of different care settings each week (Bratsch-Hines, Baker, & Vernon-Feagans, 2016; Bratsch-Hines, Mokrova, Vernon-Feagans & the FLP key investigators, 2015). For young children, this constant change in care within and across time and settings requires the child to adjust to different caregivers and often different parent work schedules each week. In the FLP sample, the number of provider changes across settings and time was negatively associated with children's social adjustment (Bratsch-Hines et al., 2015).

Childcare accessibility and quality for rural families continue to be limited by geographic isolation, parental work hours, the age of the child, and cost (Forry & Walker, 2011). Data from the FLP suggest an increase in the use of formal childcare as children get older. At the 2-month visit, 25% of children were in some form of childcare for 10 or more hours each week. Interestingly, most children at this young age were cared for in a relative's home, likely because of distance from childcare facilities, work hours, and the greater cost of infant care. Yet, 91% of not poor children were cared for in a relative's home compared to 43% of children near or in poverty, which may be due to the lack of relatives available and mothers not working in the near or in poverty group. By 36 months of age, there was a shift away from care provided in a relative's home and more children were cared for in a more formal childcare center, even if that center was some distance from the parent's work and home. In the FLP, there were very few high-quality childcare centers in the counties in which our families resided.

Quality of childcare is a major issue for families in both urban and rural settings; previous research has suggested that the quality of early childcare is important in the prediction of children's later language and school readiness skills (Crosnoe et al., 2010; NICHD ECCRN, 2005). Not surprisingly, childcare quality ratings across the first 3 years of life in the FLP sample using the HOME (Bradley, 1994), were found to be lower for poor families versus not poor families. In addition, rural African American children in the FLP sample were shown to experience lower quality childcare than their non-African American peers in toddlerhood (De Marco, Crouter, Vernon-Feagans, & FLP Key Investigators, 2009). This difference may be important in understanding some children's school readiness. One recent study of rural children's school readiness found that the quality of the pre-k classroom was an important predictor of school readiness, even though other factors such as maternal education were also important in differentiating children who were better prepared for school (Justice, Jiang, Khan & Dynia, 2017).

Some studies have speculated that language scaffolding used by parents and caregivers might be a critical aspect of high-quality caregiving that is linked to better child language and school readiness (Cabell, Justice, Konold, & McGinty, 2011; Peisner-Feinberg et al., 2001; Piasta, Justice, McGinty, & Kaderavek, 2012; Vandell et al., 2010). Indeed, an important contribution of the FLP to the childcare quality literature has been the focus on both language in the home and language in the childcare setting. Previous research has found that children at risk may benefit more from high-quality childcare than children not at risk in terms of their concurrent and later academic success (Dearing, McCartney, & Taylor, 2009). Much work to date has only speculated that the language provided by the caregiver in high-quality childcare settings might be the most important factor in buffering children from poorer outcomes. However, previous work has demonstrated that although the overall quality of childcare was important in predicting the language development of preschool children, the most salient feature of childcare quality for predicting children's language was the teacher's initiations of language to the target child and the child's verbal initiations to the teacher (McCartney, 1984). In addition, children with lower language skills seemed to benefit more from caregiver–child verbal interactions than children with higher language skills.

In the FLP study, we gathered observational data on the language mothers used with their child during a joint picture book task in the home, as well as language used during caregiver–child interactions in the childcare setting. We examined whether high levels of caregiver–child language interactions in childcare at 36 months would be of more benefit to children who came from homes with lower versus higher levels of maternal language stimulation. Unlike other studies, the FLP study controlled for a host of socioeconomic variables, such as income and maternal education, as well as earlier child language and cognition skills, structural childcare variables, and overall quality of both the home and the childcare environments using the previously mentioned HOME observation ratings (Bradley, 1994). Our findings suggested that children of mothers with low language stimulation during the picture book sharing interaction had better language at 36 months and 2 years later if these children had a childcare provider who interacted verbally with them more often

(Vernon-Feagans, Bratsch-Hines, & FLP Key Investigators, 2013). This finding held up, even after controlling for the quality of the home environment and the quality of the childcare environment. Thus, language in the childcare setting seemed to be a particularly important feature of childcare quality that could impact children's concurrent and later language, at least in the rural context.

Parenting in Rural America

Positive, sensitive, and verbally stimulating parenting is highly related to children's competence in social, emotional, cognitive, and language domains (Burchinal, Roberts, Zeisel, Hennon, & Hooper, 2006; Evans, Gonnella, Marcynyszyn, Gentile, & Salpekar, 2005; NICHD ECCRN, 2005). There is growing evidence that poverty may impact children's development, in part through its negative effect on parenting and other stressors in the home. Looked at another way, the quality of parenting may mediate the relationship between poverty/risk and child development early in life. In examining risk associated with poverty in our sample, the FLP has adopted a cumulative risk approach which considers an accumulation of 9 risk factors (i.e., parental education, income, single parenthood, health, and food insufficiency) rather than a single risk in isolation (Burchinal, Roberts, Hooper, & Zeisel, 2000; Hooper, Burchinal, Roberts, Zeisel, & Neebe, 1998). Using this approach, we have found that the overall quality of parent language and parent sensitivity is a partial mediator of the relationship between the cumulative risk indicator and children's development in language, cognition, and executive function in the first 3 years of life (Vernon-Feagans & Cox, 2013). Other studies have also found relationships between SES-related risk and parenting with implications for child language. For example, SES was related to maternal vocabulary, and in turn, mother vocabulary was related to child vocabulary as early as 20 months of age (Bornstein, Haynes, & Painter, 1998). Others have shown that maternal sensitivity and cognitive stimulation, behaviors speculated to act as proxies for maternal language stimulation, were partial mediators of the relationship between SES and child language (Raviv, Kessenich, & Morrison, 2004). Thus, this relationship between maternal language and child language and literacy has been a focus of much work in the FLP.

Maternal Language Input

Studies have consistently shown that mothers with higher education levels and higher incomes, as well as more prestigious careers, appear to use a greater amount and more diverse and complex language with their young children than mothers from lower SES backgrounds. This greater and more complex language input has been positively associated with children's early language and literacy (Hart & Risley, 1995; Hoff, 2003; Rowe, Leech, & Cabrera, 2017). A growing literature has examined whether maternal language input might be an important mediator of the relationship between SES and maternal education on child language development and other important school readiness skills (Hoff, 2003, 2013; Hoff and Naigles, 2002; Rowe, Raudenbush, & Goldin-Meadow, 2012). For example, maternal language input variables have been shown to fully mediate maternal education-related differences in 2-year-olds' vocabularies (Hoff, 2003). Maternal language input has also been shown to be a partial mediator of the relationship between SES and child language (Huttenlocher, Waterfall, Vasilyeva, Vevea, & Hedges, 2010; Rowe, Raudenbush, & Goldin-Meadow, 2012; Vernon-Feagans, Bratsch-Hines, et al., 2013).

Rural children live further from language-rich resources such as libraries, and family homes may be more isolated (Clarke, Koziolo, & Sheridan, 2017; O'Hare, 2009; Vernon-Feagans et al., 2015). Work from the FLP has argued that because of this rural geographic isolation, maternal language input may be even more important and account for more variance in child language and literacy than urban mother's language input, because urban children are exposed to more outside influences (Vernon-Feagans, Bratsch-Hines et al., 2013). The FLP has found that maternal language input over the first 3 years of life is a partial mediator of the relationship between SES-related variables and children's language development across early childhood (Vernon-Feagans, Bratsch-Hines et al., 2013). It is hard to compare our language findings to previous studies that have not used a cumulative risk framework or have not used a rural sample. Yet, while our cumulative risk variable accounted for about 10–12% of the variance in child language, the addition of maternal language more than doubled the amount of variance accounted for, increasing it to 25% to 28% (Vernon-Feagans, Bratsch-Hines et al., 2013). This larger amount of variance accounted for by maternal language input could be due to the larger influence of mothers in a rural sample, as has been mentioned previously.

Furthermore, because of the nature of the FLP sample, race differences among college-educated mothers, high school educated mothers, and non-high school-educated mothers could be examined allowing us to somewhat disentangle the influence of race and education level that has been conflated in most previous studies (Hart & Risley, 1995; Huttenlocher et al., 2010). These analyses revealed no race differences within education levels on any of the many maternal language input variables in the home language sessions at 6-, 15-, 24-, and 36-months. There were also no race differences on child language measures at school entry except for one vocabulary measure, with African American children scoring more poorly (Vernon-Feagans, Bratsch-Hines, Reynolds, & Willoughby, 2019). Thus, although our findings suggest that maternal language input could not be implicated in the child race differences on standardized vocabulary measures, it may be that poorer quality childcare available to African American families (mentioned earlier), and/or issues of discrimination and bias related to standardized vocabulary measures, are implicated in these differences. This study also found that across all race groups, maternal language input from 6 to 36 months was a partial mediator of the relationship between maternal education and child language at pre-k and in kindergarten. In addition, maternal education still had a direct impact on child language measures, even after controlling for a host of demographic and home variables. Thus, both maternal language and maternal education appear to be important predictors of child outcomes for children growing up in the context of rural poverty.

Both Mother and Father Language Input

The role of maternal language input in a child's development is clear. There is a growing emphasis on the complementary and unique contribution of fathers to a child's development. While mothers and fathers often interact with young children quite similarly, there may be language input differences worth highlighting that help explain the importance of fathers (Rowe, Coker, & Pan, 2004; Tamis-LeMonda, Baumwell, & Cristofaro, 2012). For example, fathers have been found to engage in more rough and tumble play with their children and may use different words that reflect their different interests in comparison to mothers (Cabrera, Fitzgerald, Bradley, & Roggman, 2014). Specifically, fathers have been found to encourage children to engage in more complex language interactions and use more explicit clarification questions (Leech, Salo, Rowe, & Cabrera, 2013; Rowe et al., 2004). It has also been suggested previously that since rural fathers work more nonstandard work hours, they may also play a larger role in caring for their young children when they are not working (Presser, 2007). Although less is known about fathers' language input and children's development, especially for rural fathers, there has been mounting evidence over the last 10 years on the importance of father's language interactions with their children in predicting later development (Baker, Vernon-Feagans & Family Life Project Investigators, 2015; Pancsofar & Vernon-Feagans, 2006; Pancsofar, Vernon-Feagans & FLP Investigators, 2010; Tamis-LeMonda et al., 2012).

FLP data have been used in a series of studies to examine mother and father language input across early childhood in the subsample of families with a continuously present father figure in the home (only about 500 of the nearly 1300 children in the sample). The data on language interactions came from videotaped sessions in which mothers and fathers shared a wordless picture-book with their children in separate sessions. Each book was slightly altered to be racially and culturally sensitive. This kind of book sharing by parents and children has been linked to children's later literacy skills through the enhancement of children's vocabularies and other mechanisms (Neuman, 1997; Payne, Whitehurst, & Angell, 1994; Sénéchal, LeFevre, Hudson, & Lawson, 1996).

In the FLP sample, mother and father means on the language input measures were surprisingly similar with respect to the number of different words used with their child and the mean length of utterance, which is a measure of language complexity. Despite these similarities, maternal and paternal language appears to predict child outcomes in quite different ways, with father language input being more important in predicting child outcomes than mother language input in two-parent families (Baker et al., 2015; Pancsofar et al., 2010). For example, fathers' education and number of different words used during the picture book task at 6-months were uniquely associated with more optimal language development for toddlers at 15- and 36-months, even in the presence of maternal language input; only maternal education, but not maternal language input, was uniquely predictive of child language (Panscofar et al., 2010). A second study examined father language input during the picture-book session just prior to kindergarten entry in relation to end of kindergarten literacy and math skills. There were no differences between mother and fathers in terms of language complexity or word diversity, although both mother and father language complexity were important predictors of child academic skills (Baker et al., 2015). After controlling for demographic characteristics, fathers' complexity of language predicted children's math and literacy skills above and beyond mothers' language input. Thus by 60 months, both mother and father language complexity, and maternal education, seemed to be uniquely and independently contributing to children's literacy skills, measured at the end of kindergarten year; only father language input predicted math skills.

In our more recent paper, we examined both mother and father input from 6 to 36 months in more depth in relation to kindergarten achievement (Reynolds, Vernon-Feagans, Bratsch-Hines, Baker, & the Family Life Project Key Investigators, 2019). We found that mothers' complexity of language and *wh-* questions predicted kindergarten vocabulary, while only mother's mean length of utterance predicted kindergarten math skills. Fathers' complexity of language and *wh-* questions predicted kindergarten vocabulary, while fathers' *wh-* questions also predicted math skills. Overall, these findings demonstrate that rural fathers play a critical role in their children's early language and academic success. Father's language input may be even more important than mother's language in predicting children's language and school readiness skills.

Household Chaos and Children's Development

One way to capture recent changes in rural family life attributable to work schedules, lack of transportation, geographic isolation, and poverty at the more proximal level of the household is to measure what has been termed *household chaos*. This construct has been developed over the last 20 years to describe the instability and disorganization that often characterizes households that struggle with work/family balance, especially in the context of poverty. Two major components of chaos have been identified: *disorganization* and *instability* (Sameroff, 2010; Vernon-Feagans, Garrett-Peters, De Marco, & Bratsch-Hines, 2012). *Disorganization* refers to high levels of noise, crowding, clutter, and lack of preparation for daily living. This has often been measured in the home setting but could be present at the neighborhood and community level as well. *Instability* refers to frequent changes over time; for example, numerous household moves, changes in the parental figures in the family, and changes in parental jobs and work hours. This may also include change over time in the people who live in the household. Children (and their parents) who live in poverty are often exposed to a multitude of these psychosocial stressors (Evans & Wachs, 2010). Thus, household chaos has been identified as a key mechanism by which poverty exerts an influence on children's development. For example, one of the few longitudinal studies to date in a rural sample reported that chaos mediated the relationship between poverty and children's socioemotional adjustment (child learned helplessness, psychological distress, self-regulatory behaviors) in a sample of third to fifth graders followed into seventh and eighth grade (Evans et al., 2005).

Chaotic environments have been hypothesized to interfere with children's developing attentional and regulatory processes and may be especially detrimental for young children who are learning to manage their behavior in response to their home and school environment (Li-Grining, 2007). In addition, there is now growing evidence that chaotic households provide young children with a less optimal parenting environment because it undermines parents' ability to provide the language input and scaffolding that young children need to develop optimally. Direct links have been found between household chaos, exposure to chronic noise in the neighborhood environment, and residential crowding (controlling for SES) and language development in early childhood (Evans, Maxwell, & Hart, 1999; Maxwell & Evans, 2000). These authors hypothesized that household disorganization (noise, clutter, household density) would directly influence children's language development as a result of the overstimulation of too many people and disorganization in the home that could lead young children to block out and withdraw from the chaotic environment. Further, when homes contain high levels of background noise and many people living in a small area, it may be difficult for a young child to process language directed to her/him because of the many background distractions. The ultimate result of this chaos may be that children eventually shut down processing and withdraw from joint-attentional activities and other parent–child interactions that promote language and other aspects of development.

In the FLP, we measured 10 indicators of chaos that factored into the two previously defined dimensions: *disorganization* and *instability*. Because of the longitudinal nature of our project, we were able to create chaos indicators that were aggregated across five data collection time points over the children's first 3 years of life (Vernon-Feagans, Garrett-Peters, Willoughby, Mills-Koonce, & the FLP key investigators, 2012). These indicators were used in a series of papers that demonstrated that accumulated household chaos over the first 3 years of a child's life was negatively associated with multiple aspects of children's development including language and behavioral regulation skills (Vernon-Feagans, Garrett-Peters, De Marco & Bratsch-Hines, 2012; Vernon-Feagans, Garrett-Peters, Willoughby et al., 2012; Vernon-Feagans, Willoughby, Garrett-Peters, & the FLP Key Investigators, 2016). *Disorganization,* in particular, was a significant predictor of both receptive and expressive language on standardized assessments at 36 months of age, even in the presence of important covariates such as family poverty, maternal literacy and depression, child gender and temperament, parenting behavior, and geographic isolation. We found similar results for the influence of disorganization on child socioemotional competence and problem behaviors at age five, even after controlling for important covariates such as poverty and maternal education (Vernon-Feagans, Garrett-Peters, De Marco, Bratsch-Hines, 2012). A recent study (Garrett-Peters, Mokrova, Vernon-Feagans, Willoughby, Pan, & FLP Key

Investigators, 2016) found a mediating role of early cumulative household chaos (6–58 months) in associations between early family income poverty (6 months) and children's academic achievement in kindergarten. Results revealed that in the presence of household disorganization and important covariates, poverty was no longer directly related to academic achievement in kindergarten. Income poverty was, however, positively related to household disorganization, which was in turn, associated with lower academic achievement. These results are consistent with previous research indicating that household chaos conveys some of the adverse longitudinal effects of poverty on children's basic cognitive, academic, and social-behavioral outcomes at least in this rural sample. In another recent paper, the FLP examined whether household chaos, measured across the first 3 years of life, predicted observed and teacher-rated behavioral regulation in kindergarten above and beyond poverty-related variables (Vernon-Feagans et al., 2016). In addition, this study tested whether parent responsivity and acceptance behaviors, measured during the first 3 years of life, as well as executive function (EF) skills, which were measured when children were 3–5 years of age, mediated the relationship between early household chaos and kindergarten behavioral regulation. Results suggested that household chaos disorganization indirectly predicted kindergarten behavioral regulation through intermediate impacts on parenting behaviors and children's early EF skills.

These findings suggest the detrimental impact of early household chaos disorganization and the mediating role of the parenting environment, in understanding children's early and later development at school age. As was mentioned earlier, household chaos may have a more profound impact on rural children because of the geographic isolation of homes, parents' multiple jobs, nonstandard work hours, and distance to work, that are all greater in rural communities.

Early Poverty Stressors and Brain Development

As we have outlined previously in the chapter, growing up in poverty often means being exposed to higher than average levels of a host of stressors such as infrequent or problematic parent–child interactions, high levels of conflict within the home, low-quality childcare arrangements, and suboptimal environments with increased risks and hazards (Bradley & Corwyn, 2002; Brooks-Gunn, Duncan, & Meritato, 1997; Evans, 2004; Mistry, Biesanz, Taylor, Burchinal, & Cox, 2004). Children who grow up in rural communities may experience these effects more acutely than urban children, as rural in comparison to urban communities tend to have higher poverty rates, greater isolation from key services such as high-quality schools and health care, and parents who are more likely to have service-related jobs with nonstandard work schedules (Vernon-Feagans et al., 2015).

These factors are associated with poverty, but may also have a more proximal influence on a child's development because they lead to higher than average levels of household chaos including disorganization, instability, and unpredictability (defined earlier in this chapter) Bronfenbrenner & Evans, 2000; Vernon-Feagans, Garrett-Peters, De Marco, Bratsch-Hines, 2012; Vernon-Feagans, Garrett-Peters, Willoughby et al., 2012). The result of this is home and social environments which are both impoverished (in terms of less cognitive stimulation or one-on-one interactions), but also characterized by overstimulating and overwhelming input that is chaotic, disconnected, or confusing for the developing child (Evans, 2004; Vernon Feagans, Garrett-Peters, Willoughby et al., 2012). Work from the FLP and others has shown that high levels of neighborhood and household poverty and chaos are associated with poorer child outcomes in language development, academic performance, and cognitive and socio-emotional functioning (Blair & Raver, 2012; Evans, 2006; Evans, Bullinger, & Hygge, 1998; Garrett-Peters et al., 2016; Huston et al., 2001; Maxwell & Evans, 2000) and may also have long-lasting effects on physical health (Kim et al., 2018).

Previous research has demonstrated that the presence of environmental stressors such as those associated with living in rural poverty *early* in development can be particularly harmful and have long-lasting consequences in impactful areas such as mental health and school achievement that shape the course of one's life (Duncan, Magnuson, Kalil, & Ziol-Guest, 2012; Duncan et al., 2010; Engle & Black, 2008; Evans & Kim, 2013). Importantly, in many of these studies early poverty was more predictive of negative outcomes than poverty experienced when children were older (Brooks-Gunn, Guo, & Furstenberg, 1993; Duncan & Brooks-Gunn, 2000; Duncan, Yeung, Brooks-Gunn, & Smith, 1998; Lipman & Offord, 1997; Lipman, Offord, & Boyle, 1994; Rutter, 1976). Complimentary work with adults has demonstrated that exposure to poverty in childhood has lasting impacts on psychological and physical health, even after accounting for adult exposure to poverty (Cohen, Janicki-Deverts, Chen, & Matthews, 2010; Danese & McEwen, 2012; Evans, Chen, Miller, & Seeman, 2012).

One mechanism through which the experience of poverty and associated risks early in development may have a larger and more lasting impact on development is through an influence on brain development. Neural development occurs rapidly and displays a great deal of plasticity in the first few years of life, making it especially vulnerable to input from the early environment during this period (e.g., Sanders, Stevens, Coch, & Neville, 2006; Stevens & Neville, 2013). A growing body of theoretical and empirical work has demonstrated that basic neural circuitry is being established during the first years of life. This neural circuitry lays the groundwork for later development, but is also at least partially impacted by the child's social and physical environment (De Bellis, 2001; Gunnar, Fisher, & The Early Experience, Stress and Prevention Network, 2006; Nelson, 2000; Propper & Moore, 2006; Swingler et al., 2018; Swingler, Perry, Calkins, & Bell, 2017). Experience is thought to be especially important in the first 2 years of life when a spurt in brain growth occurs. This growth is characterized by an overproduction of neural connections, and subsequent experience is thought to determine which connections are maintained and strengthened (because of use) and which are selectively eliminated (Greenough & Black, 1992; Knudsen, 2004; Nelson & Bloom, 1997; Nelson, Thomas, & de Haan, 2006; Singer, 1995).

Thus, in this way, early experiences can have a direct influence on brain development with consequences for future behavior and functioning. Extreme examples of this come from research with animals and studies of abnormal environments characterized by neglect or abuse; studies have shown repeatedly that poor environmental experiences are related to abnormal structural and functional brain development that can lead to suboptimal cognitive and behavioral functioning (Chugani et al., 2001; Curtis & Cicchetti, 2007; De Bellis, 2001; Gunnar et al., 2006; Marshall, Fox, & BEIP Core Group, 2004; McEwen, 1998; Rutter & O'Connor, 2004). Recent work has begun to demonstrate that even normative variation in environmental experiences, such as quality of caregiving, is related to different patterns of brain functioning (e.g., Bernier, Calkins, & Bell, 2016; Hane & Fox, 2006; Swingler et al., 2017; Swingler et al., 2018). Thus, the child's early environment can have a direct effect on the experience-dependent maturation and organization of neural systems which lay the groundwork for future cognitive and socio-emotional functioning.

Stress, HPA Axis, Parenting, and Brain Development

Work by FLP researchers has identified the development of stress physiology as a central component in the influence of the environment on brain development (e.g., Blair & Raver, 2012). In this model, stress hormone levels act as a primary conduit or mechanism through which cognitive and social-emotional development in early childhood is shaped by experience. Three brain regions (the amygdala, hippocampus, and medial prefrontal cortex) regulate the physiological stress systems, particularly the hypothalamus–pituitary–adrenal axis (HPA axis) and autonomic nervous system (ANS), which control physiological responses to stress (e.g., fight or flight; Ulrich, Lai, & Herman, 2009). When the HPA axis is activated by stress, a series of hormones are released by the hypothalamus. This stimulates the release of cortisol, a glucocorticoid (steroid hormone), from the adrenal glands (Mills-Koonce & Towe-Goodman, 2012). While the release of cortisol is adaptive in the short term because it facilitates the body's mobilization of resources in response to environmental demands (allostasis), chronic exposure to high levels of cortisol can cause dysfunction in the brain and associated physiological systems (allostatic load), leading to increased risks for poor psychological and physical outcomes (Kim et al., 2018; McEwen & Gianoros, 2011; Sapolsky, 1996). This is perhaps because stress hormones have been shown to change neural activity in the brain, especially in key areas involved in the control of attention and emotion (Arnsten, 2000; Yuen et al., 2009). While moderate levels of stress hormones can have a positive effect on neural activity and connections in the brain which may improve behavioral performance, very high (or very low) levels result in a dampening of activity and, consequently, poorer performance (Ramos & Arnsten, 2007; Segal, Richter-Levin, & Maggio, 2010). Repeated exposure to high levels of stress and stress hormones over time has been shown to have a lasting impact on both physiological and neural functioning, especially when the exposure happens early in development (McLaughlin, Sheridan, Tibu, Fox, Zeanah, & Nelson, 2015).

Children who grow up in poverty are more likely to experience chronic stressors that generate this "wear" (allostatic load) on stress regulatory systems including the HPA axis with hypothesized lasting implications for child functioning (Finegood, Rarick, Blair, & FLP Investigators, 2017). A growing body of literature, much of it using data from the FLP, has shown support for this hypothesis and demonstrated that poverty adversely affects children's development by altering levels of stress hormones (e.g., Blair, Granger et al., 2011; Blair, Raver et al., 2011; Evans, 2003; Lupien, King, Meaney, & McEwen, 2001). We have found in the FLP sample that living in rural poverty is associated with elevated resting or baseline levels of cortisol in infancy and into early childhood (Blair, Granger et al., 2011; Blair, Raver, Granger, Mills-Konce, Hibel, & FLP Key Investigators, 2011; Blair, Berry, Mills-Koonce, Granger, & the FLP Key Investigators, 2013). In addition, higher levels of salivary cortisol measured at three-time points across the first 2 years of life were uniquely associated with lower executive function ability and, to a lesser extent, child IQ at 3 years of life (Blair, Granger et al., 2011). This finding demonstrates potential support for the idea that higher levels of stress hormones can have lasting impacts on cognitive functioning.

While results from the FLP study have demonstrated an association between years spent living in rural poverty and baseline cortisol levels, findings have also shown that this association is mediated through characteristics of the child's household (Blair, Raver et al., 2011; Hibel, Granger, Blair, Cox, & the FLP Investigators, 2011) and through sensitive and responsive parenting behavior (Blair et al., 2008; Mills-Koonce et al., 2011). For example, instability in the number of caregivers in the home, as well as parents' perceptions of financial insecurity, were each uniquely associated with higher baseline salivary cortisol levels in infants and toddlers in the FLP sample (Blair, Raver et al., 2011). This finding is consistent with the hypothesis that living in unstable and financially insecure homes is associated with changes in the physiological functioning characteristic of those living in uncertainty and adversity (Blair & Raver, 2012).

A separate FLP paper demonstrated that maternal engagement early in development mediated the association between poverty and cortisol levels in children in the infant and toddler period (Blair et al., 2008). In these analyses, income-to-need ratio (i.e., the total household income of anyone who resided in the household divided by the federal poverty threshold for a family of that size and composition) demonstrated no independent relation with cortisol, and the effect of an index of social advantage on child cortisol was wholly accounted for by maternal engagement with the child during interaction. Infants whose primary caregivers exhibited higher levels of engagement in structured parent–child interactions were characterized by more optimal patterns of baseline cortisol and cortisol reactivity increase in response to an emotion challenge. Further, cortisol reactivity in response to challenge in toddlers was associated with maternal engagement as assessed in infancy, but not as assessed during the toddler period, emphasizing the potential importance of early parenting behavior on later child functioning. These analyses also indicated that resting level of cortisol was higher for African American (versus non-African American) children in the FLP sample, likely reflecting conditions of increased risk associated with deep poverty as African American children in the sample were from disproportionately low-income families (Blair et al., 2008; Blair, Granger, et al., 2011). The importance of maternal sensitivity for child cortisol levels, above and beyond the influence of family income, was further demonstrated in a recent FLP paper (Berry et al., 2017). Importantly, within-person changes in maternal sensitivity across the first 2 years of life were associated with coincident changes in children's baseline cortisol levels, demonstrating the strong influence of maternal behavior on stress hormone levels in development in our rural sample.

Of interest to note, thus far analyses examining the effects of maternal behavior on child cortisol in the FLP sample have found associations with positive, but not negative, aspects of *maternal* behavior (Blair, Granger et al., 2011). Conversely, in a paper examining the influence of father contributions to cortisol responses in infancy and toddlerhood in a subset of the FLP sample living with both biological parents, father negativity (harsh and controlling parenting) was found to be associated with higher cortisol levels in response to an emotion stressor in infancy and higher overall levels of cortisol in toddlerhood, both of which suggest less regulated physiological functioning and arousal (Mills-Koonce et al., 2011).

Taken together, findings from the FLP project demonstrate a clear association between living in rural poverty and elevated levels of stress hormones, both at rest and in response to a stressful event. Our results further suggest that elevated levels of stress hormones in early development have negative implications for child cognitive functioning (e.g., executive functions), with the potential to have far-reaching consequences for the child across a variety of important domains which rely on these cognitive skills (e.g., academic readiness and self-regulation) in development. Given that these cognitive skills depend on areas of the brain which are sensitive to the presence of elevated stress hormones, one hypothesis is that chronic exposure to stress and stress hormones early in development has impacted neural development in areas underlying these abilities. However, our results also demonstrate the importance (and potential protective nature) of parenting behavior and other aspects of the child's social and household environment on levels of stress hormones in the children in our sample. In particular, our findings suggest a potential buffering effect of positive maternal behavior on the negative consequences of living in rural poverty for the child's developing physiological and neural systems.

The Transition to School

Children in rural areas have also been found to experience greater risks to successful educational trajectories. Many factors are likely associated with these risks. For instance, teachers in rural areas have more experience but fewer advanced degrees. Teachers often have not had access to high-quality professional development programs that could supply them with the necessary tools to enhance children's school learning (Vernon-Feagans, 2009; Vernon-Feagans, Bratsch-Hines, Varghese, Cutrer, & Garwood, 2018). Children in rural communities are also more likely to repeat a grade in school. National data have reported that 14% of school-aged children in small rural areas and 12% of those in large rural areas have repeated a grade, compared to 8% of urban children (National Advisory Committee on Rural Health and Human Services, 2015). Rural children are also less likely than their urban peers to participate in organized activities outside of school and to read for pleasure on a typical day. Even with these challenges, national data (Showalter, Klein, Johnson, & Hartmen, 2017) have consistently found that rural children nationwide enter school at the national average with scores very similar to suburban children who are more advantaged economically. Thus, it has not been clear why rural children become at greater risk academically as they move through elementary and secondary school.

In the FLP, we have found similar trends to the national data on rural achievement in early elementary school, with the FLP children entering school with good readiness skills (Vernon-Feagans et al., 2015). This is especially impressive since the FLP sample is not a general rural sample but is specifically examining children who are from low wealth communities, many of whom live in poverty. The African American FLP children entered school with standardized scores at or above the national average (kindergarten Woodcock Johnson Letter-Word Identification, $M = 107.39$, $SD = 12.06$) and were very similar to their non-African American peers ($M = 107.29$, $SD = 12.12$). This is particularly impressive for our African American families since they were much poorer than our non-African American sample. Over time, however, the scores for both groups began to decline, with FLP African American children at the national average in third grade (third grade Woodcock Johnson Letter-Word Identification, $M = 99.92$, $SD = 11.15$) and non-African American children still somewhat above the national average ($M = 104.36$, $SD = 11.97$). These data suggest that overall these rural children should be poised to do well in school from their school entry skills, but there appears to be a downward trend over elementary school for all rural children, and especially African American children, in our sample. It seemed important to understand whether the quality of instruction might make a difference for the FLP children's achievement in literacy.

As part of the FLP, we observed classroom quality to examine whether more years of a better quality of instruction might positively impact the children's literacy and related skills. One way to conceptualize the quality of instruction in early elementary school has been to measure the kind of classroom environment that promotes learning, especially in early literacy, with a focus on how teachers support and scaffold student learning. A classroom quality measure that captures quality across early childhood and early elementary school classrooms is the Classroom Assessment Scoring System (CLASS; Pianta, La Paro, & Hamre, 2008). The CLASS contains three subscales: *Emotional Support* measures teacher's responsivity to student concerns, as well as the teacher's warmth and ability to take the perspective of different kinds of students; *Classroom Organization* measures teacher's ability to manage the productive behavior of students in the classroom to maximize learning opportunities for children; and *Instructional Support* measures teachers' ability to promote higher order thinking, give constructive feedback to students, scaffold children's skills, and use stimulating language that allows for the expansion of student ideas to promote learning (Pianta et al., 2008).

Few studies have tried to examine general classroom quality over a number of years in elementary school, especially in relation to children's early literacy, and very few studies have used a rural sample. One prior study used the CLASS to examine how classroom quality in kindergarten and first grade related to children's literacy trajectories over these two grades (Curby, Rimm-Kaufman, & Ponitz, 2009). This rural study found some support for the importance of classroom quality using each dimension separately as a continuous variable; however, there were also some contradictory findings. For instance, children who had lower initial basic letter–word identification scores grew faster in literacy in classrooms with higher quality Instructional Support. On the other hand, children with higher initial scores in letter–word identification benefitted the most from classrooms with lower quality Instructional Support. For all the findings the effect sizes were very small.

Recently, it has been suggested that children may benefit from classroom instruction/quality only when quality exceeds a certain threshold. For instance, a series of studies and a recent monograph have demonstrated that, at least in early childhood settings, there seems to be a threshold effect for classroom quality on children's emergent literacy skills (Burchinal, Vandergrift, Pianta, & Mashburn, 2010; Burchinal et al., 2014; Burchinal, Zaslow, & Tarullo, 2016).

The FLP has used a threshold approach in examining the CLASS in pre-k and over early elementary school. Using a threshold approach to categorize children according to the number of years of higher quality classrooms they experienced during pre-K and kindergarten, CLASS Emotional Support and Classroom Organization predicted better child social-emotional functioning at the end of both kindergarten and first grade (Broekhuizen, Mokrova, Burchinal, Garrett-Peters, & The FLP Key Investigators, 2016). In an extension of this initial work, FLP examined the quality of classroom environments continuously from kindergarten through third grade, while controlling for child kindergarten entry skills and demographic variables, as well as the quality of the home environment (Vernon-Feagans, Mokrova, Carr, Garrett-Peters, Burchinal, & the FLP Key Investigators, 2019). In addition, this study also examined whether there might be a compensatory effect of classroom quality, such that children with lower literacy skills before kindergarten entry might benefit even more from multiple years of better classroom quality in relation to third grade literacy skills, as compared to children with higher literacy skills before kindergarten entry. The findings from this study suggest that children who experience more years of better quality classrooms across 4 years, have better reading comprehension and general academic knowledge in third grade, even after controlling for demographic characteristics, child school entry skills, and the quality of parenting in the home. Importantly, an interaction between the years of better classroom quality and children's literacy skills prior to kindergarten entry suggested that more years of better classroom quality was more promotive of growth in reading comprehension for children who entered kindergarten with lower literacy skills (See Fig. 5). Thus, better classroom quality over time, not just during a single school year, could possibly serve as an important way to reduce the literacy gaps between children with higher and lower literacy skills at school entry.

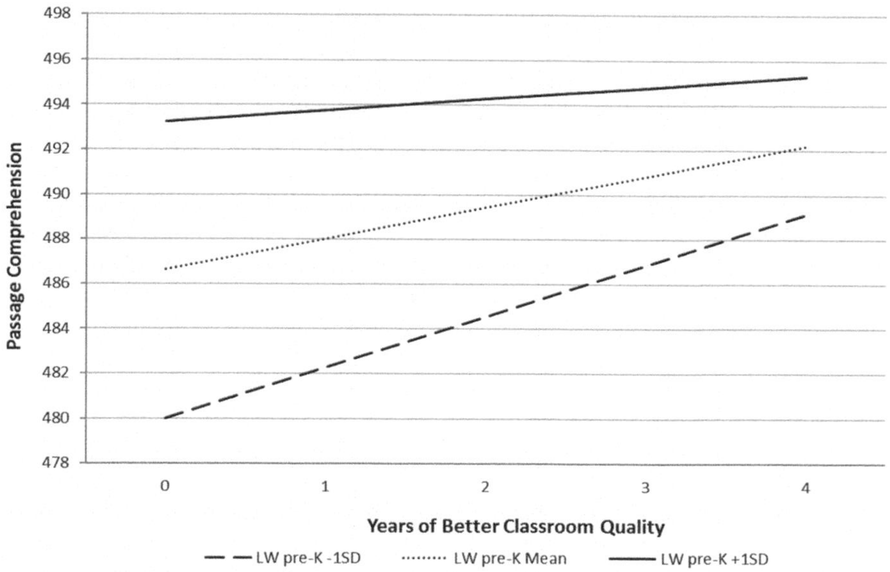

Fig. 5 Interaction of years of better classroom quality and children's Woodcock Johnson III Letter-Word ID prior to school entry predicting passage comprehension. Note: LW pre-K = Woodcock Johnson III Letter-Word ID prior to school entry. Source: Vernon-Feagans et al., 2018

In an effort to address the realities of rural schools and promote children's literacy skills, a professional development intervention for rural early elementary teachers (The Targeted Reading Intervention; TRI) was developed (Amendum, Vernon-Feagans, & Ginsberg, 2011; Vernon-Feagans, Kainz et al., 2013; Vernon-Feagans, Bratsch-Hines et al., 2018). The TRI is part of a new generation of early interventions preparing classroom teachers to use specific strategies with individual learners to prevent reading failure. The TRI is unique in that it uses literacy coaches, who can be thousands of miles away from target schools, to deliver ongoing professional development to classroom teachers in remote rural schools via webcam technology. Literacy coaches use the webcams to observe teachers weekly as they instruct an individual struggling reader in one-on-one sessions and provide immediate feedback to help classroom teachers choose the best individualized, instructional strategies. Teachers work with a struggling reader for 15 min a day for 6–8 weeks before moving on to another struggling reader. Using webcam technology is more cost effective and feasible in rural areas where geographic isolation may prevent access to high-quality professional development (Vernon-Feagans, Bratsch-Hines et al., 2018).

Effectiveness data from previous randomized controlled trials have shown effect sizes between 0.28 and 0.63 on student reading gains (Amendum et al., 2011; Vernon-Feagans, Kainz et al., 2013; Vernon-Feagans, Bratsch-Hines et al., 2018). A number of independent groups, including *What Works Clearinghouse*, have endorsed the TRI as one of only a few early professional development programs that have shown effectiveness and especially cost effectiveness. It not only works but is affordable for low wealth rural schools. Our most recent RCT study has now replicated our results that the TRI can promote rapid reading gains in a very short period on all aspects of literacy from decoding accuracy to spelling and to passage comprehension in rural low wealth schools (Vernon-Feagans, Bratsch-Hines et al., 2018).

Thus, the data from FLP and TRI suggest there may be ways to prevent the downward slope of literacy achievement in rural children through better instruction in the classroom, especially for children with the lowest skills. Further research on the FLP sample may help us to understand the other factors in children's lives that either buffer children from poorer outcomes or exacerbate poor school outcomes.

Conclusion

Young families in rural America are experiencing a more challenging environment for optimal family and work life than their parents and grandparents did. These families have been trying to adjust to the changing economic and population shifts in their communities while doing the best for their families, especially their young children. Yet, many low wealth and less educated rural families face challenges that are likely greater than similar families living in more urban areas. These challenges include two large, central shifts in rural life: the loss of good jobs in farming and other industries, and less access to higher education. These shifts have been associated with working nonstandard work hours, living further from work with little access to public transportation, and being far from many supportive family services and institutions of higher education. The impact of these shifts has been a decrease in the amount and quality of family time, despite parents' desire for more family time. Rural families, and especially young families, struggle to be the best parents they can be, but many young families are left with very few options to provide their children with the best homes and schools.

Despite these formidable challenges, the FLP has found that parenting and good instruction in childcare and school can make a difference in the biological, cognitive, and academic functioning of young children living in rural areas. For instance, the FLP found that more caregiver–child verbal interactions in a childcare setting could buffer the effects of less frequent and complex linguistic input in the home. FLP has also found that the parenting behavior of both mothers and fathers in rural families makes a difference for their children's biological functioning and academic readiness and achievement, even if their time with children is limited. We have shown specific effects for the role of linguistic input from both parents, but especially fathers. FLP is one of the only projects to show that father language is an especially important predictor of children's language and early math skills, over and above the influence of mother language. Instead, the mother's contribution in early development may be more strongly conveyed through her education level rather than her language input in early childhood, although mother language does become more important at school age. For instance, our most recent paper (Reynolds et al., 2019) shows that both mothers' and fathers' language input predicts children's kindergarten achievement, beyond a host of demographic controls that includes the quality of the home environment. This finding points to the importance of both mother and father language input, beyond just good parenting, in predicting child outcomes in rural communities.

FLP has also contributed to the literature on rural families by examining the role of household chaos for understanding the development of children from rural households. Household chaos has likely increased in rural and low wealth families because of the rise of nonstandard work hours for noncollege educated parents, long distances to work and childcare, and the lack of public transportation that together impact the ability to have predictable schedules and the time needed for optimal parenting. In many of our papers on chaos we have demonstrated the wide-ranging impact of household chaos but also the positive mediating role of parenting, on children's language, behavior, and academics. Our results have demonstrated that increased stress in the home environment, like that associated with greater chaos and disorganization, has the potential to disrupt children's biological functioning. However, we have also shown that sensitive and engaged parenting behavior has the potential to mediate this relationship. While growing up in poverty does appear to put children at increased risk for elevated stress responses and stress hormones, more work is needed to examine the potential mechanisms through which this may impact neural development and associated cognitive functioning, as well as what factors my help mediate this process.

Results from the FLP study also suggest that the rural children in our sample were well prepared at school entry. Both African American and non-African American children in our sample began school with reading and academic skills at or above the national average. This is quite remarkable, given the greater poverty levels and much lower parental education levels compared to other rural studies and most urban studies. These good outcomes for children may be because their families have sacrificed other pleasures and personal resources to provide their children with a good and enriching family life and childcare. These findings are particularly impressive for the African American families. For instance, despite the fact that African American mothers in the FLP live in much deeper poverty than non-African American mothers, across maternal education levels linguistic input during mother–child interactions are of the same quantity and quality as non-African American mothers. In addition, we only see lower scores for African American children on standardized vocabulary measures at school entry, not on naturalistic language samples or on teacher ratings. Findings from the FLP mirror other studies showing that maternal education and changes in maternal education are important drivers of parenting behavior and children's development in multiple areas of functioning (Magnuson, 2007; Rowe, Denmark, Harden & Stapleton, 2016).

Finally, FLP data has demonstrated that more years of better classroom quality can make a difference for all children in reading abilities and general academic knowledge by third grade. In addition, children who come into school with the lowest academic readiness skills profit the most from more years of better quality classroom instruction. Even though teachers in rural communities tend to have less education than more urban teachers, they also tend to have more experience than urban teachers. This experience may be a marker of commitment to place and demonstrate a dedication to make a difference in children's lives by promoting better academic achievement. Their lack of access to high-quality professional development may have prevented many rural teachers from becoming effective teachers. Our intervention studies of the Targeted Reading Intervention implemented in low wealth rural communities have shown that most rural teachers are eager to learn new skills and instructional strategies that promote child reading and achievement in early elementary school. The teachers in our intervention rapidly promoted large reading gains for struggling readers, using our webcam coaching model. Part of what these rural teachers may convey, besides good instruction, is their commitment to their community and the families and children who live there.

Future studies beyond FLP need to delve more deeply into the role of extended family, religious institutions, and other sources of support that may be unique to rural communities and help children succeed. Other factors such as peers and less formal community resources should also be studied, especially as children get older. With the FLP, we hope to better understand what happens to the children as they enter middle school and high school by exploring factors associated with later academic and social success, and pursuit of higher education. Further work should also examine how parents and their children see their future opportunities, and how some children go on to access good jobs and/or higher education that keep them in their community and lead to better lives for them and for future generations in rural America.

References

Amendum, S. J., Vernon-Feagans, L., & Ginsberg, M. C. (2011). The effectiveness of a technologically facilitated classroom-based early reading intervention: The targeted reading intervention. *The Elementary School Journal, 112*(1), 107–131.

Arnsten, A. F. T. (2000). Through the looking glass: Differential noradrenergic modulation of prefrontal cortical function. *Neural Plasticity, 7*(1–2), 133–146. https://doi.org/10.1155/NP.2000.133

Baker, C. E., Vernon-Feagans, L., & Family Life Project Investigators. (2015). Fathers' language input during shared book activities: Links to children's kindergarten achievement. *Journal of Applied Developmental Psychology, 36*, 53–59. https://doi.org/10.1016/j.appdev.2014.11.009

Bernier, A., Calkins, S. D., & Bell, M. A. (2016). Longitudinal associations between the quality of mother–infant interactions and brain development across infancy. *Child Development, 87*(4), 1159–1174. https://doi.org/10.1111/cdev.12518

Berry, D., Blair, C., Willoughby, M., Granger, D. A., Mills-Koonce, W. R., & Family Life Project Key Investigators. (2017). Maternal sensitivity and adrenocortical functioning across infancy and toddlerhood: Physiological adaptation to context? *Development and Psychopathology, 29*(1), 303–317. https://doi.org/10.1017/S0954579416000158

Blair, C., Berry, D., Mills-Koonce, R., Granger, D., & Family Life Project Investigators. (2013). Cumulative effects of early poverty on cortisol in young children: Moderation by autonomic nervous system activity. *Psychoneuroendocrinology, 38*(11), 2666–2675. https://doi.org/10.1016/j.psyneuen.2013.06.025

Blair, C., Granger, D. A., Kivlighan, K. T., Mills-Koonce, R., Willoughby, M., Greenberg, M. T., … Fortunato, C. K. (2008). Maternal and child contributions to cortisol response to emotional arousal in young children from low-income, rural communities. *Developmental Psychology, 44*(4), 1095–1109. https://doi.org/10.1037/0012-1649.44.4.1095

Blair, C., Granger, D. A., Willoughby, M., Mills-Koonce, R., Cox, M., Greenberg, M. T., … The FLP Investigators. (2011). Salivary cortisol mediates effects of poverty and parenting on executive functions in early childhood. *Child Development, 82*(6), 1970–1984. https://doi.org/10.1111/j.1467-8624.2011.01643.x

Blair, C., & Raver, C. C. (2012). Child development in the context of adversity: Experiential canalization of brain and behavior. *American Psychologist, 67*(4), 309–318. https://doi.org/10.1037/a0027493

Blair, C., Raver, C. C., Granger, D., Mills-Koonce, R., Hibel, L., & Family Life Project Key Investigators. (2011). Allostasis and allostatic load in the context of poverty in early childhood. *Development and Psychopathology, 23*(3), 845–857. https://doi.org/10.1017/S0954579411000344

Bornstein, M. H., Haynes, M. O., & Painter, K. M. (1998). Sources of child vocabulary competence: A multivariate model. *Journal of Child Language, 25*(2), 367–393.

Bradley, R. H. (1994). The HOME Inventory: Review and reflections. *Advances in Child Development and Behavior, 25*, 241–288.

Bradley, R. H., & Corwyn, R. F. (2002). Socioeconomic status and child development. *Annual Review of Psychology, 53*, 371–399. https://doi.org/10.1146/annurev.psych.53.100901.135233

Bratsch-Hines, M., Baker, C., & Vernon-Feagans, L. (2016). Minority families in the rural United States: Family processes, child care, and early schooling. In L. J. Crockett & G. Carlo (Eds.), *Rural ethnic minority youth and families in the United States: Theory, research, and applications* (pp. 143–164). Cham, Switzerland: Springer. https://doi.org/10.1007/978-3-319-20976-0_9

Bratsch-Hines, M. E., Mokrova, I., Vernon-Feagans, L., & The Family Life Project Key Investigators. (2015). Child care instability from 6 to 36 months and the social adjustment of children in prekindergarten. *Early Childhood Research Quarterly, 30*(PA), 106–116. https://doi.org/10.1016/j.ecresq.2014.09.002

Broekhuizen, M. L., Mokrova, I. L., Burchinal, M. R., Garrett-Peters, P. T., & Family Life Project Key Investigators. (2016). Classroom quality at pre-kindergarten and kindergarten and children's social skills and behavior problems. *Early Childhood Research Quarterly, 36*, 212–222. https://doi.org/10.1016/j.ecresq.2016.01.005

Bronfenbrenner, U., & Evans, G. W. (2000). Developmental science in the 21st century: Merging questions, theoretical models, research designs, and empirical findings. *Social Development, 9*(1), 115–125. https://doi.org/10.1111/1467-9507.00114

Brooks-Gunn, J., & Duncan, G. J. (1997). The effects of poverty on children. *Future of Children, 7*(2), 55–71. https://doi.org/10.2307/1602387

Brooks-Gunn, J., Duncan, G. J., & Meritato, N. (1997). Poor families, poor outcomes: The well-being of children and youth. In G. J. Duncan & J. Brooks-Gunn (Eds.), *Consequences of growing up poor* (pp. 1–17). New York: Russell Sage Foundation.

Brooks-Gunn, J., Guo, G., & Furstenberg, F. F., Jr. (1993). Who drops out of and who continues beyond high school? A 20-year follow-up of black urban youth. *Journal of Research on Adolescence, 3*(3), 271–294.

Burchinal, M., Roberts, J. E., Zeisel, S. A., Hennon, E. A., & Hooper, S. (2006). Social risk and protective child, parenting, and child care factors in early elementary school years. *Parenting: Science and Practice, 6*(1), 79–113.

Burchinal, M., Vandergrift, N., Pianta, R., & Mashburn, A. (2010). Threshold analysis of association between child care quality and child outcomes for low-income children in pre-kindergarten programs. *Early Childhood Research Quarterly, 25*(2), 166–176.

Burchinal, M., Vernon-Feagans, L., Vitiello, V., Greenberg, M., & The Family Life Project Key Investigators. (2014). Thresholds in the association between child care quality and child outcomes in rural preschool children. *Early Childhood Research Quarterly, 29*(1), 41–51. https://doi.org/10.1016/j.ecresq.2013.09.004

Burchinal, M., Zaslow, M., & Tarullo, L. (Eds.). (2016). *Quality thresholds, features, and dosage in early care and education: Secondary data analyses of child outcomes*. Hoboken, NJ: Wiley.

Burchinal, M. R., Roberts, J. E., Hooper, S., & Zeisel, S. A. (2000). Cumulative risk and early cognitive development: A comparison of statistical risk models. *Developmental Psychology, 36*(6), 793–807. https://doi.org/10.1037/0012-1649.36.6.793

Cabell, S. Q., Justice, L. M., Konold, T. R., & McGinty, A. S. (2011). Profiles of emergent literacy skills among preschool children who are at risk for academic difficulties. *Early Childhood Research Quarterly, 26*(1), 1–14.

Cabrera, N. J., Fitzgerald, H. E., Bradley, R. H., & Roggman, L. (2014). The ecology of father-child relationships: An expanded model. *Journal of Family Theory and Review, 6*(4), 336–354. https://doi.org/10.1111/jftr.12054

Carnevale, A. P., Smith, N., & Strohl, J. (2010). *Help wanted: Projections of jobs and education requirements through 2018*. Georgetown University, Center on Education and the Workforce, McCourt School of Public Policy. Retrieved from https://cew.georgetown.edu/cew-reports/help-wanted/

Chugani, H. T., Behan, M. E., Muzik, O., Juhász, C., Nagy, F., & Chugani, D. C. (2001). Local brain functional activity following early deprivation: A study of postinstitutionalized Romanian orphans. *NeuroImage, 14*(6), 1290–1301.

Clarke, B. L., Koziol, N. A., & Sheridan, S. M. (2017). The effects of rurality on parents' engagement in children's early literacy. In G. C. Nugent, G. M. Kunz, S. M. Sheridan, T. A. Glover, & L. L. Knoche (Eds.), *Rural education research in the United States* (pp. 231–250). Switzerland: Springer, Cham. https://doi.org/10.1007/978-3-319-42940-3_12

Cohen, S., Janicki-Deverts, D., Chen, E., & Matthews, K. A. (2010). Childhood socioeconomic status and adult health. *Annals of the New York Academy of Sciences, 1186*(1), 37–55. https://doi.org/10.1111/j.1749-6632.2009.05334.x

Crosnoe, R., Leventhal, T., Wirth, R. J., Pierce, K. M., Pianta, R. C., & NICHD Early Child Care Research Network. (2010). Family socioeconomic status and consistent environmental stimulation in early childhood. *Child Development, 81*(3), 972–987. https://doi.org/10.1111/j.1467-8624.2010.01446.x

Curby, T. W., Rimm-Kaufman, S. E., & Ponitz, C. C. (2009). Teacher–child interactions and children's achievement trajectories across kindergarten and first grade. *Journal of Educational Psychology, 101*(4), 912–925. https://doi.org/10.1037/a0016647

Curtis, W. J., & Cicchetti, D. (2007). Emotion and resilience: A multilevel investigation of hemispheric electroencephalogram asymmetry and emotion regulation in maltreated and nonmaltreated children. *Development and Psychopathology, 19*(3), 811–840. https://doi.org/10.1017/S0954579407000405

Danese, A., & McEwen, B. S. (2012). Adverse childhood experiences, allostasis, allostatic load, and age-related disease. *Physiology & Behavior, 106*(1), 29–39. https://doi.org/10.1016/j.physbeh.2011.08.019

De Bellis, M. D. (2001). Developmental traumatology: The psychobiological development of maltreated children and its implications for research, treatment, and policy. *Development and Psychopathology, 13*(3), 539–564. https://doi.org/10.1017/S0954579401003078

De Marco, A., Crouter, A. C., Vernon-Feagans, L., & The Family Life Project Key Investigators. (2009). The relationship of maternal work characteristics to childcare type and quality in rural communities. *Community, Work & Family, 12*(4), 369–387. https://doi.org/10.1080/13668800802528249

Dearing, E., McCartney, K., & Taylor, B. A. (2009). Does higher quality early child care promote low-income children's math and reading achievement in middle childhood. *Child Development, 80*(5), 1329–1349. https://doi.org/10.1111/j.1467-8624.2009.01336.x

Dimitri, C., Effland, A., & Conklin, N. (2005). *The 20th century transformation of US agriculture and farm policy (No. 3)*. Washington, DC: United States Department of Agriculture, Economic Research Service.

Donnermeyer, J. (1994). Crime and violence in rural communities. In J. Blaser (Ed.), *Perspectives on violence and substance use in rural America*. North Central Regional Educational Laboratory: Oak Brook, IL.

Duncan, C. M. (1999). *Worlds apart: Why poverty persists in rural America*. New Haven, CT: Yale University Press.
Duncan, G. J., & Brooks-Gunn, J. (2000). Family poverty, welfare reform, and child development. *Child Development, 71*(1), 188–196. https://doi.org/10.1111/1467-8624.00133
Duncan, G. J., Magnuson, K., Kalil, A., & Ziol-Guest, K. (2012). The importance of early childhood poverty. *Social Indicators Research, 108*(1), 87–98. https://doi.org/10.1007/s11205-011-9867-9
Duncan, G. J., & Murnane, R. J. (Eds.). (2011). *Whither opportunity: Rising inequality, schools, and children's life chances*. New York: Russell Sage Foundation.
Duncan, G. J., Yeung, W. J., Brooks-Gunn, J., & Smith, J. R. (1998). How much does childhood poverty affect the life chances of children? *American Sociological Review, 63*(3), 406–423.
Duncan, G. J., Ziol-Guest, K. M., & Kalil, A. (2010). Early-childhood poverty and adult attainment, behavior, and health. *Child Development, 81*(1), 306–325. https://doi.org/10.1111/j.1467-8624.2009.01396.x
Enchautegui, M. E. (2013). *Nonstandard work schedules and the well-being of low-income families* (Paper 26). Washington, DC: Urban Institute, Low Income Working Families Project. Retrieved from https://www.urban.org/sites/default/files/publication/32696/412877-Nonstandard-Work-Schedules-and-the-Well-being-of-Low-Income-Families.PDF
Engle, P. L., & Black, M. M. (2008). The effect of poverty on child development and educational outcomes. *Annals of the New York Academy of Sciences, 1136*(1), 243–256. https://doi.org/10.1196/annals.1425.023
Evans, G. W. (2003). A multimethodological analysis of cumulative risk and allostatic load among rural children. *Developmental Psychology, 39*(5), 924–933.
Evans, G. W. (2004). The environment of childhood poverty. *American Psychologist, 59*(2), 77–92. https://doi.org/10.1037/0003-066X.59.2.77
Evans, G. W. (2006). Child development and the physical environment. *Annual Review of Psychology, 57*(10), 423–451. https://doi.org/10.1146/annurev.psych.57.102904.190057
Evans, G. W., Bullinger, M., & Hygge, S. (1998). Chronic noise exposure and physiological response: A prospective study of children living under environmental stress. *Psychological Science, 9*(1), 75–77. https://doi.org/10.1111/1467-9280.00014
Evans, G. W., Chen, E., Miller, G., & Seeman, T. (2012). How poverty gets under the skin: A life course perspective. In V. Maholmes & R. King (Eds.), *The Oxford handbook of poverty and child development* (pp. 13–36). New York: Oxford University Press.
Evans, G. W., Gonnella, C., Marcynyszyn, L. A., Gentile, L., & Salpekar, N. (2005). The role of chaos in poverty and children's socioemotional adjustment. *Psychological Science, 16*(7), 560–565. https://doi.org/10.1111/j.0956-7976.2005.01575.x
Evans, G. W., & Kim, P. (2013). Childhood poverty, chronic stress, self-regulation, and coping. *Child Development Perspectives, 7*(1), 43–48. https://doi.org/10.1111/cdep.12013
Evans, G. W., Maxwell, L. E., & Hart, B. (1999). Parental language and verbal responsiveness to children in crowded homes. *Developmental Psychology, 35*(4), 1020–1023.
Evans, G. W., & Wachs, T. D. (2010). *Chaos and its influence on children's development*. Washington, DC: American Psychological Association.
Finegood, E. D., Rarick, J. R. D., Blair, C., & Family Life Project Investigators. (2017). Exploring longitudinal associations between neighborhood disadvantage and cortisol levels in early childhood. *Development and Psychopathology, 29*(5), 1649–1662.
Forry, N. D., & Walker, S. K. (2011). Child care in rural America. In K. E. Smith & A. R. Tickamyer (Eds.), *Economic restructuring and family well-being in rural America* (pp. 256–272). University Park, PA: The Pennsylvania State University Press.
Garrett-Peters, P. T., Mokrova, I., Vernon-Feagans, L., Willoughby, M., Pan, Y., & The Family Life Project Key Investigators. (2016). The role of household chaos in understanding relations between early poverty and children's academic achievement. *Early Childhood Research Quarterly, 37*, 16–25. https://doi.org/10.1016/j.ecresq.2016.02.004

Greenough, W. T., & Black, J. E. (1992). Induction of brain structure by experience: Substrates for cognitive development. In M. R. Gunnar & C. A. Nelson (Eds.), *The Minnesota Symposium on Child Psychology* (Vol. 24,. *Developmental behavioral neuroscience*, pp. 155–200). Hillsdale, NJ: Lawrence Erlbaum Associates.

Grosswald, B. (2004). The effects of shift work on family satisfaction. *Families in Society, 85*(3), 413–423. https://doi.org/10.1606/1044-3894.1503

Gunnar, M. R., Fisher, P. A., & The Early Experience, Stress, and Prevention Network. (2006). Bringing basic research on early experience and stress neurobiology to bear on preventive interventions for neglected and maltreated children. *Development and Psychopathology, 18*(3), 651–677. https://doi.org/10.1017/S0954579406060330

Han, W.-J. (2005). Nonstandard work schedules and child care decisions: Evidence from the NICHD Study of Early Child Care. *Early Childhood Research Quarterly, 19*(2), 231–256. https://doi.org/10.1016/j.ecresq.2004.04.003

Hane, A., & Fox, N. A. (2006). Ordinary variations in maternal caregiving influence human infants' stress reactivity. *Psychological Science, 17*(6), 550–556. https://doi.org/10.1111/j.1467-9280.2006.01742.x

Hart, B., & Risley, T. R. (1995). *Meaningful differences in the everyday experience of young American children*. Baltimore, MD: Brookes Publishing.

Heath, S. B. (1983). *Ways with words: Language, life and work in communities and classrooms*. New York, NY: Cambridge University Press.

Hibel, L. C., Granger, D. A., Blair, C., Cox, M. J., & Family Life Project Key Investigators. (2011). Maternal sensitivity buffers the adrenocortical implications of intimate partner violence exposure during early childhood. *Development and Psychopathology, 23*(2), 689–701. https://doi.org/10.1017/S0954579411000010

Hoff, E. (2003). The specificity of environmental influence: Socioeconomic status affects early vocabulary development via maternal speech. *Child Development, 74*(5), 1368–1378. https://doi.org/10.1111/1467-8624.00612

Hoff, E. (2013). Interpreting the early language trajectories of children from low-SES and language minority homes: Implications for closing achievement gaps. *Developmental Psychology, 49*(1), 4–14. https://doi.org/10.1037/a0027238

Hoff, E., & Naigles, L. (2002). How children use input to acquire a lexicon. *Child Development, 73*(2), 418–433. https://doi.org/10.1111/1467-8624.00415

Hooper, S. R., Burchinal, M. R., Roberts, J. E., Zeisel, S., & Neebe, E. C. (1998). Social and family risk factors for infant development at one year: An application of the cumulative risk model. *Journal of Applied Developmental Psychology, 19*(1), 85–96. https://doi.org/10.1016/S0193-3973(99)80029-X

Huston, A. C., Duncan, G. J., Granger, R., Bos, J., McLoyd, V., Mistry, R., … Ventura, A. (2001). Work-based antipoverty programs for parents can enhance the school performance and social behavior of children. *Child Development, 72*(1), 318–336. https://doi.org/10.1111/1467-8624.00281

Huttenlocher, J., Waterfall, H., Vasilyeva, M., Vevea, J., & Hedges, L. V. (2010). Sources of variability in children's language growth. *Cognitive Psychology, 61*(4), 343–365. https://doi.org/10.1016/j.cogpsych.2010.08.002

Jaure, R., Rapoza, R. A., & Swesnik, D. (2000). *Opening doors to rural homeownership: Outcomes from the National Rural Housing Coalition*. Rural Homeownership Symposium. National Rural Housing Coalition. Washington, DC.

Joshi, P., & Bogen, K. (2007). Nonstandard schedules and young children's behavioral outcomes among working low-income families. *Journal of Marriage and Family, 69*(1), 139–156. https://doi.org/10.1111/j.1741-3737.2006.00350.x

Justice, L. M., Jiang, H., Khan, K. S., & Dynia, J. M. (2017). Kindergarten readiness profiles of rural, Appalachian children from low-income households. *Journal of Applied Developmental Psychology, 50*, 1–14. https://doi.org/10.1016/j.appdev.2017.02.004

Kannapel, P. J., & DeYoung, A. J. (1999). The rural school problem in 1999: A review and critique of the literature. *Journal of Research in Rural Education, 15*(2), 67–79.

Kim, P., Evans, G. W., Chen, E., Miller, G., & Seeman, T. (2018). How socioeconomic disadvantages get under the skin and into the brain to influence health development across the lifespan. In N. Halfon, C. B. Forrest, R. M. Lerner, & E. M. Faustman (Eds.), *Handbook of life course health development* (pp. 463–497). Cham, Switzerland: Springer. https://doi.org/10.1007/978-3-319-47143-3_19

Knudsen, E. I. (2004). Sensitive periods in the development of the brain and behavior. *Journal of Cognitive Neuroscience, 16*(8), 1412–1425. https://doi.org/10.1162/0898929042304796

Leech, K. A., Salo, V. C., Rowe, M. L., & Cabrera, N. J. (2013). Father input and child vocabulary development: The importance of Wh questions and clarification requests. *Seminars in Speech and Language, 34*(4), 249–259. https://doi.org/10.1055/s-0033-1353445

Li-Grining, C. P. (2007). Effortful control among low-income preschoolers in three cities: Stability, change, and individual differences. *Developmental Psychology, 43*(1), 208–221. https://doi.org/10.1037/0012-1649.43.1.208

Lipman, E. L., & Offord, D. R. (1997). Psychosocial morbidity among poor children in Ontario. In G. J. Duncan & J. Brooks-Gunn (Eds.), *Consequences of growing up poor* (pp. 239–287). New York: Russell Sage Foundation.

Lipman, E. L., Offord, D. R., & Boyle, M. H. (1994). Relation between economic disadvantage and psychosocial morbidity in children. *Canadian Medical Association Journal, 151*(4), 431–437.

Lupien, S. J., King, S., Meaney, M. J., & McEwen, B. S. (2001). Can poverty get under your skin? Basal cortisol levels and cognitive function in children from low and high socioeconomic status. *Development and Psychopathology, 13*(3), 653–676. https://doi.org/10.1017/S0954579401003133

Magnuson, K. (2007). Maternal education and children's academic achievement during middle childhood. *Developmental Psychology, 43*(6), 1497–1512. https://doi.org/10.1037/0012-1649.43.6.1497

Marshall, P. J., Fox, N. A., & BEIP Core Group. (2004). A comparison of the electroencephalogram between institutionalized and community children in Romania. *Journal of Cognitive Neuroscience, 16*(8), 1327–1338. https://doi.org/10.1162/0898929042304723

Mattingly, M. J., & Stransky, M. L. (2010). *Young child poverty in 2009: Rural poverty rate jumps to nearly 29 percent in second year of recession* (Issue Brief No. 17). Durham, NH: Carsey School of Public Policy. Retrieved from https://scholars.unh.edu/carsey/120/

Maxwell, L. E., & Evans, G. W. (2000). The effects of noise on preschool children's prereading skills. *Journal of Environmental Psychology, 20*(1), 91–97. https://doi.org/10.1006/jevp.1999.0144

McCartney, K. (1984). Effect of quality of day care environment on children's language development. *Developmental Psychology, 20*(2), 244–260. https://doi.org/10.1037/0012-1649.20.2.244

McEwen, B. S. (1998). Stress, adaptation, and disease: Allostasis and allostatic load. *Annals of the New York Academy of Sciences, 840*(1), 33–44. https://doi.org/10.1111/j.1749-6632.1998.tb09546.x

McEwen, B. S., & Gianaros, P. (2011). Stress- and allostasis-induced brain plasticity. *Annual Review of Medicine, 62*, 431–445. https://doi.org/10.1146/annurev-med-052209-100430

McLaughlin, K. A., Sheridan, M. A., Tibu, F., Fox, N. A., Zeanah, C. H., & Nelson, C. A., III. (2015). Causal effects of the early caregiving environment on development of stress response systems in children. *Proceedings of the National Academy of Sciences, 112*(18), 5637–5642. https://doi.org/10.1073/pnas.1423363112

McLoyd, V. C. (1998). Socioeconomic disadvantage and child development. *American Psychologist, 53*(2), 185–204. https://doi.org/10.1037/0003-066X.53.2.185

Mills-Koonce, W. R., Garrett-Peters, P., Barnett, M., Granger, D., Blair, C., & Cox, M. J. (2011). Father contributions to cortisol responses in infancy and early childhood. *Developmental Psychology, 47*(2), 388–395. https://doi.org/10.1037/a0021066

Mills-Koonce, W. R., & Towe-Goodman, N. (2012). Poverty and HPA functioning in young children. In V. Maholmes & R. B. King (Eds.), *The Oxford handbook of poverty and child development* (pp. 387–403). New York, NY: Oxford University Press. https://doi.org/10.1093/oxfordhb/9780199769100.013.0022

Mistry, R. S., Biesanz, J. C., Taylor, L. C., Burchinal, M., & Cox, M. J. (2004). Family income and its relation to preschool children's adjustment for families in the NICHD study of early child care. *Developmental Psychology, 40*(5), 727–745.

National Advisory Committee on Rural Health and Human Services. (2015, December). *Child poverty in rural America* (Policy Brief). Washington, DC: Health Resources and Services Administration Retrieved from https://www.hrsa.gov/advisorycommittees/rural/publications/childpoverty1215.pdf

National Center for Education Statistics (NCES). (2006). *The condition of education 2006* (NCES 2006–071). Washington, DC: U.S. Department of Education. Retrieved from https://nces.ed.gov/pubs2006/2006071.pdf

National Center for Education Statistics (NCES). (2017). *The condition of education 2017* (NCES 2017–144). Washington, DC: U.S. Department of Education. Retrieved from https://nces.ed.gov/pubs2017/2017144.pdf

Nelson, C. A., III. (2000). The neurobiological bases of early intervention. In J. P. Shonkoff & S. J. Meisels (Eds.), *Handbook of early childhood intervention* (2nd ed., pp. 204–227). New York, NY: Cambridge University Press.

Nelson, C. A., III, & Bloom, F. E. (1997). Child development and neuroscience. *Child Development, 68*(5), 970–987. https://doi.org/10.1111/j.1467-8624.1997.tb01974.x

Nelson, C. A., III, Thomas, K. M., & de Haan, M. (2006). Neural bases of cognitive development. In D. Kuhn, R. S. Siegler, W. Damon, & R. M. Lerner (Eds.), Handbook of child psychology: Cognition, perception, and language (6th ed., Vol. 2, pp. 3–57). Hoboken, NJ: John Wiley & Sons, Inc.

Neuman, S. B. (1997). Guiding young children's participation in early literacy development: A family literacy program for adolescent mothers. *Early Child Development and Care, 127*(1), 119–129. https://doi.org/10.1080/0300443971270110

NICHD Early Child Care Research Network (ECCRN). (2005). Duration and developmental timing of poverty and children's cognitive and social development from birth through third grade. *Child Development, 76*(4), 795–810. https://doi.org/10.1111/j.1467-8624.2005.00878.x

Odom, E. C., Vernon-Feagans, L., & Crouter, A. C. (2013). Nonstandard maternal work schedules: Implications for African American children's early language outcomes. *Early Childhood Research Quarterly, 28*(2), 379–387. https://doi.org/10.1016/j.ecresq.2012.10.001

O'Hare, W. P. (2009). *The forgotten fifth: Child poverty in rural America*. Durham, N.H.: Carsey Institute, University of New Hampshire. Retrieved from https://scholars.unh.edu/cgi/viewcontent.cgi?article=1075&context=carsey

Pancsofar, N., & Vernon-Feagans, L. (2006). Mother and father language input to young children: Contributions to later language development. *Journal of Applied Developmental Psychology, 27*(6), 571–587.

Pancsofar, N., Vernon-Feagans, L., & The Family Life Project Investigators. (2010). Fathers' early contributions to children's language development in families from low-income rural communities. *Early Childhood Research Quarterly, 25*(4), 450–463. https://doi.org/10.1016/j.ecresq.2010.02.001

Payne, A. C., Whitehurst, G. J., & Angell, A. L. (1994). The role of home literacy environment in the development of language ability in preschool children from low-income families. *Early Childhood Research Quarterly, 9*(3–4), 427–440. https://doi.org/10.1016/0885-2006(94)90018-3

Peisner-Feinberg, E. S., Burchinal, M. R., Clifford, R. M., Culkin, M. L., Howes, C., Kagan, S. L., & Yazejian, N. (2001). The relation of preschool child-care quality to children's cognitive and social developmental trajectories through second grade. *Child Development, 72*(5), 1534–1553. https://doi.org/10.1111/1467-8624.00364

Pianta, R. C., La Paro, K. M., & Hamre, B. K. (2008). Classroom Assessment Scoring System™: Manual K-3. Baltimore, MD: Brookes Publishing.

Piasta, S. B., Justice, L. M., McGinty, A. S., & Kaderavek, J. N. (2012). Increasing young children's contact with print during shared reading: Longitudinal effects on literacy achievement. *Child Development, 83*(3), 810–820. https://doi.org/10.1111/j.1467-8624.2012.01754.x

Presser, H. B. (2003). *Working in a 24/7 economy: Challenges for American families*. New York, NY: Russell Sage Foundation.
Presser, H. B. (2004). Employment in a 24/7 economy: Challenges for the family. In A. C. Crouter & A. Booth (Eds.), *Work-family challenges for low-income parents and their children* (pp. 83–105). Mahwah, NJ: Lawrence Erlbaum Associates.
Presser, H. B. (2007). Toward a 24-hour economy: Implications for the temporal structure and functioning of family life. In J. Vérnon, S. Pennac, & J. Légaré (Eds.), *Ages, generations and the social contract* (pp. 325–342). https://doi.org/10.1007/978-1-4020-5973-5_15
Propper, C., & Moore, G. A. (2006). The influence of parenting on infant emotionality: A multilevel psychobiological perspective. *Developmental Review, 26*(4), 427–460. https://doi.org/10.1016/j.dr.2006.06.003
Provasnik, S., Kewal Ramani, A., Coleman, M. M., Gilbertson, L., Herring, W., & Xie, Q. (2007). *Status of education in rural America* (NCES 2007-040). Washington, DC: U.S. Department of Education. Retrieved from https://nces.ed.gov/pubs2007/2007040.pdf
Ramos, B. P., & Arnsten, A. F. T. (2007). Adrenergic pharmacology and cognition: Focus on the prefrontal cortex. *Pharmacology & Therapeutics, 113*(3), 523–536. https://doi.org/10.1016/j.pharmthera.2006.11.006
Raviv, T., Kessenich, M., & Morrison, F. J. (2004). A mediational model of the association between socioeconomic status and three-year-old language abilities: The role of parenting factors. *Early Childhood Research Quarterly, 19*(4), 528–547.
Reardon, S. (2011). The widening academic achievement gap between the rich and the poor: New evidence and possible explanations. In G. J. Duncan & R. J. Murnane (Eds.), *Whither opportunity? Rising inequality, schools, and children's life chances* (pp. 91–116). New York, NY: Russell Sage Foundation.
Reynolds, E., Vernon-Feagans, L., Bratsch-Hines, M., Baker, C. E., & The Family Life Project Key Investigators. (2019). Mothers' and fathers' language input from 6 to 36 months in rural two-parent families: Relations to children's kindergarten achievement. *Early Childhood Research Quarterly, 47*, 385–395. https://doi.org/10.1016/j.ecresq.2018.09.002
Rivers, K. (2005). *Rural southern children falling behind in well-being indicators*. Washington, DC: Population Reference Bureau. Retrieved from https://www.prb.org/ruralsouthernchildrenfallingbehindinwellbeingindicators/
Rowe, M. L., Coker, D., & Pan, B. A. (2004). A comparison of fathers' and mothers' talk to toddlers in low-income families. *Social Development, 13*(2), 278–291. https://doi.org/10.1111/j.1467-9507.2004.000267.x
Rowe, M. L., Denmark, N., Harden, B. J., & Stapleton, L. M. (2016). The role of parent education and parenting knowledge in children's language and literacy skills among white, black, and Latino families. *Infant and Child Development, 25*(2), 198–220. https://doi.org/10.1002/icd.1924
Rowe, M. L., Leech, K. A., & Cabrera, N. (2017). Going beyond input quantity: Wh-questions matter for toddlers' language and cognitive development. *Cognitive Science, 41*(S1), 162–179. https://doi.org/10.1111/cogs.12349
Rowe, M. L., Raudenbush, S. W., & Goldin-Meadow, S. (2012). The pace of vocabulary growth helps predict later vocabulary skill. *Child Development, 83*(2), 508–525. https://doi.org/10.1111/j.1467-8624.2011.01710.x
Rutter, M. (1976). *Helping troubled children*. New York: Plenum.
Rutter, M., & O'Connor, T. G. (2004). Are there biological programming effects for psychological development? Findings from a study of Romanian adoptees. *Developmental Psychology, 40*(1), 81–94. https://doi.org/10.1037/0012-1649.40.1.81
Saenz, R. (2009). *Rural workers more likely to work nontraditional shifts* (Issue Brief No. 5). Durham, NH: Carsey Institute, University of New Hampshire. Retrieved from https://scholars.unh.edu/cgi/viewcontent.cgi?article=1073&context=carsey
Sameroff, A. (2010). A unified theory of development: A dialectic integration of nature and nurture. *Child Development, 81*(1), 6–22. https://doi.org/10.1111/j.1467-8624.2009.01378.x

Sanders, L. D., Stevens, C., Coch, D., & Neville, H. J. (2006). Selective auditory attention in 3-to 5-year-old children: An event-related potential study. *Neuropsychologia, 44*(11), 2126–2138.

Sapolsky, R. M. (1996). Why stress is bad for your brain. *Science, 273*(5276), 749–750. https://doi.org/10.1126/science.273.5276.749

Segal, M., Richter-Levin, G., & Maggio, N. (2010). Commentary: Stress-induced dynamic routing of hippocampal connectivity: A hypothesis. *Hippocampus, 20*(12), 1332–1338. https://doi.org/10.1002/hipo.20751

Sénéchal, M., LeFevre, J.-A., Hudson, E., & Lawson, E. P. (1996). Knowledge of storybooks as a predictor of young children's vocabulary. *Journal of Educational Psychology, 88*(3), 520–536. https://doi.org/10.1037/0022-0663.88.3.520

Showalter, D., Klein, R., Johnson, J., & Hartman, S. L. (2017). *Why rural matters 2015–2016: Understanding the changing landscape*. Washington, DC: Rural School and Community Trust.

Singer, W. (1995). Development and plasticity of cortical processing architectures. *Science, 270*(5237), 758–764. https://doi.org/10.1126/science.270.5237.758

Smith, K. E., & Tickamyer, A. R. (2011). Introduction. In K. E. Smith & A. R. Tickamyer (Eds.), *Economic restructuring and family well-being in rural America* (pp. 1–21). University Park, PA: Penn State University Press.

Stack, C. (1996). *Call to home: African Americans reclaim the rural South*. New York, NY: Basic Books.

Stevens, C., & Neville, H. (2013). Specificity of experiential effects in neurocognitive development. In M. S. Gazzaniga (Ed.), *The new cognitive neurosciences* (5th ed., pp. 2–21). Cambridge, MA: The MIT Press.

Strong, D. A., Del Grosso, P., Burwick, A., Jethwani, V., & Ponza, M. (2005). *Rural research needs and data sources for selected human services topics: Volume 1: Research needs*. Washington, DC: Assistant Secretary for Planning and Evaluation, U.S. Department of Health and Human Services.

Swingler, M. M., Isbell, E., Zeytinoglu, S., Calkins, S. D., & Leerkes, E. M. (2018). Maternal behavior predicts neural underpinnings of inhibitory control in preschoolers. *Developmental Psychobiology, 60*(6), 692–706.

Swingler, M. M., Perry, N. B., Calkins, S. D., & Bell, M. A. (2017). Maternal behavior predicts infant neurophysiological and behavioral attention processes in the first year. *Developmental Psychology, 53*(1), 13–27. https://doi.org/10.1037/dev0000187

Tamis-LeMonda, C. S., Baumwell, L., & Cristofaro, T. (2012). Parent–child conversations during play. *First Language, 32*(4), 413–438. https://doi.org/10.1177/0142723711419321

Ulrich-Lai, Y. M., & Herman, J. P. (2009). Neural regulation of endocrine and autonomic stress responses. *Nature Reviews Neuroscience, 10*(6), 397–409. https://doi.org/10.1038/nrn2647

USDA Economic Research Service (ERS). (2017). Report to the President of the United States from the Task Force on Agriculture and Rural Prosperity. Retrieved from https://www.usda.gov/sites/default/files/documents/rural-prosperity-report.pdf

USDA Economic Research Service (ERS). (2018). *Rural education at a glance*. Washington, DC: Economic Research Service. Retrieved from https://www.ers.usda.gov/webdocs/publications/90556/eib-200.pdf?v=5899.2

Vandell, D. L., Belsky, J., Burchinal, M., Steinberg, L., Vandergrift, N., & NICHD Early Child Care Research Network. (2010). Do effects of early child care extend to age 15 years? Results from the NICHD study of early child care and youth development. *Child Development, 81*(3), 737–756. https://doi.org/10.1111/j.1467-8624.2010.01431.x

Vernon-Feagans, L. (1996). *Children's talk in communities and classrooms*. Cambridge, MA: Wiley-Blackwell.

Vernon-Feagans, L. (2009). School readiness. In R. A. Shweder, T. R. Bidell, A. C. Dailey, S. D. Dixon, P. J. Miller, & J. Modell (Eds.), *The child: An encyclopedic companion* (pp. 860–862). Chicago, IL: University of Chicago Press.

Vernon, F. L., Bratsch, H. M., Reynolds, E., & Willoughby, M. (2019). How early maternal language input varies by race and education and predicts later child language. Child Development. https://doi.org/10.1111/cdev.13281

Vernon-Feagans, L., Bratsch-Hines, M., Varghese, C., Cutrer, E. A., & Garwood, J. D. (2018). Improving struggling readers' early literacy skills through a tier 2 professional development program for rural classroom teachers: The Targeted Reading Intervention. *The Elementary School Journal, 118*(4), 525–548. https://doi.org/10.1086/697491

Vernon-Feagans, L., Bratsch-Hines, M. E., & The Family Life Project Key Investigators. (2013). Caregiver–child verbal interactions in child care: A buffer against poor language outcomes when maternal language input is less. *Early Childhood Research Quarterly, 28*(4), 858–873. https://doi.org/10.1016/j.ecresq.2013.08.002

Vernon-Feagans, L., Burchinal, M., & Mokrova, I. (2015). Diverging destinies in rural America. In P. Amato, A. Booth, S. McHale, & J. Van Hook (Eds.), *Families in an era of increasing inequality: Diverging destinies* (pp. 35–49). New York: Springer. https://doi.org/10.1007/978-3-319-08308-7_3

Vernon-Feagans, L., & Cox, M. (2013). The Family Life Project: An epidemiological and developmental study of young children living in poor rural communities: I. Poverty, rurality, parenting, and risk: An introduction. *Monographs of the Society for Research in Child Development, 78*(5), 1–23. https://doi.org/10.1111/mono.12047

Vernon-Feagans, L., Gallagher, K. C., & Kainz, K. (2010). The transition to school in rural America. In J. L. Meece & J. S. Eccles (Eds.), *Handbook of research on schools, schooling, and human development* (pp. 163–184). New York, NY: Routledge.

Vernon-Feagans, L., Garrett-Peters, P., De Marco, A., & Bratsch-Hines, M. (2012). Children living in rural poverty: The role of chaos in early development. In V. Maholmes & R. B. King (Eds.), *The Oxford handbook of poverty and child development* (pp. 448–466). New York, NY: Oxford University Press.

Vernon-Feagans, L., Garrett-Peters, P., Willoughby, M., Mills-Koonce, R., & The Family Life Project Key Investigators. (2012). Chaos, poverty, and parenting: Predictors of early language development. *Early Childhood Research Quarterly, 27*(3), 339–351. https://doi.org/10.1016/j.ecresq.2011.11.001

Vernon-Feagans, L., Kainz, K., Hedrick, A., Ginsberg, M., & Amendum, S. (2013). Live webcam coaching to help early elementary classroom teachers provide effective literacy instruction for struggling readers: The Targeted Reading Intervention. *Journal of Educational Psychology, 105*(4), 1175–1187.

Vernon-Feagans, L., Mokrova, I. L., Carr, R. C., Garrett-Peters, P. T., Burchinal, M. R., & Family Life Project Key Investigators. (2019). Cumulative years of classroom quality from kindergarten to third grade: Prediction to children's third grade literacy skills. *Early Childhood Research Quarterly, 47*, 531–540. https://doi.org/10.1016/j.ecresq.2018.06.005

Vernon-Feagans, L., Willoughby, M., Garrett-Peters, P., & The Family Life Project Key Investigators. (2016). Predictors of behavioral regulation in kindergarten: Household chaos, parenting, and early executive functions. *Developmental Psychology, 52*(3), 430–441. https://doi.org/10.1037/dev0000087

Yuen, E. Y., Liu, W., Karatsoreos, I. N., Feng, J., McEwen, B. S., & Yan, Z. (2009). Acute stress enhances glutamatergic transmission in prefrontal cortex and facilitates working memory. *Proceedings of the National Academy of Sciences, 106*(33), 14075–14079. https://doi.org/10.1073/pnas.0906791106

Latino Prosocial Development in the Rural U.S.

Gustavo Carlo, Madison Memmott-Elison, and Lisa J. Crockett

Families and children residing in rural communities in the U.S. are facing a number of challenges. Across the country, many rural communities are experiencing chronic and rapidly changing dynamics, which place rural children and families at risk. According to recent data, 16.9% of individuals living in poverty reside in nonmetro areas; educational attainment is lowest in rural areas as compared to urban areas; and rates of problem behaviors in rural areas (e.g., major depression and suicide rates) are significantly higher in rural rather than urban areas (Fontanella et al., 2015). In the midst of these challenging circumstances, some rural communities are experiencing rapid demographic changes resulting from immigrants seeking economic opportunities. Although trends of out-migration to urban areas continue to exist, nearly 20% of the U.S. population (or approximately 60 million) still reside in rural areas (U.S. Census Bureau, 2010). In light of current circumstances and changing demographics in the rural U.S., examining and understanding social, contextual, interpersonal, and intrapersonal processes linked to rural children's development is of great importance.

For several decades, scholars have conducted research on rural families in the U.S. Studies of rural families in Midwest U.S., such as the research on rural Iowa families (Elder & Conger, 2000), have yielded rich understanding of the challenges of rural poverty and its impact on children's and families' health and maladjustment. Such research, for example, demonstrated that loss of social capital and lack of community resources can undermine children's health and well-being (Elder & Conger, 2000). Other research affirms the presence of additional risk factors (e.g., toxicant exposure from well water, pesticides, and herbicides; sparsely structured

G. Carlo (✉) · M. Memmott-Elison
University of Missouri, Columbia, MO, USA
e-mail: carlog@missouri.edu

L. J. Crockett
University of Nebraska-Lincoln, Lincoln, NE, USA

J. E. Glick et al. (eds.), *Rural Families and Communities in the United States*,
National Symposium on Family Issues 10, https://doi.org/10.1007/978-3-030-37689-5_9

adult-supervised activities) that can exacerbate physical and psychological maladjustment in rural children and youth (Janicke & Davis, 2011; National Advisory Committee on Rural Health and Human Services, 2008; Nelson et al., 2013; Wickrama, Elder, & Abraham, 2007). Of particular importance, substantive evidence exists on the long-term consequences of economic strain, poverty, and family stress on youth maladjustment, prevalent in rural areas (Conger, Rueter, & Conger, 2000; McCubbin & Patterson, 1983). That parents' mental health can be disrupted by exposure to such stress, leading to less effective parenting, and in turn to psychological and behavioral problems, has illuminated pathways to maladjustment in children from these communities. This is referred to as the Family Stress Model (FSM; Conger et al., 2000). Many of these findings have been replicated across different rural (and urban) areas in the U.S. (e.g., Conger et al., 2002).

Other researchers have extended this earlier work to examine factors that can mitigate such negative developmental outcomes (Masten, 2001). In these studies, scholars have focused on identifying resilience factors that can buffer individuals against adversity. Investigators have demonstrated the buffering effects of close family relationships and social support (Armstrong, Birnie-Lefcovitch, & Ungar, 2005; Murry, Butler-Barnes, Mayo-Gamble, & Inniss-Thompson, 2018). These studies suggest possible avenues for intervention and policy efforts aimed at enhancing such resilience, ultimately mitigating negative developmental outcomes and maladjustment. Although the research on resilience shows possible avenues for overcoming adversity and reducing maladjustment, there is still a need to examine factors that can promote positive developmental outcomes, health, and well-being.

In recent years, there has been a burgeoning interest in studying prosocial behaviors (i.e., actions intended to benefit others; Eisenberg, Fabes, & Spinrad, 2006). Prosocial behaviors reflect a wide array of actions including volunteerism, helping and comforting others, sharing or donating resources, heroism, and charitable commitments. These behaviors are frequently exhibited in homes, schools, and communities and may target individuals or groups. Most parents and citizens deem these behaviors as desirable and worthy actions that promote interpersonal harmony and cooperation. Indeed, prosocial behaviors, especially altruistic actions (i.e., conduct exhibited with the primary intention of benefiting others rather than one's self), are one important element of morality and a central aspect of moral character (Carlo, 2014). However, prosocial behaviors are multifaceted and there might be different motives (e.g., selfless or selfish) for engaging in prosocial actions. Furthermore, and perhaps of greater relevance to the present essay, prosocial behaviors are markers of socioemotional and sociobehavioral health and well-being (Carlo, 2006).

Over several decades, investigators have shown that children who frequently express prosocial behaviors also demonstrate healthy sociocognitive and socioemotive characteristics. Higher levels of prosocial behaviors have been linked to good self-regulation skills and higher levels of perspective taking, theory of mind, moral reasoning, empathy, and sympathy (Carlo, 2006; Eisenberg, Hofer, Sulik, & Liew, 2014). Moreover, these actions are positively related to higher levels of trustworthiness, better quality parent and peer relationships, higher peer status, and better academic outcomes. Perhaps more importantly, prosocial behaviors are associated with lower anxiety symptoms, improved physical health, less aggression, less delinquency, less illegal substance use, and even longer life expectancy (Carlo, 2006, 2014). In short, prosocial behaviors are correlated with several indices of physical and psychological health and markers of healthy social and interpersonal functioning.

Although the accumulating evidence suggests that prosocial behaviors are markers of health and well-being, it is important to note that some prosocial behaviors are linked to negative adjustment and unhealthy outcomes. For example, prosocial actions motivated by self-interest (such as behaviors to gain the approval of others, social trust, or status) are associated with more aggression and delinquency, and lower levels of sociocognitive (e.g., moral reasoning, perspective taking), and socioemotive (e.g., sympathy) tendencies (Carlo, 2014). Furthermore, prosocial behaviors might be enacted more frequently to in-group (versus out-group) members, which could create or exacerbate social injustice or inequities. Indeed, as scholars have noted, prosocial behaviors could be enacted effectively as a means to take advantage of others or to harm others (Carlo, 2014; Hawley, 2003). In addition, as with many other human behaviors, there may be a personal cost (psychological burden or physical risk) to extremely high levels of prosocial behaviors. Thus, it is important to examine specific forms and motives of prosocial actions to more accurately assess sociobehavioral functioning.

Despite the promise of the study of prosocial behaviors as a marker of healthy social functioning and well-being, studies of these actions in rural children and youth are sparse. This is unfortunate because too much focus on pathology and maladjustment in rural children and youth presents a skewed perspective on the functioning of these populations. Research that examines both positive and negative developmental outcomes could lead to more balanced perspectives on rural populations and inspire efforts to promote and foster positive healthy social functioning rather than only efforts to reduce pathology and maladjustment.

The present chapter reviews existing theories and research on youth prosocial development, with a particular focus on rural populations. We begin with a brief overview of major theoretical frameworks on prosocial development. Then we present a synopsis of research on prosocial development in rural youth, briefly discuss relevant conceptual and cultural considerations, and posit an adapted, culturally sensitive model to guide future research in this area. The chapter concludes by identifying gaps in research, methodological challenges, and theoretical and applied implications.

Theories and Research of Prosocial Development

The study of prosocial behaviors has a long history across varied scholarly disciplines, with a particularly strong focus on social and developmental psychology. We briefly present three primary general theories that have greatly influenced research in this area. Research on select influences of prosocial development is subsequently reviewed.

An early influential theory of prosocial development was based on the cognitive-developmental theory (Kohlberg, 1969; Piaget, 1970). This perspective emphasized advances in cognitive skills across childhood and adolescence as predictors of prosocial traits (e.g., empathy and sympathy) and prosocial behaviors. In particular, increases in prosocial behaviors could be accounted for by corresponding increases in perspective taking and moral reasoning (Eisenberg & Fabes, 1998). There is overall support for this notion such that perspective taking and moral reasoning have both been linked to higher levels of prosocial behaviors (Carlo, 2006; Carlo, Knight, McGinley, Goodvin, & Roesch, 2010). Furthermore, prosocial behaviors have been shown to increase with age during childhood and early adolescence, though prosocial behaviors appear to decrease somewhat during middle adolescence until late adolescence and young adulthood (Eisenberg & Fabes, 1998).

Socialization theorists, in contrast, highlight the roles of social agents such as parents, peers, media, and significant others as primary influences on prosocial behaviors (Grusec, Goodnow, & Kuczynski, 2000; Hoffman, 2008; see Carlo, 2014, for a review). According to these scholars, socialization agents engage in practices and model behaviors that foster or discourage prosocial behaviors in children and adolescents. Furthermore, prosocial traits, such as empathy (i.e., feeling the same as another) and sympathy (i.e., feelings of sorrow or concern for others), are facilitated by warm and nurturing caregivers and experiences. For example, parents who use inductive disciplining practices foster perspective taking, effective self-regulation skills, and concern for others, which results in subsequent prosocial tendencies. In contrast, power assertive disciplining practices foster emotion dysregulation and self-oriented emotions (e.g., anger), which reduce subsequent prosocial tendencies. Other studies show that observing prosocial models can induce more prosocial behaviors in children (see Eisenberg & Valiente, 2002). Taken together, there is substantive supportive evidence for links between socialization practices and empathy-related processes and prosocial behaviors (Eisenberg & Valiente, 2002; Hoffman, 2008).

A third major influential theory borrows from both cognitive-developmental and socialization theories. Social cognitive theorists acknowledge the interplay of socialization and cognitive mechanisms as influences of children's development (Bandura, 1989; Carlo, 2006; Eisenberg, 1986). These mechanisms are posited to be impacted by reciprocal processes such that behavioral outcomes affect personal attributes (Carlo & Randall, 2001). These broad notions facilitate the compatibility of social cognitive theory with a wide range of biological- and socialization-based perspectives. Indeed, several lines of research support the tenets of social cognitive theory. For example, scholars have demonstrated the influence of parents, peers, and media on children's moral development (Bandura, 1989; Carlo, 2006; Eisenberg et al., 2006). Other researchers have shown that biological and cognitive processes (e.g., attributions, temperament) are linked to such outcomes. There is also recent growing evidence on reciprocal relations between parenting, sociocognitive, and socioemotive characteristics and prosocial behaviors (Carlo, Mestre, Samper, Tur, & Armenta, 2010; Newton, Laible, Carlo, Steele, & McGinley, 2014; Padilla-Walker, Carlo, Christensen, & Yorgason, 2012).

In general, these theories and the extant research yield evidence of the importance of socialization agents, and sociocognitive and socioemotive traits in predicting prosocial outcomes. However, the predominance of research on prosocial development has focused on white, European American children and youth. Moreover, urban children and youth have been the social context of most of this research. Research on prosocial development in children and adolescents from rural communities is sparse.

Theory and Research on Prosocial Development in Rural Populations

There are a number of theoretical frameworks and conceptual notions that we can draw from in order to explain prosocial development in rural populations. For instance, some research discusses the notion of youth bulges, which include "large youth cohorts relative to the adult population" (Urdal, 2004). Youth bulges are most commonly noted in poor rural communities and nations (e.g., Assaad & Roudi-Fahimi, 2007; Urdal, 2004. This concept may be particularly relevant to the study of Latino/a youth residing in the U.S., since this demographic tends to report a lower socioeconomic status than other prominent racial/ethnic groups (Office of Health Disparities and Health Equity, 2015) and increasingly reside in rural communities (Kandel & Cromartie, 2004). The concept of a *youth bulge* has been conceptually tied to limited adult–child interactions (McIntosh, Hart, & Youniss, 2007), and in other studies, limited parent–adolescent interactions (i.e., premature parental disengagement) have been linked to increases in behavioral problems such as youth deviancy (Dishion, Nelson, & Bullock, 2004). Although youth bulges have historically been applied to antisocial development, this framework has also recently been applied to prosocial development. Youth whose economic surroundings are characterized by a youth bulge tend to engage in less civic engagement because their parents have fewer resources (e.g., time and political knowledge) to invest in each youth (Hart, Atkins, Markey, & Youniss, 2004). Synthesizing these findings, we suggest that rural adolescents and young adults may report fewer prosocial behaviors due to the existence of youth bulges in their communities.

Additionally, scholars recently commented on the link between the availability of family resources in rural communities and the association with youth development. Youth who follow a "resourceful pathway," or youth who have a supportive relational environment in terms of parent-, sibling-, extended family-, and even neighbor-, child interactions, will be enabled to engage in more productive behaviors, including prosocial behaviors (Elder & Conger, 2000). Because Latino/a adolescents and young adults place a salient emphasis on family and community cohesion (Kopak, Chen, Haas, & Gillmore, 2012), this perspective may be especially applicable (further discussion on this topic will follow). Therefore, there is more than one perspective that suggests rural youth are able or socially emotionally capable of engaging in prosocial behaviors. These individuals simply have fewer resources to support their prosocial development due to the limited social infrastructure of their rural communities.

The Need for Ecology and Culture in Rural Youth Development

Historically, rural communities in the U.S. have been fairly homogeneous in terms of racial/ethnic makeup, where the majority of community members are European American (Flora, Flora, & Gastmeyer, 2016). Because of this, research and theory investigating development in rural communities have largely omitted diverse subpopulations such as Latino/as. Granted, Latino/as entering rural communities not only experience youth bulges and limited resources, but also must deal with culture-related stress/stressors associated with assimilation into the broader rural U.S. culture (Finch, Frank, & Vega, 2004; Gonzales, Knight, Morgan-Lopez, Saenz, & Sirolli, 2002). With this intersectionality in mind, there are a number of important nuances that researchers and theorists should be aware of when investigating the rural integration experiences of Latino/as' and other racial/ethnic minorities. For example, how do rural communities view the integration of diverse individuals? Is migration viewed by the standing community as a threat, and if so, how is integration impacted? What contributes to negative views of migration? How do community perceptions of Latino/a's integration into rural communities influence Latino/a members' prosocial development? Researchers should avoid taking a pathological approach to ethnic/racial minority members' development, and instead, highlight the assets that Latino/a populations bring with them (e.g., familism, strong moral values, and religious orientation) that may buffer the effect of limited resources, youth bulges, and/or assimilation to broader U.S. rural culture.

Studies of Prosocial Behaviors in Rural Adolescents

To our knowledge, two published studies exist on prosocial development in rural youth, using one longitudinal dataset (Carlo, Crockett, Randall, & Roesch, 2007; Carlo, Crockett, Wilkinson, & Beal, 2011). In the first study, investigators examined the trajectory of prosocial behaviors in mostly white European adolescents from rural communities in Pennsylvania, U.S., across early to late adolescence (Carlo et al., 2007). The findings yielded evidence that prosocial behavior levels decreased gradually until late adolescence wherein there was a slight rebound. Moreover, increases in the quality of peer relationships predicted decreases in prosocial behavior for girls but not boys. These findings are in accord with suggestions by scholars that many rural communities lack adequate opportunities for engagement in prosocial activities and possibly have low resourced schools and community support agencies. The slight rebound in prosocial behaviors in late adolescence might also reflect the associated responsibilities, maturity, and changes in a social context (e.g., transition from school to career and family) that occur for many individuals during this period.

Interestingly, that increases in the quality of peer relationships accounted for decreases in prosocial behaviors for girls but not boys, suggests the somewhat greater influence of negative peer relationships on rural girls' prosocial behaviors. This finding is consistent with other research, which suggests that girls might be particularly prone to negative peer influence (Crick & Grotpeter, 1995). However, we would note that some of this effect might also reflect the overall greater frequency of prosocial behaviors in girls relative to boys. Boys' levels of prosocial behavior remained relatively stable across time. Although girls' prosocial behavior levels were relatively high in early adolescence, their levels were declining to the level of boys' prosocial behaviors by late adolescence. This suggests that rural girls might be relatively more vulnerable to factors that undermine prosocial behaviors during adolescence.

In the other published study using the same longitudinal dataset, researchers investigated the links between prosocial behaviors in middle adolescence and subsequent substance use in young adulthood (Carlo et al., 2011). Rural adolescents who frequently exhibited prosocial behaviors were less likely to engage in substance use in young adulthood than those who exhibited relatively low levels of prosocial behaviors. These researchers reported significant, negative relations between earlier prosocial behaviors and substance use (i.e. getting drunk and marijuana use). Ironically, earlier prosocial behavior negatively predicted subsequent cigarette smoking via substance use in adolescence. These findings demonstrate protective effects of exhibiting prosocial behaviors in adolescence on substance use problems in young adulthood. The findings are consistent with previous research that shows mitigating effects of prosocial behaviors on later maladjustment and antisocial outcomes (see Carlo, 2014). In other words, prosocial behaviors can be conceptualized not only as a marker of health and well-being but also as a protective factor that inhibits negative symptomatology.

Research on rural adolescents suggests protective factors that mitigate against negative symptomatology. For example, rural adolescents who have higher levels of school bonding (Shears, Edwards, & Stanley, 2006), academic achievement (Kostelecky, 2005), positive peer relationships (Dunn, Kitts, Lewis, Goodrow, & Scherzer, 2011), and parental attachment (Kostelecky, 2005) are less likely to consume alcohol, use marijuana and other drugs, and engage in sexual behavior. Some perspectives on morality argue that prosocial behaviors and problem behaviors, such as substance use and risky sexual behavior, are incongruous (see Carlo, 2006). These studies, though not focused on prosocial development, suggest that resiliency factors can prevent problem outcomes for rural youth.

The Latino/a Youth Development (LYD) Model

A theoretical model that has sought to take a culturally sensitive approach to understanding and studying rural Latino/as' adjustment (including their moral/prosocial development) is the Latino/a Youth Development (LYD) model (Carlo & Conejo, 2019; Carlo & de Guzman, 2009; Raffaelli, Carlo, Carranza, & Gonzalez-Kruger, 2005). This model suggests that individuals' contextual experiences (such as residing in a rural community) affect the development of their interpersonal traits and stressors (Fig. 1). According to the LYD model, interpersonal traits are generic (e.g., appraisals and coping), moral (e.g., emotions and values), and culture-specific (e.g., cultural values), while stressors are specifically culture-related, such as discrimination or language barriers. Traits and culture-related stressors influence one another in the LYD model, and in turn, each contributes to individuals' moral and prosocial behaviors. Thus, this framework proposes indirect associations between contextual experiences and characteristics (e.g., family, peers, poverty, life stressors) and individuals' prosocial behaviors via relevant and culture-specific interpersonal traits and culture-related stress.

Applied specifically to rural U.S. Latino/a adolescents and young adults' prosocial moral development, it is possible that Latino/a youth experience life history stressors such as migration and immigration status, which might be compounded with residing in a rural community context characterized by youth bulges, limited diversity, and a lack of bilingual family and school resources. As a result, it is possible that these youth experience additional culture-related stress (e.g., discrimination and marginalization) that forces them to cope with the challenges of integration

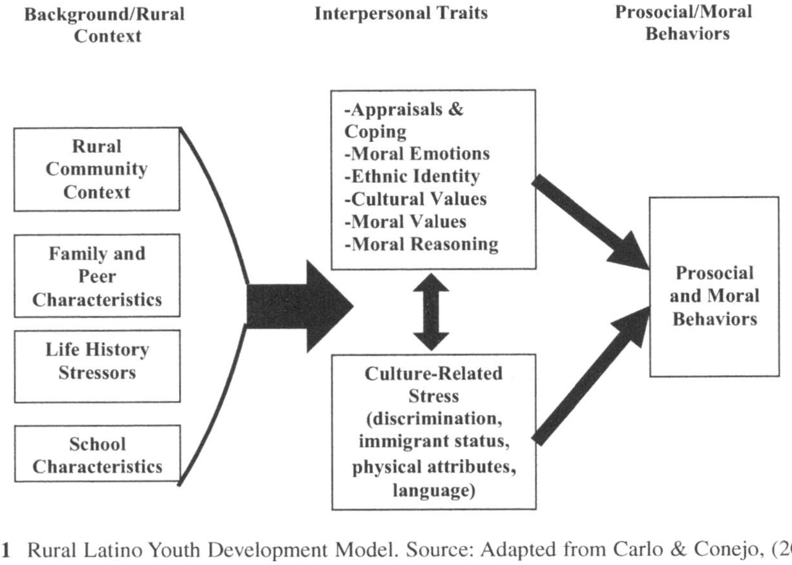

Fig. 1 Rural Latino Youth Development Model. Source: Adapted from Carlo & Conejo, (2019); Carlo & de Guzman, (2009); Raffaelli et al., (2005)

into their community. However, cultural strengths and resources (e.g., strong ethnic identity, family, and cultural values) and sociocognitive/socioemotive traits (e.g., moral reasoning, empathy, coping, and appraisals) can influence the way that Latino/a youth perceive and respond to culture-related stressors. In turn, these inter- and intra-personal traits and culture-related mechanisms can mitigate negative symptomatology and enhance positive symptomatology (e.g., prosocial behaviors). Thus, the model demonstrates a culturally sensitive and process-oriented approach to better understand U.S. Latino/a rural youth that is compatible with traditional theoretical perspectives on prosocial development.

Research on the LYD Model

While the LYD model suggests that background contexts such as family, peer, and neighborhood characteristics, life stressors, and school climate affect *rural* adolescents' prosocial development (Carlo & Conejo, 2019; Carlo & de Guzman, 2009; Raffaelli et al., 2005), the empirical evidence with diverse populations for this model is still in its infancy. In an ongoing study, researchers conducted a study of U.S. Latino/a families and youth in the Northern Great Plains (see Carlo, Crockett, Streit, & Cardenas, 2016). Although this study was not conducted with a rural sample, the characteristics of the Northern Great Plains communities in which the sample resides closely parallels the characteristics of rural communities (see Carlo et al., 2016, for a discussion of the sociodemographics of the sample).

In one study, investigators showed support for the generalizability of social cognitive theory to a sample of U.S. Latino/a youth from the Northern Great Plains (Carlo, Streit, & Crockett, 2018). Specifically, U.S. Latino/a youth who reported high levels of parental support were more likely to report high levels of prosocial moral reasoning, and in turn, report higher levels of altruistic prosocial behaviors and lower levels of public prosocial behaviors. Moreover, higher levels of parental support were associated with higher levels of empathic concern, which was linked to higher levels of prosocial moral reasoning, altruistic prosocial behaviors, and lower levels of public prosocial behaviors. These findings are in accord with social cognitive theory and the LYD model that accords importance on parental support, empathic concern, and moral reasoning as facilitators of altruistic prosocial behaviors (and mitigating selfishly motivated, public prosocial behaviors).

From the perspective of the LYD model, it is possible that during early and middle adolescence, youth acquire newfound social and emotional resources, which can result in more effective coping mechanisms to deal with culturally relevant stressors (Carlo & Conejo, 2019; Carlo & de Guzman, 2009; Raffaelli et al., 2005). In one study using the same sample of U.S. Latino/a youth sample (Davis, Carlo, Streit, & Crockett, 2018), researchers show support for the Family Stress Model (FSM; Conger et al., 2000; Conger et al., 2002). That is, those caregivers who reported high levels of economic stress were more likely to report higher depressive symptoms, which in turn predicted less parental warmth and lower levels of youth compliant prosocial behaviors. In other words, exposure to economic strain in the family could undermine youth prosocial behaviors.

Interestingly, however, there was also evidence that such stress was positively linked to altruistic prosocial behaviors. Although this latter finding might be counterintuitive, moral scholars have noted that altruistic tendencies may sometime emerge from demanding and stressful contexts. This notion has been referred to as *altruism born of suffering* (Staub, 2005). Conceptually, exposure to trauma or stress can sometimes result in greater motivation to overcome the challenges and transform into a strong desire to alleviate similar suffering in others. A greater emotional sensitivity and empathic tendencies to suffering can emerge from direct or close contact with trauma or stress (Carlo, Fabes, Laible, & Kupanoff, 1999). The findings are promising and provide a basis to examine whether U.S. Latino/a youth are accessing specific coping mechanisms that foster altruistic prosocial behaviors in spite of exposure to family stressors.

Taken together, there is preliminary support for the utility of the LYD model. However, more empirical work that examines resilience and enhancing factors in relation to prosocial development in samples of rural Latino/a (and other ethnic and racial minorities) adolescents is needed.

Conclusions and Directions for Research

Despite the growing interest in studying positive youth development and adjustment, research on prosocial development in rural youth is sparse. A few studies focus on this area and reveal evidence of changes in prosocial behaviors across adolescence and into young adulthood, but more research is needed. The research demonstrates that changes in prosocial behavior are linked to changes in quality of peer relationships for girls (but not boys). Furthermore, there is support for the notion that frequently exhibited prosocial behaviors in earlier adolescence predict subsequent substance use in young adulthood. These studies are in accord with scholars' suggestions that rural contexts could contribute to reported declines in prosocial behaviors among rural adolescents. On the other hand, the research findings also provide a window of opportunity such that early prosocial behaviors can mitigate problem behaviors (e.g., substance use problems) in later life.

Our recent efforts to investigate prosocial development in U.S. Latino/a youth, though quite limited, suggest support for traditional social cognitive models and FSM. Moreover, the findings are consistent with the LYD model and speak to the importance of examining the interplay of parenting, personal characteristics, and culture-related mechanisms as predictors of prosocial behaviors. Such work is needed to redress the skewed emphases on pathology and deficit-based approaches of previous research among rural and ethnic-racial minority youth.

Research Gaps and Challenges

Future investigations are needed to further our understanding of prosocial development in rural youth and particular directions are recommended. First, longitudinal studies specifically designed to examine prosocial outcomes in rural youth are needed. Understanding changes in prosocial behaviors across time require study designs that can explain such changes in both boys and girls, as well as, across the varied and diverse populations of youth in rural areas. Second, basic information regarding the biological- and environment-based processes that contribute to prosocial behaviors in rural youth is missing. For example, studies that examine macro-level contextual influences on rural youth prosocial development are lacking. Given the continuing rapidly changing sociodemographics in rural areas, studies that can adequately account for these changes are needed. Third, the increased ethnic-racial diversity in many rural areas in the U.S. necessitates a coordinated effort to examine prosocial development among minority youth that reside in rural areas. One would expect that the lack of adequate access to resources and services for ethnic-racial minority populations and the potential for added culture-related stressors (e.g., discrimination, immigration-related stress, and language difficulties) in many rural areas will result in relatively high levels of risk for these youth. And fourth, there are several barriers to accessing and recruiting rural U.S. Latino/as. Immigration status-related fears and stress, distance and transportation challenges, high mobility, and issues of building trust and rapport are difficulties that hamper efforts to conduct longitudinal and rigorous research with this population. Well-funded, coordinated multisite projects will be needed to conduct investigations that can illuminate influential mechanisms of health and well-being for U.S. Latino/as in rural communities.

Importance and Significance of Work

In light of the rapidly growing U.S. Latino/a population in rural communities, understanding prosocial development and well-being in youth is worthwhile and critical. Thus far, the predominance of our understanding of U.S. Latino/a youth development is based on urban (mostly East Coast, West Coast, and Southwest) populations. However, communities in urban cluster areas have distinct features not often found in rural areas. Therefore, research on U.S. Latino/a families in rural areas provides an important test of applying existing theories to a distinct social context. Ecologically valid theories that are pertinent to such areas are needed. Finally, research on prosocial development and well-being in these understudied regions of the U.S. is vital to the development of effective intervention programs and policies that will benefit Latino/as, as well as, all who reside in the rural U.S.

References

Armstrong, M. I., Birnie-Lefcovitch, S., & Ungar, M. T. (2005). Pathways between social support, family well being, quality of parenting, and child resilience: What we know. *Journal of Child and Family Studies, 14*(2), 269–281.

Assaad, R., & Roudi-Fahimi, F. (2007). *Youth in the Middle East and North Africa: Demographic opportunity or challenge*? Washington, DC: Population Reference Bureau. Retrieved from https://www.prb.org/youthinmena/

Bandura, A. (1989). Regulation of cognitive processes through perceived self-efficacy. *Developmental Psychology, 25*(5), 729–735.

Carlo, G. (2006). Care-based and altruistically-based morality. In M. Killen & J. G. Smetana (Eds.), *Handbook of moral development* (pp. 551–579). Mahwah, NJ: Erlbaum.

Carlo, G. (2014). The development and correlates of prosocial moral behaviors. In M. Killen & J. G. Smetana (Eds.), *Handbook of moral development* (2nd ed., pp. 208–234). New York, NY: Psychology Press.

Carlo, G., & Conejo, L. D. (2019). Traditional and culture-specific parenting of prosociality in U.S. Latino/as. In D. Laible, G. Carlo, & L. Padilla-Walker (Eds.), *Oxford handbook of parenting and moral development*. New York: Oxford University Press.

Carlo, G., Crockett, L. J., Randall, B. A., & Roesch, S. C. (2007). A latent growth curve analysis of prosocial behavior among rural adolescents. *Journal of Research on Adolescence, 17*(2), 301–324.

Carlo, G., Crockett, L. J., Streit, C., & Cardenas, R. (2016). Rural Latino/a youth and parents on the Northern Great Plains: Preliminary findings from the Latino Youth Care Project (LYCP). In L. J. Crockett & G. Carlo (Eds.), *Rural ethnic minority youth and families in the United States: Theory, research, and applications* (pp. 165–183). New York: Springer.

Carlo, G., Crockett, L. J., Wilkinson, J. L., & Beal, S. J. (2011). The longitudinal relationships between rural adolescents' prosocial behaviors and young adult substance use. *Journal of Youth and Adolescence, 40*(9), 1192–1202.

Carlo, G., & de Guzman, M. R. T. (2009). Theories and research on prosocial competencies among U.S. Latinos/as. In F. Villaruel, G. Carlo, J. M. Grau, M. Azmitia, N. J. Cabrera, & T. J. Chahin (Eds.), *Handbook of U.S. Latino psychology* (pp. 191–211). Thousand Oaks, CA: Sage Publications.

Carlo, G., Fabes, R. A., Laible, D., & Kupanoff, K. (1999). Early adolescence and prosocial/moral behavior II: The role of social and contextual influences. *The Journal of Early Adolescence, 19*(2), 133–147.

Carlo, G., Knight, G. P., McGinley, M., Goodvin, R., & Roesch, S. C. (2010). Understanding the developmental relations between perspective taking and prosocial behaviors: A meta-analytic review. In J. Carpendale, G. Iarocci, U. Muller, B. Sokol, & A. Young (Eds.), *Self- and social-regulation: Exploring the relations between social interaction, social cognition, and the development of executive functions* (pp. 234–269). Oxford, UK: Oxford University Press.

Carlo, G., Mestre, M. V., Samper, P., Tur, A., & Armenta, B. E. (2010). The longitudinal relations among dimensions of parenting styles, sympathy, prosocial moral reasoning and prosocial behaviors. *International Journal of Behavioral Development, 35*(2), 116–124.

Carlo, G., & Randall, B. A. (2001). Are all prosocial behaviors equal? A socioecological developmental conception of prosocial behavior. In F. Columbus (Ed.), *Advances in psychology research* (Vol. II, pp. 151–170). Huntington, NY: Nova Science Publishers.

Carlo, G., Streit, C., & Crockett, L. (2018). Generalizability of a traditional social cognitive model of prosocial behaviors to U.S. Latino/a youth. *Cultural Diversity and Ethnic Minority Psychology, 24*(4), 596–604.

Conger, K. J., Rueter, M. A., & Conger, R. D. (2000). The role of economic pressure in the lives of parents and their adolescents: The Family Stress Model. In L. J. Crockett & R. K. Silbereisen (Eds.), *Negotiating adolescence in times of social change* (pp. 201–223). New York, NY: Cambridge University Press.

Conger, R. D., Wallace, L. E., Sun, Y., Simons, R. L., McLoyd, V. C., & Brody, G. H. (2002). Economic pressure in African American families: A replication and extension of the family stress model. *Developmental Psychology, 38*(2), 179–193.
Crick, N. R., & Grotpeter, J. K. (1995). Relational aggression, gender, and social psychological adjustment. *Child Development, 66*(3), 710–722.
Davis, A. N., Carlo, G., Streit, C., & Crockett, L. (2018). Considering economic stress and empathic traits in predicting prosocial behaviors among U.S. Latino adolescents. *Social Development, 27*(1), 58–72.
Dishion, T. J., Nelson, S. E., & Bullock, B. M. (2004). Premature adolescent autonomy: Parent disengagement and deviant peer process in the amplification of problem behaviour. *Journal of Adolescence, 27*(5), 515–530.
Dunn, M. S., Kitts, C., Lewis, S., Goodrow, B., & Scherzer, G. D. (2011). Effects of youth assets on adolescent alcohol, tobacco, marijuana use, and sexual behavior. *Journal of Alcohol and Drug Education, 55*(3), 23–40.
Eisenberg, N. (1986). *Altruistic cognition, emotion, and behavior*. Hillsdale, NJ: Erlbaum.
Eisenberg, N., & Fabes, R. A. (1998). Prosocial development. In W. Damon (Series Ed.) & N. Eisenberg (Vol. Ed.), *Handbook of child psychology, Vol. 3: Social, emotional, and personality development* (5th ed., pp. 701–778). New York: John Wiley.
Eisenberg, N., Fabes, R. A., & Spinard, T. L. (2006). Prosocial development. In W. Damon, R. M. Lerner, & N. Eisenberg (Eds.), *Handbook of child psychology, Vol. 3. Social, emotional, and personality development* (6th ed., pp. 646–718). Hoboken, NJ: Wiley.
Eisenberg, N., Hofer, C., Sulik, M. J., & Liew, J. (2014). The development of prosocial moral reasoning and a prosocial orientation in young adulthood: Concurrent and longitudinal correlates. *Developmental Psychology, 50*(1), 58–70. https://doi.org/10.1037/a0032990
Eisenberg, N., & Valiente, C. (2002). Parenting and children's prosocial and moral development. In M. H. Bornstein (Ed.), *Handbook of parenting: Vol. 5. Practical issues in parenting* (2nd ed., pp. 111–142). Mahwah, NJ: Erlbaum.
Elder, G. H., Jr., & Conger, R. D. (2000). *Children of the land: Adversity and success in rural America*. University of Chicago Press.
Finch, B. K., Frank, R., & Vega, W. A. (2004). Acculturation and acculturation stress: A social-epidemiological approach to Mexican migrant farmworkers' health. *International Migration Review, 38*(1), 236–262.
Flora, C. B., Flora, J. L., & Gasteyer, S. P. (2016). *Rural communities: Legacy and change* (5th ed.). Boulder, CO: Westview Press.
Fontanella, C. A., Hiance-Steelesmith, D. L., Phillips, G. S., Bridge, J. A., Lester, N., Sweeney, H. A., & Campo, J. V. (2015). Widening rural-urban disparities in youth suicides, United States, 1996-2010. *JAMA Pediatrics, 169*(5), 466–473. https://doi.org/10.1001/jamapediatrics.2014.3561
Gonzales, N. A., Knight, G. P., Morgan-Lopez, A. A., Saenz, D., & Sirolli, A. (2002). Acculturation and the mental health of Latino youths: An integration and critique of the literature. In J. M. Contreras, K. A. Kerns, & A. M. Neal-Barnett (Eds.), *Praiger series in applied psychology. Latino children and families in the United States: Current research and future directions* (pp. 45–76). Westport, CT: Praeger.
Grusec, J. E., Goodnow, J. J., & Kuczynski, L. (2000). New directions in analyses of parenting contributions to children's acquisition of values. *Child Development, 71*(1), 205–211.
Hart, D., Atkins, R., Markey, P., & Youniss, J. (2004). Youth bulges in communities: The effects of age structure on adolescent civic knowledge and civic participation. *Psychological Science, 15*(9), 591–597.
Hawley, P. H. (2003). Prosocial and coercive configurations of resource control in early adolescence. *Merrill-Palmer Quarterly, 49*(3), 279–309.
Hoffman, M. L. (2008). Empathy and prosocial behavior. In M. Lewis, J. M. Haviland-Jones, & L. F. Barrett (Eds.), *Handbook of emotions* (3rd ed., pp. 440–455). New York: The Guilford Press.
Janicke, D. M., & Davis, A. M. (2011). Introduction to the special section: Rural health issues in pediatric psychology. *Journal of Pediatric Psychology, 36*(6), 647–651.

Kandel, W., & Cromartie, J. (2004). *New patterns of Hispanic settlement in rural America*. Washington, DC: U.S. Department Agriculture, Economic Research Service. Retrieved from https://www.ers.usda.gov/publications/pub-details/?pubid=47091

Kohlberg, L. (1969). Stage and sequence: The cognitive–developmental approach to socialization. In D. A. Goslin (Ed.), *Handbook of socialization theory and research* (pp. 347–480). Chicago: Rand McNally.

Kopak, A. M., Chen, A. C. C., Haas, S. A., & Gillmore, M. R. (2012). The importance of family factors to protect against substance use related problems among Mexican heritage and white youth. *Drug and Alcohol Dependence, 124*(1), 34–41.

Kostelecky, K. L. (2005). Parental attachment, academic achievement, life events and their relationship to alcohol and drug use during adolescence. *Journal of Adolescence, 28*(5), 665–669.

Masten, A. S. (2001). Ordinary magic: Resilience processes in development. *American Psychologist, 56*(3), 227–238.

McCubbin, H. I., & Patterson, J. M. (1983). The family stress process: The double ABCX model of adjustment and adaptation. *Marriage & Family Review, 6*(1–2), 7–37.

McIntosh, H., Hart, D., & Youniss, J. (2007). The influence of family political discussion on youth civic development: Which parent qualities matter? *PS: Political Science & Politics, 40*(3), 495–499.

Murry, V. M., Butler-Barnes, S. T., Mayo-Gamble, T. L., & Inniss-Thompson, M. N. (2018). Excavating new constructs for family stress theories in the context of everyday life experiences of black American families. *Journal of Family Theory & Review, 10*(2), 384–405.

National Advisory Committee on Rural Health and Human Services (NACRHHS). (2008). The 2008 report to the secretary: Rural Health and Human Services issues. Washington, DC: U.S. Department of Health and Human Services. Retrieved from https://www.hrsa.gov/advisorycommittees/rural/2008secreport.pdf

Nelson, T. D., Kidwell, K. M., Armenta, B. E., Crockett, L. J., Carlo, G., & Whitbeck, L. B. (2013). Rural Latino adolescent health: Preliminary examination of health risks and cultural correlates. *Journal of Health Psychology, 19*(6), 802–808.

Newton, E. K., Laible, D., Carlo, G., Steele, J. S., & McGinley, M. (2014). Do sensitive parents foster kind children, or vice versa? Bidirectional influences between children's prosocial behavior and parental sensitivity. *Developmental Psychology, 50*(6), 1808–1817.

Office of Health Disparities and Health Equity. (2015). *Nebraska health disparities report: Health equity for all Nebraskans*. Nebraska: Department of Health and Human Services. Retrieved Accessed October 2, 2018, from http://dhhs.ne.gov/Reports/Health%20Disparities%20Report%20-%202015.pdf

Padilla-Walker, L. M., Carlo, G., Christensen, K. J., & Yorgason, J. B. (2012). Bidirectional relations between authoritative parenting and adolescents' prosocial behaviors. *Journal of Research on Adolescence, 22*(3), 400–408.

Piaget, J. (1970). Piaget's theory. In P. H. Mussen (Ed.), *Carmichael's manual of child psychology* (Vol. 1, 3rd ed., pp. 703–732). New York: Wiley.

Raffaelli, M., Carlo, G., Carranza, M. A., & Gonzalez-Kruger, G. E. (2005). Understanding Latino children and adolescents in the mainstream: Placing culture at the center of developmental models. *New Directions for Child and Adolescent Development, 2005*(109), 23–32.

Shears, J., Edwards, R. W., & Stanley, L. R. (2006). School bonding and substance use in rural communities. *Social Work Research, 30*(1), 6–18.

Staub, E. (2005). The roots of goodness: The fulfillment of basic human needs and the development of caring, helping and nonaggression, inclusive caring, moral courage, active bystandership, and altruism born of suffering. In G. Carlo & C. P. Edwards (Eds.), *Vol. 51 of the Nebraska Symposium on motivation: Moral motivation through the life span* (pp. 33–72). Lincoln, NE: University of Nebraska Press.

U.S. Census Bureau. (2010). American Community Survey. Washington, DC. Retrieved from https://www.census.gov/programs-surveys/acs/guidance/which-data-tool/data-tools-chart.html

Urdal, H. (2004, July). *The devil in the demographics: The effect of youth bulges on domestic armed conflict, 1950–2000* (Working Paper No. 29740). Washington, DC: The World Bank. Retrieved from http://documents.worldbank.org/curated/en/794881468762939913/The-devil-in-the-demographics-the-effect-of-youth-bulges-on-domestic-armed-conflict-1950-2000
Wickrama, K. A., Elder, G. H., Jr., & Abraham, W. T. (2007). Rurality and ethnicity in adolescent physical illness: Are children of the growing rural Latino population at excess health risk? *Journal of Rural Health, 23*(3), 228–237.

Rural Families in the U.S.: Theory, Research, and Policy

Matthew M. Brooks and Sabrina T. Voltaire

Why Focus on the Rural U.S.?

The U.S. is a large multiethnic country with highly varying conditions of work, family, and community life. Yet, research historically has compared urban versus rural areas with limited attention to the variation in composition and disparities in health and demographic trends across and within rural areas themselves (Greene, Murphy, & Rossheim, 2018; Lichter & Brown, 2011; van Dis, 2002). Relying solely on the rural–urban dichotomy can limit research by assuming population and geographic homogeneity at the expense of potential within-group variation. The rural U.S., which is often viewed as ethnically homogenous, certainly include counties that are predominantly non-Hispanic white. The rural U.S. also includes the counties of the Mississippi Delta that are majority African American and Native American Reservation counties as well as an increasing prevalence of other ethnic groups in rural counties that are becoming new destinations for recent immigrants. In a similar vein, rural areas are often viewed as economically homogenous. Although some rural counties are indeed dependent on agriculture, this encompasses only 22% of counties with another 16% dependent on manufacturing, and 30% classified as nonspecialized (Economic Research Service, 2017). This chapter aims to highlight the need for research that compares the living conditions and demographic trends across these rural communities and explores the mechanisms by which these contextual factors influence rural families, while bringing rural diversity to the forefront.

An emphasis on the rural U.S. is needed in research and practice today given the unique experiences and challenges faced by individuals and families living in rural

M. M. Brooks (✉)
Penn State, University Park, State College, PA, USA
e-mail: mfb5341@psu.edu

S. T. Voltaire
Penn State, University Park, PA, USA

J. E. Glick et al. (eds.), *Rural Families and Communities in the United States*,
National Symposium on Family Issues 10, https://doi.org/10.1007/978-3-030-37689-5_10

communities. Without a careful investigation, both negative and positive assumptions can paint an incomplete picture of the rural reality. Research on the rural U.S. can help to identify strengths and weaknesses while separating facts from longstanding assumptions. Moreover, to the extent that conditions in rural communities may lead to health and economic disadvantages, there is a need for further investigation of the impact on costs associated with public health and public assistance initiatives. Thus, these investigations allow for a better understanding of risks and protective factors that inform policy and intervention targets.

Additionally, research on the rural U.S.' communities can highlight the diversity and complexity of the population of interest while accounting for changes in the immediate environment, particularly if it goes beyond comparisons to urban communities and instead focuses on within-rural regions or groups. It is also important to consider changes in geographical boundaries and challenges associated with such reclassifications as they may influence residents' access to resources as well as interfere with ongoing research and practice initiatives. Researchers who consider these changes may be better equipped to incorporate both the historical and the current contexts in terms of sociodemographic factors relevant for explaining variations in individual outcomes and for identifying appropriate and contemporary targets for interventions. This chapter reviews the research presented in this volume and the new directions it points to for further investigation, policy, and interventions.

The Hard Life and Unique Challenges in Rural Areas

Poverty

As outlined by Tickamyer (chapter "Rural Poverty: Research and Policy for U.S. Families") persistent poverty may be the single most significant social issue facing rural communities in the U.S. and, therefore, poverty must be at the forefront of any overview of challenges in these areas. There is a significant rural–urban disparity in poverty, with consistently higher poverty in rural counties since the 1970s. Many rural counties, particularly those with significant populations of minority groups, have had poverty rates of over 20% for decades, often accompanied by oppressive local political economies that make improvements difficult (Duncan, 2015; Weber & Miller, 2017).

Much has been written about persistent poverty in rural areas, but most relevant to rural families are the challenges posed by the intergenerational transmission of poverty and limited opportunities for upward socioeconomic mobility. The good news is that research suggests that children from nonmetro counties have much higher levels of upward mobility than those from metro counties (Chetty, Hendren, Kline, & Saez, 2014; Weber, Fannin, Miller, & Goetz, 2018;); those who are from the most remote counties have the highest levels of upward mobility. This rural advantage is not evenly distributed throughout the country. Children from rural southern counties, often those with majority African American populations, have the lowest upward mobility and highest levels of child poverty (Call & Voss, 2016; Voss, Long, Hammer, & Friedman, 2006; Weber et al., 2018). Many of the reasons cited for the rural advantage in upward mobility are primarily economic; however, the role the family plays in this mobility for rural youth remains unexplored (Vernon-Feagans & Swingler, chapter "Early Development and Family Life in Rural America").

Demographic Trends

In the past few decades, rural areas in the U.S. have experienced changes in age composition. The general out-migration of young adults from rural communities is noted by Mattingly (chapter "Changes in Work and Family Across the Rural U.S."). In many communities, fertility rates have declined which leads to a natural decrease that is exacerbated by negative net migration (Johnson, 2011; Johnson & Fuguitt, 2000; Johnson & Lichter, 2008). Such out-migration is not evenly distributed. Although the pattern and magnitude of migration vary based on county characteristics (Johnson & Winkler, 2015), outmigration of recent high school graduates to college towns and metro areas—in what has been dubbed a brain drain—has damaged local economies and schools through a growing absence of those with high levels of human capital (Carr & Kefalas, 2009). Young people from families lower on the socioeconomic ladder often stay in their origin communities because they lack human and social capital needed to find and secure jobs outside of their own rural community (Fitchen, 1994, 1995).

At the other end of the life course, there are two significant demographic trends that shape older populations: (1) a larger population of individuals *aging in place* along with out-migration of younger family members and (2) a growing movement, particularly among wealthier older adults, to move to rural retirement destinations (Cromartie, chapter "Demographic Components of Aging in the Nonmetropolitan U.S., 1980–2017"; Glasgow & Brown, 2012). Aging in place at the community level refers to counties where the median age is increasing due to a large aging elderly population and, as mentioned earlier, the out-migration of youth. Elderly individuals who remain in these communities may experience social isolation and lack social support from family members no longer living in the same local community (i.e., adult children and grandchildren). Many communities experiencing a population that is largely aging in place lack the health services needed to provide care to this vulnerable group (Chan, Hart, & Goodman, 2006; Himes & Rutrough, 1994).

Other rural communities, extensively documented by Cromartie (chapter "Demographic Components of Aging in the Nonmetropolitan U.S., 1980–2017"), have experienced an influx of retirees creating an aging dynamic that differs from those we have described. In some areas, older in-migrants often have considerable wealth and resources and are attracted to these destination communities to take advantage of natural and cultural amenities available only in nonmetropolitan areas.

A typical rural retirement destination is within proximity to a metro area, near natural amenities, and has cultural amenities such as festivals or golf courses that may have previously attracted these retirees for vacations before they decided to relocate and retire in these communities (Brown, Bolender, Kulcsar, Glasgow, & Sanders, 2011). Research has highlighted the negative consequences that may accrue for increasingly popular retirement destinations, including increases in the cost of living and conflicts with long-term residents (Hunter, Boardman, & Saint Onge, 2005; Sherman, 2018). These demographic dynamics may exacerbate inequality across rural communities.

Rural Families

The economic and demographic challenges in rural contexts may be further demonstrated by their effects on families and intergenerational relationships. Family life in the rural U.S. indeed reflects these unique challenges through the constraints and opportunities parents regularly experience in their attempt to raise and provide for their children. First, the increase in shift work may reduce predictability and stability in the homes of rural families. When combined with other concerning trends, such as school consolidation or rising costs of child care, rural parents are in a particularly precarious position of balancing work and family demands. The increasing pressure on time and finances tends to affect parenting practices and parenting quality with immediate and long-term repercussions for parent and child well-being (Murry, Cooper, Burnett, & Inniss-Thompson, chapter "Rural African Americans' Family Relationships and Well-Being"). Though shift work may be advantageous to some families by allowing parents to align their schedules to their children's needs, in most cases, shift work is more likely linked to fluctuating hours week to week. Thus, irregular work schedules create an unpredictable environment while severely limiting the amount and quality of time parents can spend with their children. The highly variable work schedule for hourly wage jobs may also restrict parents' ability to establish and maintain routine activities such as family meals and bedtime or to attend community and school events. Shift work paid at the minimum wage may place additional strain on family life as family members take on as many work hours as possible in order to afford a minimal standard of living (Mattingly, chapter "Changes in Work and Family Across the Rural U.S.").

Moreover, activities and tasks related to parenting may be significantly more strenuous for single-parent households compared to those with two or more providers since caregiving, household labor, and other resources such as time and money are derived from one parent. With increasing rates of divorce and decreasing rates of marriage, the number of single adults with children is on the rise in rural areas placing even greater pressure on one individual to provide and care for the household (Mattingly, chapter "Changes in Work and Family Across the Rural U.S."). This demographic trend directly relates to the quality of parenting based on how much time a parent can devote to child-centered activities and parent's emotional availability during play and instructional interactions with their children. Indeed, there are well-established linkages between parenting stress, emotional availability, and child outcomes with higher stress associated with more hostile (McMahon & Meins, 2012) and less sensitive parenting (Sutherland, Altenhofen, & Biringen, 2012). Challenges to sufficient parenting time and the quality of the parent–child relationship also have implications for limit setting and monitoring which in turn affect child's academic outcomes (Lowe & Dotterer, 2013; Malczyk & Lawson, 2017) and likelihood of engaging in risky behaviors (Abar, Jackson, Colby, & Barnett, 2015; DiClemente et al., 2001; Gentile, Reimer, Nathanson, Walsh, & Eisenmann, 2014).

Rural parents have limited access to resources such as childcare, extracurricular activities, and afterschool programs for their children. When available, these resources may provide support to parents as well as opportunities for other adults in the community to contribute to child care and socialization. There is evidence that youth involvement in such programs may limit exposure and access to negative influences while promoting positive development (Eccles, Barber, Stone, & Hunt, 2003). By virtue of their remote location, rural families may have less access to community resources that are important to youth well-being such as leisure activities, academic tutoring, and adult supervision. Furthermore, opportunities for post-secondary education are few and distant to those interested in obtaining a degree. Pursuing a college education can be burdensome in terms of tuition costs, but the distance also removes students from other supportive resources such as friends and family members left behind in rural communities. Yet, educational achievement is important because it creates access to career opportunities and access to the resources that often come with full-time employment such as health benefits. Gaps in wages based on education level perpetuate poverty rates with numerous families stuck in this restrictive cycle for many generations (Partridge, Pérez-Silva, & Schreiner, chapter "Employment and Wages in the Places Left Behind").

Limited family resources lead to educational disadvantages for children, evident in early childhood and compounded over time with deficits at the school and community levels (Vernon-Feagans & Swingler, chapter "Early Development and Family Life in Rural America"). Children living in poverty, a common fate in the rural U.S., show deficits in language acquisition and cognitive and regulatory skills associated with school readiness. These limitations may be intensified by low quality of care and education. Parents and caregivers would potentially be able to diminish disparities in child outcomes by providing more structured and stimulating educational environments such as having children participate in formalized preschool or head start programs. However, their efforts are likely to miss the mark or lose their effect over time because of a larger system characterized by a low quality of education in schools and limited access to other instructional settings such as libraries, museums, and parks (Vernon-Feagans & Swingler, chapter "Early Development and Family Life in Rural America").

For these reasons, unfavorable patterns tend to persist across generations with noticeable differences in educational attainment, employment opportunities, and financial security. A focus on the intergenerational transmission of poverty has led to a much-needed understanding of the mechanisms by which family and community disadvantages and stressors lead to adverse outcomes in children. However, knowledge is still lacking concerning factors associated with positive outcomes and well-being (Carlo, Memmott-Elison, & Crockett, chapter "Latino Prosocial Development in the Rural U.S."). More research is needed on social and individual determinants of well-being in childhood and middle adulthood, with well-being defined and measured as more than the absence of problematic behaviors or psychopathologies. Such consideration may lead to a better understanding of the complexity and diversity of the rural U.S. by accounting for lifestyle dispositions and cultural norms and traditions as potential protective factors that promote well-being (e.g., the value placed on hard work and being a steward of the land).

Much of the work presented in this volume has viewed the problems facing rural families and communities as primarily economic. Certainly, many rural communities have faced economic problems in the past but a few specific challenges are looming larger today. First, jobs once considered *good jobs,* because they allowed one to support the family, have been eliminated over time. Automation and offshoring have led to the decline of many manufacturing jobs (Devaraj, Wornell, Faulk, & Hicks, chapter "Rural Job Loss to Offshoring and Automation"), and low-skill rural workers are the most vulnerable to these changes, particularly automation. The loss of manufacturing jobs has been felt primary by men (Partridge et al., chapter "Employment and Wages in the Places Left Behind"). Running parallel to this is the growing prevalence of jobs that offer inconsistent hours, limited benefits, and are short-term in nature (McLaughlin & Coleman-Jensen, 2008; Slack, 2010). Uncertainty regarding employment has direct negative consequences for families with limited childcare in rural areas multiplying the effects of loss of good jobs (Liu, 2013; Powell, 1997). Another unique economic challenge is decreasing participation in the labor force (Mattingly, chapter "Changes in Work and Family Across the Rural U.S."; Partridge et al., chapter "Employment and Wages in the Places Left Behind"). Decreasing labor force participation can significantly destabilize families not only through the loss of income, but also through increased risk of suicide (Monnat, 2017), impacts on children's education outcomes, and lower rates of participation in a variety of community organizations (Devaraj et al., chapter "Rural Job Loss to Offshoring and Automation").

In addition to the economic and demographic strains discussed, many rural families and communities are also facing a significant burden on their limited resources due to the opioid crisis. Although the opioid epidemic, the rise in opioid dependence and addiction in the U.S., is not disproportionately rural (Monnat, chapter "Opioid Crisis in the Rural U.S."), it has manifested itself in unique ways in rural America. Monnat describes how segments of the rural population are especially vulnerable to opioid addiction. The impacts of opioid addiction on health outcomes, particularly on infant health, are much larger in rural areas and have larger regional variation within rural America when compared to more urban areas. Limited access to health care in many rural areas, particularly in the most remote of counties (Haggerty, Roberge, Lévesque, Gauthier, & Loignon, 2014; Rigg & Monnat, 2015) is likely a factor that further compounds these problems. The opioid crisis has also put intense strain on local police and child welfare systems, and has created employment shortages in some places (Monnat, chapter "Opioid Crisis in the Rural U.S."; National Advisory Committee on Rural Health and Human Services, 2016). These different impacts beg the question, what is the role of policy, particularly state-level policy, in addressing the issues?

Future Directions

The work exemplified in this volume highlights the complexity of the rural U.S. and the challenges facing the families who live there. More such interdisciplinary efforts are needed to share resources and lessons learned in the study of rural families. Collaborative research may lead to more comprehensive findings that inform theories and identify gaps in knowledge. To this end, we identify several areas that could benefit from a multidisciplinary approach and recognition of the complexity of rural life in the U.S.:

Theory

There is a clear need for revisions and specifications of existing theories that consider factors and pathways unique to rural populations (Tickamyer, chapter "Rural Poverty: Research and Policy for U.S. Families"). For example, theoretical frameworks like Bronfenbrenner's ecological systems theory (1979) and family stress theory (McCubbin, 1983) provide a necessary foundation and roadmap for research on rural communities. But these broad perspectives are often applied without consideration for the diversity of rural populations and families. Researchers should incorporate these long-standing theoretical frameworks with an eye to adjusting them for the unique conditions within rural areas that shape family processes and subsequent family and child well-being. This requires including rural conditions specifically rather than a more typical strategy of combining rural areas as one to compare to urban populations and settings.

Measurement

Too often, research in the U.S. divides the nation into two groups: (1) metropolitan or urban counties and (2) nonmetropolitan or rural counties. Metropolitan counties are typically defined as those that contain a city of more than 50,000 people or have strong economic ties to a county with a city of the needed size. Nonmetropolitan or rural areas of the country are a classification residual or the leftover group of counties that are not designated as metropolitan. Rather than leaving nonmetropolitan areas as one catch-all category, research should consider rural areas based on the unique demographic, economic, and social conditions within.

Addressing many of the social and economic problems facing rural families and communities requires incorporating such detail in the data analyzed. Currently, this is difficult for several reasons. Rural individuals and households are underrepresented in primary social science data sources such as the Current Population Survey (CPS), the Survey of Income and Program Participation (SIPP), and the Panel Study of Income Dynamics (PSID). Almost all recurring national surveys censor geographic information about participants to some extent. This is particularly true of rural or nonmetropolitan individuals who often do not even have county identifiers provided. For example, in the CPS, many nonmetro individuals do not have their county provided and are instead grouped in an undisclosed nonmetro county. This geographic censoring is done to provide needed confidentiality for participants and is likely to remain in place for data collection. However, the practice makes it difficult for researchers to compare rural areas and promotes comparisons between metro and nonmetro individuals alone.

One potential step is a rural-specific national data collection project. A longitudinal study of rural America would ensure that researchers can make a within-rural-areas comparison, and ask rural respondents about important social issues in their lives that would not be applicable to ask in urban settings, such as school consolidation, and would illuminate rural issues that are evident at smaller levels of geography than the county. An ideal national rural survey would, in addition to the traditional battery of survey questions, gather information on income earned from both formal and informal work, on material hardship, on access to services, and on use of charitable or government services.

A second way to improve the collection of rural data is through more precise statistical categorization of rural areas. By far the most common categorization of rural areas is the metro–nonmetro county-level classification produced by the Office of Budget and Management. In many cases, however, counties are not the best level of geography for capturing data from rural areas (Isserman, 2005). Many of the chapters in this volume echo this critique. Even classification schemes that go beyond a binary metro–nonmetro classification scheme, such as the Rural-Urban Continuum Codes or the Urban Influence Codes, can be applied only to counties. Importantly, the classification of county means different things in different parts of the country in terms of size, population, and the governmental functions they serve. However, at present, the county is the smallest level of geography for which the U.S. Census provides yearly estimates based on the American Community Survey. As such, scholarly and policy research will continue to use county as the unit of analysis for the rural U.S. A complete account of the limitations associated with data on rural communities goes beyond this chapter, but we emphasize that new classification schemes and data sets must be developed if we are to understand and promote the well-being of rural communities.

The difficulties around data collection in the rural U.S. seem confounded with the fact that targeted participants are already overworked and often distrustful of researchers who have the reputation, real, or perceived, of being judgmental and demanding (Hochschild, 2016). Although the need to study individuals and families in their full context is evident, the logistics of collecting data on multiple levels often conflict with participants' work and family demands as discussed throughout this volume. For example, workers with a nonstandard schedule from an isolated neighborhood will undoubtedly find it difficult to complete lengthy questionnaires, visit the university research lab, or find transportation to community events where data may be collected. Furthermore, stereotypes and assumptions on either side may hinder the ability to recruit and maintain participation over time. Researchers are left to battle the tension between the need for intensive longitudinal designs and undeniably limited time and resources at the individual and community level. Possible solutions to this dilemma will need to consider approaches that maximize each contact with individuals and families in terms of the amount of data collected for a relatively low cost to participants. Some examples might include the use of wearable technology and GPS tracking that are automatically recurring and nonintrusive.

Sampling

Another study design challenge stems from the fact that most research samples in the current literature are still falling short of being representative of the rural population in terms of its ethnic, cultural, political, and economic diversity (Carlo et al., chapter "Latino Prosocial Development in the Rural U.S."; Murry et al., chapter "Rural African Americans' Family Relationships and Well-Being"). There is a need for continuing and increasing effort, as well as proven strategies, for participant recruitment and retention in those contexts including but not limited to community partnerships, incentives, and multisite collaboration.

One of the most challenging tasks concerns the ability to follow rural individuals and families longitudinally considering the variability and instability of measures and definitions of geographical boundaries. Rapid changes in the workforce may lead to relocations and the inability to track participants in and out of rural communities. Migration related to agricultural labor demands, though an essential contributor to the diversity of rural communities, emphasizes the difficulties for longitudinal research since participants move in response to job availability. Moreover, boundaries and classifications separating urban from rural areas are quite fluid. Thus, research populations may arbitrarily change from rural to urban or vice versa depending on exact boundaries or investigator decisions.

Community Partnerships

Some of the work in this volume highlights another strategy to improve the quality of information about rural communities—recruiting and training local residents as long-term research staff for projects that address needs at the local level (Murry et al., chapter "Rural African Americans' Family Relationships and Well-Being"; Vernon-Feagans & Swingler, chapter "Early Development and Family Life in Rural America"). Similarly, community agencies can help introduce research and intervention programs with more familiarly than researchers from institutions outside the communities. These groups can be important partners as they host informational group sessions and conduct interviews and lab visits. Such partnerships reduce transportation and time burdens on individual participants and provide local capacity for ongoing research and program implementation. Local organizations and agencies often have administrative data that could appropriately inform research. More discussion and initiative are needed in order to facilitate long-term partnerships between academic research institutions and rural communities. A strengths-based approach to research may be beneficial in combatting stereotypes while facilitating and maintaining positive community partnerships with organizations that often provide research and intervention initiatives. A long-term goal would be to share lessons learned during such engagement and research by focusing on community-level characteristics that could hinder or facilitate such extensive and continuous collaboration.

Community partnerships can also aid in improving the lives of rural residents. If loss of stable jobs and labor force participation are sources of many of the challenges facing rural families, then one question that emerges is, can new good jobs be brought back to rural areas? Much has been written on how individual communities have attracted new firms to their area, but individual success stories do not provide a universal answer. Many rural communities lack the necessary human capital or built infrastructure to attract the types of business that have relocated to rural area in the past, and continued international economic integration has left much of the rural U.S. directly competing with low wage labor across the globe (Devaraj et al., chapter "Rural Job Loss to Offshoring and Automation"). Although the answer to the question of how to bring better jobs to rural communities remains unknown, one answer may be found in interdisciplinary research between those who study rural families and communities. This problem-solving research will likely need to involve partnerships between policymakers, community development extensions, residents, businesses, and local governments.

Interventions

Despite these challenges to research on rural communities, it is clear that some aspects of rural life are in need of intervention to improve well-being and break the intergenerational cycle of disadvantage. Poverty, unemployment, social isolation, and low quality of child care and education are widespread, and the repercussions for individual and family well-being are well-established. It is indeed challenging to design and deliver interventions to rural communities. In the short term, efforts are needed to alleviate unfavorable circumstances through public assistance programs. But the research presented in this volume also calls for long-term investment and commitment to providing interventions among rural families. For example, early child-centered programs might yield some progress toward breaking intergenerational patterns of poverty and disadvantage in rural communities. However, these programs cannot simply be transferred from those designed to strengthen and aid urban families. Instead, a high priority for prevention and intervention effort should be to look at how unique family structure and dynamics found within rural communities can be leveraged to be beneficial and protective for children's well-being.

Policy

As advocated by Tickamyer (chapter "Rural Poverty: Research and Policy for U.S. Families"), a critical future direction for rural research is how national policies, such as welfare reform, have uniquely impacted rural communities. Many of the assumptions regarding welfare reform during the 1990s only took into account issues associated with poverty in big cities, specifically that of recipients of public benefits who are unemployed (Tickamyer, chapter "Rural Poverty: Research and Policy for U.S. Families"). Although this assumption has many flaws in its own right, it is particularly problematic in rural areas where working poverty is prevalent, and therefore, work requirements to receive assistance would have little effect (Jensen & Slack, 2003). To further compound this issue, receiving public assistance has a significant negative stigma in rural areas (Sherman, 2009).

With many rural counties and municipal governments lacking the financial resources and tax base to address a variety of local economic and social issues (Lobao & Kraybill, 2005), including challenges of the opioid crisis, national, or state level rural-specific policy may be needed to address these issues. However, two long-term policy challenges stand in the way. First, the process of devolution, or the transfer of governmental responsibility from higher levels of government to local governments (Lobao & Kraybill, 2005; Sharp & Parsi, 2003; Tickaymer, White, Tadlock, & Henderson, 2007), has created the situation whereby local governments face increased responsibilities without sufficient financial or legal resources to solve problems. Second, many scholars would argue that there is minimal rural-specific policy in the U.S., and what rural policy exists is primarily focused on agricultural areas and economies (Browne & Swanson, 1995; Isserman, 2007). Lack of rural-specific policy in the nation means that many policies aimed at addressing families' challenges do not account for key differences between urban and rural communities and economies. A need for unique rural-specific policies encompasses all family and socioeconomic issues, and a movement toward place-based policies that address place-specific problems may dramatically improve the lives of rural families and communities.

Policies should also be designed to reduce the stigmatization of public assistance that offers much needed relief to the working poor who populate many rural communities. There are pathways to breaking the intergenerational cycle of poverty in the rural U.S. (Weber et al., 2018). Many welfare programs have been designed to promote marriage and reduce single parenthood (Edin & Schafer, 2015), which historically was not viewed as a problem in rural areas. However, at a time when the rural family may be facing more challenges, policies need to be adapted to find ways of strengthening rural families. Overall social science and policy researchers need to continue to explore how government programs at all levels can aid rural families and communities.

The success of these initiatives is dependent on the larger setting. Some needs related to employment and community resources are better addressed by organizations from private and public sectors, other than government. There is a significant need for businesses to create incentives for in-migration by raising human capital and community appeal. Policies instituted at the state and county level could encourage and monitor businesses to be "good citizens" in terms of their involvement in community projects, long-term commitment, and wages offered. Similarly, universities, religious organizations, and other nonprofit agencies could contribute by consistently offering recreational and educational services that attract families and individuals who may consider moving to, instead of away from rural communities in order to pursue better career and life opportunities. These public–private partnerships can also lead to improvements in the health outcomes of rural families through increased access to clinics and health services.

Conclusion

The chapters presented in this volume provide overwhelming evidence of the consistent disadvantages for families and children living in contemporary rural communities in the U.S. whether the focus is on health, economic, or other social outcomes. Though incomplete, these findings are sufficient to warrant the need for prevention and intervention programs that aim to alleviate stressors and improve outcomes over time. Initiatives should target impacts that span across generations, especially for family assistance and child development programs. Programs that increase the financial stability and/or the social capital in rural communities have the potential for creating positive changes for current residents while also attracting new employers and employees. Creating new opportunities for rural youth to participate in higher education and the skilled labor force may deter migration and build a new type of rural community with intergenerational mobility once again possible. Clearly no single policy will ameliorate all of the problems facing rural families and communities in part because they are not monolithic and the challenges they face vary across the country. But working to implement evidence-based practices at the individual, family, and community level designed for many different challenges would certainly improve lives and reduce poverty and marginalization overall in many rural areas.

References

Abar, C. C., Jackson, K. M., Colby, S. M., & Barnett, N. P. (2015). Parent–child discrepancies in reports of parental monitoring and their relationship to adolescent alcohol-related behaviors. *Journal of Youth and Adolescence, 44*(9), 1688–1701. https://doi.org/10.1007/s10964-014-0143-6

Bronfenbrenner, U. (1979). *The ecology of human development*. Cambridge, MA: Harvard University Press.

Brown, D. L., Bolender, B. C., Kulcsar, L. J., Glasgow, N., & Sanders, S. (2011). Intercounty variability of net migration at older ages as a path-dependent process. *Rural Sociology, 76*(1), 44–73. https://doi.org/10.1111/j.1549-0831.2010.00034.x

Browne, W. P., & Swanson, L. E. (1995). Living with the minimum: Rural public policy. In E. N. Castle (Ed.), *The changing American countryside: Rural people and places* (pp. 481–492). Lawrence, KS: University of Kansas Press.

Call, M. A., & Voss, P. R. (2016). Spatio-temporal dimensions of child poverty in America, 1990–2010. *Environment and Planning A, 48*(1), 172–191. https://doi.org/10.1177/0308518X15597907

Carr, P. J., & Kefalas, M. J. (2009). *Hollowing out the middle: The rural brain drain and what it means for America*. Boston, MA: Beacon Press.

Chan, L., Hart, L. G., & Goodman, D. C. (2006). Geographic access to health care for rural Medicare beneficiaries. *Journal of Rural Health, 22*(2), 140–146. https://doi.org/10.1111/j.1748-0361.2006.00022.x

Chetty, R., Hendren, N., Kline, P., & Saez, E. (2014). Where is the land of opportunity? The geography of intergenerational mobility in the United States. *The Quarterly Journal of Economics, 129*(4), 1553–1623. https://doi.org/10.1093/qje/qju022

DiClemente, R. J., Wingood, G. M., Crosby, R., Sionean, C., Cobb, B. K., Harrington, K., … Oh, M. K. (2001). Parental monitoring: Association with adolescents' risk behaviors. *Pediatrics, 107*(6), 1363–1368. https://doi.org/10.1542/peds.107.6.1363

Duncan, C. M. (2015). *Worlds apart: Poverty and politics in rural America* (2nd ed.). New Haven, CT: Yale University Press.

Eccles, J. S., Barber, B. L., Stone, M., & Hunt, J. (2003). Extracurricular activities and adolescent development. *Journal of Social Issues, 59*(4), 865–889. https://doi.org/10.1046/j.0022-4537.2003.00095.x

Economic Research Service. (2017). *ERS county typology codes, 2015 edition*. Washington, DC: United States Department of Agriculture. Retrieved from https://www.ers.usda.gov/data-products/county-typology-codes/

Edin, K., & Shaefer, H. L. (2015). *$2.00 a day: Living on almost nothing in America*. New York, NY: Houghton Mifflin Harcourt.

Fitchen, J. M. (1994). Residential mobility among the rural poor. *Rural Sociology, 59*(3), 416–436. https://doi.org/10.1111/j.1549-0831.1994.tb00540.x

Fitchen, J. M. (1995). Spatial redistribution of poverty through migration of poor people to depressed rural communities. *Rural Sociology, 60*(2), 181–201. https://doi.org/10.1111/j.1549-0831.1995.tb00568.x

Gentile, D. A., Reimer, R. A., Nathanson, A. I., Walsh, D. A., & Eisenmann, J. C. (2014). Protective effects of parental monitoring of children's media use: A prospective study. *JAMA Pediatrics, 168*(5), 479–484.

Glasgow, N., & Brown, D. L. (2012). Rural ageing in the United States: Trends and contexts. *Journal of Rural Studies, 28*(4), 422–431. https://doi.org/10.1016/j.jrurstud.2012.01.002

Greene, K. M., Murphy, S. T., & Rossheim, M. E. (2018). Context and culture: Reasons young adults drink and drive in rural America. *Accident Analysis and Prevention, 121*, 194–201. https://doi.org/10.1016/j.aap.2018.09.008

Haggerty, J. L., Roberge, D., Lévesque, J.-F., Gauthier, J., & Loignon, C. (2014). An exploration of rural–urban differences in healthcare-seeking trajectories: Implications for measures of accessibility. *Health & Place, 28*, 92–98. https://doi.org/10.1016/j.healthplace.2014.03.005

Himes, C. L., & Rutrough, T. S. (1994). Differences in the use of health services by metropolitan and nonmetropolitan elderly. *The Journal of Rural Health, 10*(2), 80–88. https://doi.org/10.1111/j.1748-0361.1994.tb00214.x

Hochschild, A. R. (2016). *Strangers in their own land: Anger and mourning on the American right*. New York: The New Press.

Hunter, L. M., Boardman, J. D., & Saint Onge, J. M. (2005). The association between natural amenities, rural population growth, and long-term residents' economic well-being. *Rural Sociology, 70*(4), 452–469. https://doi.org/10.1526/003601105775012714

Isserman, A. M. (2005). In the national interest: Defining rural and urban correctly in research and public policy. *International Regional Science Review, 28*(4), 465–499. https://doi.org/10.1177/0160017605279000

Isserman, A. M. (2007). Getting state rural policy right: Definitions, growth, and program eligibility. *The Journal of Regional Analysis and Policy, 37*(1), 72–79.

Jensen, L., & Slack, T. (2003). Underemployment in America: Measurement and evidence. *American Journal of Community Psychology, 32*(1–2), 21–31. https://doi.org/10.1023/A:1025686621578

Johnson, K. M. (2011). The continuing incidence of natural decrease in American counties. *Rural Sociology, 76*(1), 74–100.

Johnson, K. M., & Fuguitt, G. V. (2000). Continuity and change in rural migration patterns, 1950–1995. *Rural Sociology, 65*(1), 27–49. https://doi.org/10.1111/j.1549-0831.2000.tb00341.x

Johnson, K. M., & Lichter, D. T. (2008). Natural increase: A new source of population growth in emerging Hispanic destinations in the United States. *Population and Development Review, 34*(2), 327–346. https://doi.org/10.1111/j.1728-4457.2008.00222.x

Johnson, K. M., & Winkler, R. L. (2015). Migration signatures across the decades: Net migration by age in U.S. counties, 1950-2010. *Demographic Research, 32*(1), 1065–1080. https://doi.org/10.4054/DemRes.2015.32.38

Lichter, D. T., & Brown, D. L. (2011). Rural America in an urban society: Changing spatial and social boundaries. *Annual Review of Sociology, 37*, 565–592. https://doi.org/10.1146/annurev-soc-081309-150208

Liu, M. (2013). An ecological review of literature on factors influencing working mothers' child care arrangements. *Journal of Child and Family Studies, 24*(1), 161–171. https://doi.org/10.1007/s10826-013-9822-2

Lobao, L., & Kraybill, D. S. (2005). The emerging roles of county governments in metropolitan and nonmetropolitan areas: Findings from a national survey. *Economic Development Quarterly, 19*(3), 245–259. https://doi.org/10.1177/0891242405276514

Lowe, K., & Dotterer, A. M. (2013). Parental monitoring, parental warmth, and minority youths' academic outcomes: Exploring the integrative model of parenting. *Journal of Youth and Adolescence, 42*(9), 1413–1425. https://doi.org/10.1007/s10964-013-9934-4

Malczyk, B. R., & Lawson, H. A. (2017). Parental monitoring, the parent-child relationship and children's academic engagement in mother-headed single-parent families. *Children and Youth Services Review, 73*(C), 274–282. https://doi.org/10.1016/j.childyouth.2016.12.019

McCubbin, H. I., & Patterson, J. M. (1983). The family stress process: The double ABCX model of adjustment and adaptation. *Marriage & Family Review, 6*(1–2), 7–37. https://doi.org/10.1300/J002v06n01_02

McLaughlin, D. K., & Coleman-Jensen, A. J. (2008). Nonstandard employment in the nonmetropolitan United States. *Rural Sociology, 73*(4), 631–659.

McMahon, C. A., & Meins, E. (2012). Mind-mindedness, parenting stress, and emotional availability in mothers of preschoolers. *Early Childhood Research Quarterly, 27*(2), 245–252. https://doi.org/10.1016/j.ecresq.2011.08.002

Monnat, S. M. (2017, April). *Deaths of despair from the cities to the hollers: Explaining spatial differences in US drug, alcohol, and suicide mortality rates*. Paper presented at the annual meeting of Population Association of America, Chicago, IL.

National Advisory Committee on Rural Health and Human Services. (2016). *Families in crisis: The human service implications of the rural opioid misuse* (Policy Brief, July). Retrieved from https://www.hrsa.gov/advisorycommittees/rural/publications/opioidabuse.pdf

Powell, L. M. (1997). The impact of child care costs on the labour supply of married mothers: Evidence from Canada. *The Canadian Journal of Economics, 30*(3), 577–594. https://doi.org/10.2307/136234

Rigg, K. K., & Monnat, S. M. (2015). Urban vs. rural differences in prescription opioid misuse among adults in the United States: Informing region specific drug policies and interventions. *International Journal of Drug Policy, 26*(5), 484–491. https://doi.org/10.1016/j.drugpo.2014.10.001

Sharp, J. S., & Parisi, D. (2003). Devolution: Who is responsible for rural America. In D. L. Brown & L. E. Swanson (Eds.), *Challenges for rural America in the twenty-first century* (pp. 353–362). University Park, PA: Penn State University Press.

Sherman, J. (2009). *Those who work, those who don't: Poverty, morality, and family in rural America*. Minneapolis, MN: University of Minnesota.

Sherman, J. (2018). "Not allowed to inherit my kingdom": Amenity development and social inequality in the rural west. *Rural Sociology, 83*(1), 174–207. https://doi.org/10.1111/ruso.12168

Slack, T. (2010). Working poverty across the metro-nonmetro divide: A quarter century in perspective, 1979–2003. *Rural Sociology, 75*(3), 363–387.

Sutherland, K. E., Altenhofen, S., & Biringen, Z. (2012). Emotional availability during mother-child interactions in divorcing and intact married families. *Journal of Divorce & Remarriage, 53*(2), 126–141. https://doi.org/10.1080/10502556.2011.651974

Tickamyer, A., White, J., Tadlock, B., & Henderson, D. (2007). The spatial politics of public policy: Devolution, development, and welfare reform. In L. M. Labao, G. Hooks, & A. R. Tickamyer (Eds.), *The sociology of spatial inequality* (pp. 113–139). Albany, NY: SUNY Press.

Van Dis, J. (2002). Where we live: Health care in rural vs urban America. *JAMA: The Journal of the American Medical Association, 287*(1), 108–108. https://doi.org/10.1001/jama.287.1.108

Voss, P. R., Long, D. D., Hammer, R. B., & Friedman, S. (2006). County child poverty rates in the US: A spatial regression approach. *Population Research and Policy Review, 25*(4), 369–391. https://doi.org/10.1007/s11113-006-9007-4

Weber, B., Fannin, J. M., Miller, K., & Goetz, S. (2018). Intergenerational mobility of low-income youth in metropolitan and non-metropolitan America: A spatial analysis. *Regional Science Policy & Practice, 10*(2), 87–101. https://doi.org/10.1111/rsp3.12122

Weber, B., & Miller, K. (2017). Poverty in rural America then and now. In A. Tickamyer, J. Sherman, & J. Warlick (Eds.), *Rural Poverty in the United States* (pp. 28–64). New York: Columbia University Press.

Index

A
Adaptive racial socialization, 185
Additional Child Tax Credit (ACTC), 17
Adult–child interactions, 241
African American adolescents
  developmental pathways, 182
  F.A.M.I.L.Y, 188
  income, 178
  orientations, 185
  risk behavior engagement, 181
African American parenting, 176, 181, 188
African Americans families
  culturally tailored programs, 193
  ecological frameworks (*see* Ecological frameworks)
  educational opportunities, 171
  environmental changes, 170
  historical pattern, 170–172
  population shifts, 190–192
  positive relationships and well-being, 170
  post-civil rights era, 169
  vestiges of slavery, 170
Age and racial-ethnic structure
  children, 32
  Hispanic population, 35
  population pyramids, 32
  rural areas, 35
  sex distribution, 35
  United States, 35
Agglomeration forces, 91
Aging
  aging trends (*see* Nonmetro aging)
  aspects, 145
  baby boomers, 163
  causes, 164
  county-level aging, 146
  decomposition techniques, 162
  demographic components, 147
  fertility and mortality, 162
  historical engines, 145
  improvements, 145
  migration, 146
  regions, 157
  research, 147
  rural, 163
  young-adult out-migration, 162
Aging-in-place, 146, 255
Agriculture and manufacturing, 30, 39
Aid to Families with Dependent Children (AFDC), 16
Alcohol
  deaths and suicides, 123, 137
  suicide mortality, 125
  use disorders, 123
Allostatic load, 218, 219
American Community Survey (ACS), 28, 30, 32, 35, 37, 38, 68, 93, 94, 130
Appalachian poverty, 13
Appalachia's rural communities, 126
Appalachian Regional Commission (ARC), 18
Autonomic nervous system (ANS), 218

B
Bartik instrument, 63
Benzodiazepines, 125
Bifurcation of jobs, 90
Bureau of Labor Statistics (BLS), 68

J. E. Glick et al. (eds.), *Rural Families and Communities in the United States*,
National Symposium on Family Issues 10, https://doi.org/10.1007/978-3-030-37689-5

C
Caregivers, 177
Causes of opioid crisis
kindling, 127–131
spark, 126, 127
Causes of rural poverty
Appalachian poverty, 13
globalization, 13
individual *vs.* structural level theories, 12
inequality, 14
people *vs.* place, 11
spatial factors, 13
The People Left Behind, 13
Center for Economic Policy Research (CEPR), 67
Child care, 10, 16, 21
Child language, 210–212, 214
Child literacy, 211–214, 221, 222
Children in rural families, 201, 204, 224
Children's school learning, 220
Chronic obstructive pulmonary disease (COPD), 123
Chronic pain, 126, 128, 132, 133
Classroom instruction/quality, 222, 225
Cocaine, 120, 125
Cognitive-developmental theory, 240
Community partnerships, 262
Community resources, 237
Cultural amenities, 256
Cultural-ecological perspectives
child well-being, 174, 176
discrimination experiences, 176
economic conditions/racial discrimination, 174
economic risk, 173
macrolevel factors, 174
macrolevel processes, 174
marital relationship, 174
mental health care system, 173
parent well-being, 174
PVEST, 175
race-/economic-related experiences, 175
racial socialization/identity, 176
Cultural strength, 245
Cultural strengths-based assets, 179–181
efficacy and effectiveness trials, 185–187
family-based preventive interventions, 183–185
F.A.M.I.L.Y study, 187–189
Culture of poverty theory, 12
Culture-related stressors, 244, 245, 247
Cumulative risk, 211, 212
Current Population Survey (CPS), 38, 67, 260

D
Data collection, 260, 261
Deaths of despair, 117, 123, 128
Decennial Census, 28, 30, 33, 34, 36–38
Deep poverty, 3, 10, 17, 171, 190
Definitions of rural, 202
Demographic changes, 237
Demographic transition, 145
Depressed economies, 136
Disability payments, 47
Disorganization, 215
Drug mortality, 125, 130, 131
Drug overdose, 136, 137

E
Early childhood
children's language development, 212, 215
classroom quality measure, 221
cognitive skills, 208
cognitive/social-emotional development, 218
cortisol levels, 219
language input, 224
poverty, 207
Early poverty stressors
behavior and functioning, 218
factors, 216
FLP, 217
host, 216
HPA axis/parenting/brain development, 218–220
impactful areas, 217
neural development, 217
overproduction, 217
Earned Income Tax Credit (EITC), 17, 42
Earnings disadvantage, 31
Eastern Kentucky region, 158, 161
Ecological frameworks
cultural–ecological perspectives, 173–176
family process and stress coping, 176, 177
risk and resilience, 177–179
stress integrative model, 179–183
Economic activity, 91, 107
Economic determinants, 128, 137
Economic development programs, 164
Economic distress, 3, 131
Economic performance, 89, 91
Economic problems, 258
Economic Research Service (ERS), 5
Economic shocks, 105, 110, 111
Educational attainment, 89, 90, 92, 101, 103, 104, 106, 112, 237

Education levels, 206, 211, 212, 224, 225
Emergency department (ED), 117, 120
Employment polarization, 104
Employment risk, 94, 95, 101
Employment-to-population ratio
  education, 77
  educational groups, 68, 69, 72, 73
  employment industries, 73
  gender differences, 74
  places left behind, 76–81
  postrecession, 81, 82
  wages, 47
Ethnic/racial minority, 242
Executive function (EF), 216
Extended family, 202–204, 226

F
Family life, 256
Family Life Project (FLP)
  college-educated mothers, 212
  contribution, 210
  cortisol levels, 219
  families, 206
  high-quality childcare centers, 209
  household chaos, 216
  mothers, 208
  physiological well-being, 201
  representative sample, 205
  rural geographic isolation, 212
  socioeconomic variables, 210
Family processes
  economic impact, 172
  intergenerational influences, 188
  parenting, 174
  research, 170
  well-being, 172
Family resources, 241
Family work, 201
Fatal opioid overdose rates, 119–122, 128, 129
Fathers and Mothers in the Lives of Youth (F.A.M.I.L.Y), 188
  African American fathers, 188, 189
  economic-/race-related factors, 189
  ethnic–racial socialization practices, 188
  preventive interventions, 189
  race-related barriers, 188
  rural families, 188
Federal Reserve Bank of St. Louis data (FRED), 48
Fentanyls, 117
Fifth vital sign, 126
Food deserts, 10
Future directions, rural US
  Bronfenbrenner's ecological systems theory, 259
  community partnerships, 262
  interventions, 262, 263
  measurement, 259–261
  policies, 263, 264
  sampling, 261

G
Generational poverty, 12
Geographic trends in opioid mortality, 117, 118, 120, 121
Geographic variation, 89
Geography of aging, 146
Good economic policy, 136
Good jobs, 258, 262
Government, 260, 262–264
Great Recession, 14, 17, 18, 47, 49, 51, 53, 55, 74, 77, 81, 82, 136
Greyhound welfare, 8

H
Hard life/challenges, rural US
  demographic trends, 255, 256
  poverty, 254, 255
  rural families, 256–259
Health care, 10, 13
Healthy food, 169
Hepatitis C Virus (HCV), 134
High-quality professional development programs, 220
High school graduates, 69, 72, 73, 76, 77, 90
Hillbilly heroin, 129
Hispanics, 29, 30, 32, 35, 127
Hopelessness, 128, 131, 133
Hourly wage jobs, 256
Household chaos
  academic achievement, 216
  chaotic environments, 215
  components, 214
  definition, 214
  disorganization, 215, 216
  EF skills, 216
  FLP, 215
  mediating role, 216
  psychosocial stressors, 214
Hypothalamus–pituitary–adrenal axis (HPA axis), 218, 219

I
Income inequality, 14
Income to needs ratio (INR), 206
Integration, 242, 244
Intergenerational transmission of rural poverty, 254

J
Job displacement, 104–107, 109, 110
Job instability, 105, 106
Job loss
- agglomeration forces, 91
- autocorrelation, 98
- automation and trade, 91
- automation/offshoring, 100, 101
- degree of concentration, 96
- due to automation, 96, 101
- educational attainment, 101
- employment growth, 92
- implications, 92
- income mobility, 91
- labor market adjustments, 101
- limitations, 111
- policy (*see* Policy)
- regional economies, 91
- regional variation, 96, 101
- relative risk measure, 95
- risk, 103
- statistical measurement, 92

Job-loss risk, 110

K
Kindergarten Woodcock Johnson Letter-Word Identification, 221
Kindling
- all-drug overdoses, 130
- *deaths of despair*, 128
- economic and family factors, 131
- economic disadvantage, 130
- economic distress, 131
- economic restructuring, 127
- factor-weighted index, 129
- family distress, 131
- fatal opioid overdose rates, 128
- geographic differences, 128
- out-migration, 128
- slow-moving stressors, 128
- social integration, 131

L
Labor force participation, 28, 29
- CPS, 67
- employment-to-population ratio, 47, 66, 74, 80
- places left behind, 76
- skill-based technological change, 51
- wages, 67

Labor market composition, 47
Labor market framework
- employment/population rate, 66
- equilibrium, 65
- labor demand/supply, 67
- skill-based technological change, 65
- theoretical underpinnings, 64

Labor markets
- geographic volatility, 90
- high-income workers, 90
- issues, 89
- urbanization effects, 89

Labor market segmentation, 48
Labor market shocks, 89, 95, 106, 109, 110, 112
Labor supply
- curve, 64, 66
- out-migration, 51
- reductions, 66, 72
- unemployment insurance benefits, 51

Language scaffolding, 210, 215
Large-scale place-based programs, 18
Latino/a adolescents, 241
Latino/a population, 247
Latino/a rural youth, 245
Latino/as. Immigration, 247
Latino/a youth, 247
Latino/a Youth Development (LYD) model, 244
- adolescence, 245
- basic information, 247
- culture-related mechanisms, 246
- ethnic-racial diversity, 247
- longitudinal studies, 247
- prosocial development, 247
- social cognitive theory, 245
- sociocognitive/socioemotive traits, 245
- trauma/stress, 246
- young adults, 244

Living in poverty, 201, 204–206
Low-wealth communities, 205
Low wage labor, 30

M
Maladjustment, 237–239, 243
Manufacturing
employment, 90, 92
exchange rate fluctuations, 61
industry composition, 76
jobs, 90–92
mining, 82
nonmetro employment, 48
rural, 59
Married couples, 37, 38
Marshall Plan, 136, 137
Maternal education, 206, 210, 212, 214, 225
Maternal language, 210–212
Medicaid, 126
Medication Assisted Treatment (MAT), 135
Mental health care, 132
Metro counties, 254
Metro/nonmetro classification scheme, 260
Metropolitan manufacturing, 48
Metro poverty, 6
Mexico, 123
Migration, 242, 244
Minority groups, 254
Mississippi Delta, 157, 158
Moving to Opportunity (MTO) program, 18

N
Narcan®, 135
Neighborhoods, 204, 214, 215, 217
Neonatal abstinence syndrome (NAS), 134
New rural order, 127
NICHD-funded project, 201
Nonmetro aging
demographic trend, 148
in-migration growth areas, 148
older-age counties, 149
older-age distribution, 147
scenarios (*see* Rural aging scenarios)
socioeconomic indicators, 150
US Senate Special Committee, 147
young-adult out-migration, 148
Nonmetropolitan areas, 47
Nonstandard schedule, 261
Nonstandard work hours, 39, 203, 207–209, 213, 216, 224, 225
Nonunionized, 30
North Carolina, 201, 205

O
Office of Management and Budget (OMB), 5, 202
Official poverty measure (OPM), 6, 9, 10
Offshorability risk, 94, 96, 109
Offshoring automation risk, 89
Older-age counties, 146, 149, 150, 156
Older in-migrants, 255
Older populations, 255
On-demand work scheduling, 30
Opioid addiction, 137
Opioid crisis, 258
all-cause mortality, 123
causes (*see* Causes of opioid crisis)
COPD, 123
fatal overdose rate, 125
geographic variation, 125
media and political attention, 123
methamphetamine, 123
rural health, 122
rural United States
abuse disorders, 133
emotional and behavioral problems, 134
emotional trauma, 134
HCV, 134
health crises, 134
implications, 133
parental drug addiction, 134
strategies, 135–137
substance use problems, 123
Opioid overdose
county-level fatal, 129
deaths, 127
middle-aged non-Hispanic whites, 121
mining industry, 128
Naloxone, 135
working-age adults, 122
Opioids, 117
OxyContin®, 126, 129

P
Pain advocates, 126
Pain clinics, 126
Panel Study of Income Dynamics (PSID), 260
Parenting, 201, 207
Parenting, rural America
children's competence, 211
FLP, 211
maternal language input, 211, 212
mother and father language input, 213, 214

Parents' mental health, 238
Pathways for African American Success (PAAS)
  parenting protective processes, 186, 187
  RCT, 184
  youth protective processes, 187
Peer relationships, 238, 242, 243, 246
Pennsylvania, 201, 205
Perceptions of rural US, 3
Permanent Normal Trading Relations (PNTR), 92
Persistent poverty counties, 6, 7
Persistent poverty locations, 13, 20–21
Personal Responsibility and Work Opportunity Reconciliation Act (PRWORA), 16, 18
Persons who inject drugs (PWID), 134
Perspective taking, 238–240
Pharmaceutical companies, 126
Pharmaceutical regulatory policies, 136
Phenomenological variant of ecological systems theory (PVEST), 175
Physicians, 118, 126, 127
Place-based approaches, 4
Places left behind
  nonmetro areas
    educational groups, 76, 79
    employment industries, 80
    gender differences, 80
    high school graduates, 77
    interaction, 76
    recession, 76
Policy
  analysis, 109, 110
  federal state, 107
  state/local state, 107–109
Policy agendas
  diversity and intersectionality, 20
  future visioning, 21, 22
  links across space and place, 19
  links, macro and microlevels, 20
  methods and data, 21
  policy and public opinion, 19, 20
Policy/program, rural poverty
  assistance effort, 15
  evidence-based programs, 18
  family assistance programs, 17
  federal system, 15
  incentives and sanctions, 15
  MTO program, 18
  place-based policies, 15
  PRWORA and TANF, 16
  social welfare, 15
  structural level approaches, 17, 18
Population aging, 146
Population growth, 35, 55–59
Population pyramids, 32–34, 38
Population shifts
  detrimental consequences, 192
  macrolevel systems, 191
  macrosystem approach, 191
  plasticity and flexibility, 192
  race-related interactions, 190
  racial discrimination, 191
  rural communities, 190
  stressors, 192
  traditional models, 192
Population trend data, 170
Post-secondary education, 90
Poverty rates, 6, 8–11, 16, 39
Poverty theory, 12
Prescription opioids, 126, 127
Problem behaviors, 243, 246
Programs to address rural poverty, 15, 18
Prosocial development
  influential theory, 240
  rural populations, 241, 242
Prosocial traits, 240
PROSPER Program, 136
Psychological health, 239
Psychological maladjustment, 238
Public opinion about poverty, 19
Purdue Pharma, 126

Q

Quality of parenting, 256

R

Racial discrimination, 174, 177, 180, 188
Real wages, 49, 65, 68, 69, 73, 76
Reliable high-speed Internet, 164
Resource extraction, 52
Retirement-related in-migration, 162–164
Rural adolescents, 242, 243, 245, 246
Rural African American, 210
Rural aging
  components, 147
  geographical reach, 148
  migration, 146
  narratives, 150
  net in-migration, 148
  older-age counties, 146
  primary cause, 147
  research agenda, 147

Rural aging scenarios
- county-level age-specific population, 151
- decennial census, 151
- demographic components, 151–153
- Eastern Kentucky region, 158, 161
- Mississippi Delta, 157, 158
- Nonmetro trends, 153
- older-age in-migration regions, 155, 156
- out-migration regions, 154, 155

Rural children's development, 237
Rural communities, 41, 42, 169
- adolescents, 242
- conditions, 254
- contemporary, 264
- demographic trends, 253
- design and deliver interventions, 263
- economic problems, 258
- foundation and roadmap, 259
- Latino/a's communities, 242
- out-migration, 255
- peer relationships, 243
- protective factors, 243
- racial/ethnic minorities, 242
- schemes and data, 260
- social issue, 254
- strengths-based approach, 262
- supportive resources, 257
- young adulthood, 243

Rural counties, 253, 254, 259, 263
Rural diversity, 253
Rural economic development, 133
Rural economies, 10
Rural employment
- labour force attachment, 28, 29
- work's changing nature, 30, 31

Rural families
- age and racial-ethnic structure, 32–36
- change, 28
- childcare, 257
- data limitations, 38, 39
- economic challenge, 258
- economic/demographic strains, 258
- educational achievement, 257
- family composition, 36–38
- family resources, 257
- geography, 41
- incomes, 40
- life, 201, 203, 214
- opioid addiction, 258
- parenting activities and tasks, 256
- racially and ethnically diverse, 32
- safety net programs, 42
- shift work, 256
- unfavorable patterns, 257
- work schedule, 256

Rural gentrification, 8
"Rural idyll", 3
Rural Latino/a immigrants, 237
Rural life
- child poverty, 205–207
- children development, 209–211
- parenting and work schedules, 207–209

Rural opioid misuse, 118, 127, 128, 131, 137
Rural opioid mortality
- demographic differences, 121, 122
- rural–urban differences, 118
- within-region variation, 121

Rural places
- agriculture and manufacturing, 30
- changes, 27
- data classification, 39
- employment patterns, 31
- Hispanics, 32
- households, 32, 36
- implications, 36
- issues, 31
- married couples, 37
- men's employment, 29
- resource-/amenity-rich, 41
- service-based economy, 30
- women's employment, 29

Rural poor, 3, 6, 8, 13, 20
Rural population, 6, 13
Rural poverty
- causes (*see* Causes of rural poverty)
- economies, 10
- education, 10
- issues, 4
- measures and figures, 6, 8
- OPM, 8, 10
- policy agendas (*see* Policy agendas)
- policy and program (*see* Policy/program, rural poverty)
- RSS, 4
- Rural Policy Research Institute, 4
- rural residents, 10
- SPM, 9
- *The People Left Behind*, 3
- US geography and demography, 5, 6

Rural poverty research, 19
Rural Sociological Society (RSS), 4
Rural-specific national data collection project, 260
Rural south, 170, 172, 174, 190
Rural United States, 27
- challenges, 259
- counties, 253

Rural United States (*cont.*)
data collection, 261
diversity and complexity, 254, 258
future directions (*see* Future directions, rural US)
hard life/challenges (*see* Hard life/ challenges, rural US)
intergenerational cycle, 264
language acquisition, 257
living conditions, 253
research and practice, 253
rural–urban dichotomy, 253
Rural/urban America's economy
conditions, 52–54
industry composition, 63, 64
industry mix, 59, 61, 63
metropolitan areas, 52
places left behind, 55–57, 59
Rural–urban continuum, 135
Rural-Urban Continuum Codes (RUCCs), 97

S
Safety net programs, 10, 16, 17
Salivary cortisol, 219
Schooling
childhood settings, 222
child social-emotional functioning, 222
classroom organization, 221
emotional support measures, 221
FLP African American children, 221
FLP classroom quality, 221
general academic knowledge, 222, 223
general classroom quality, 222
instructional support, 222
National data, 221
randomized controlled trials, 223
rural children, 201
teachers, 220
TRI, 223, 224
Self-regulation skills, 238, 240
Service industry, 203
Sexual behavior, 243
Shift-share analysis, 63
Shift work, 256
Single-family homes, 202
Single parenthood, 211
Single-parent households, 256
Skill-based technological change, 51
Small business development, 63
Social agents, 240
Social cognitive theory, 240, 245
Social determinants of health, 131
Social isolation, 255, 262
Socialization, 240, 241
Social problems, 8, 13, 118
Social safety net programs, 39
Social science data, 260
Social Security Disability Insurance (SSDI), 17
Social services, 8, 10, 13, 21
Social support, 255
Social welfare, 18
Sociobehavioral health, 238
Sociocognitive/socioemotive traits, 245
Socioeconomic status (SES), 175
Spatial clustering, 163
Special rural challenges
disproportionate shares, 132
opioid addiction, 133
preventive health interventions, 132
unintended consequence, 133
Standard of living, 6, 256
Strategies of opioid crisis
education and community, 135
good economic policy, 136
interventions, 135
Marshall Plan, 136
MAT, 135
pharmaceutical regulatory policies, 136
prevention programs, 136
promoting opportunities, 136
rural–urban continuum, 135
Stress integrative model
community settings, 181–183
cultural strength-based coping assets, 179–181
ordinary magic, 179
stressors, 179
Strong African American Families (SAAF)
caregiving practices, 185
parent-level processes, 185
RCT, 184
youth-level processes, 186
Structural theories, 12
Substance use, 239, 243, 246
Supplemental Assistance for Needy Families (SNAP), 107
Supplemental Nutrition Assistance Program (SNAP), 17, 42
Supplemental poverty measurement (SPM) data, 9, 39, 40
Supplemental Security Income (SSI), 17
Survey of Income and Program Participation (SIPP), 260
Synthetic opioids, 117, 118, 120

T
Targeted Reading Intervention (TRI), 223
Temporary Assistance to Needy Families (TANF), 16, 18, 42, 107
Tennessee Valley Authority (TVA), 18
The People Left Behind
  research conference, 4
Trade Adjustment Assistance (TAA), 107
Traditional business hours, 30
Trauma/stress, 246
24-hour economy, 30

U
Unions, 30
Unpredictable schedules, 30
Upstream strategies, 135
Upward socioeconomic mobility, 254
Urban crowding, 3
Urban places
  agriculture, 27
  American Community Survey, 35
  full-time employment, 29
  households, 37
  implications, 35
  marital status, 29
  minority population, 35
  U.S., 28
Urban poverty, 3, 10, 19
Urban/rural America, trends
  employment-to-population ratio, 49, 51
  export-based industries, 48
  farming, 48
  Great Recession, 49, 51
  industrial composition, 48
  manufacturing employment, 48
  mom-and-pop shops, 51
  negative trade balances, 48
Urban *vs.* rural, 253
US Census Bureau, 5, 9
USDA Economic Research Service (ERS), 5
USDA housing programs, 163
US rural life
  criteria, 202
  Department of Education, 202
  OMB, 202
  Pennsylvania, 201
  twenty-first century
    changes, 203
    farming, 203
    Great Depression, 203
    higher education, 204
    less-educated population, 203
    rural families, 204
    rural/urban places, 204
    sense of belonging, 203
  U.S. Federal Agencies, 202

V
Variable work hours, 30
Vulnerable populations, 110

W
Women, Infants, and Children (WIC), 17
Work hours, 30, 31

X
Xalisco drug network, 127

Y
Young-adult out-migration, 146, 147, 154, 162, 164
Youth bulges, 241, 242, 244

The manufacturer's authorised representative in the EU is Springer Nature Customer Service Centre GmbH, Europaplatz 3, 69115 Heidelberg, Germany. If you have any concerns regarding our products, please contact ProductSafety@springernature.com

Printed and bound by CPI Group (UK) Ltd, Croydon, CR0 4YY
30/09/2026
02225458-0013